S0-BPI-534

**Fundamental
Aspects of
Neoplasia**

Fundamental Aspects of Neoplasia

edited by

A. Arthur Gottlieb
Otto J. Plescia
David H. L. Bishop

RC268.57
A1
F86
1975

Springer-Verlag

New York   Heidelberg   Berlin

1975

312760

Proceedings of a Symposium held
May 20–22, 1974 at the
Waksman Institute of Microbiology of
Rutgers, the State University of New Jersey

Library of Congress Cataloging in Publication Data

Main entry under title:

Fundamental aspects of neoplasia.

Includes index.
1. Oncogenic viruses—Congresses. 2. Tumors—
Immunological aspects—Congresses. 3. Immunological
deficiency—Congresses. I. Gottlieb, A(braham) Arthur,
1937-   II. Plescia, Otto J. III. Bishop, David H. L.
IV. Rutgers University, New Brunswick, N.J.
Institute of Microbiology. [DNLM: 1. Neoplasms—
Congresses. 2. Oncogenic viruses—Congresses. BF698
G297p]
RC268.57.F86   616.9′92′071   75-4792

All rights reserved

No part of this book may be translated or reproduced
in any form without written permission from
Springer-Verlag.

© 1975 by Springer-Verlag New York Inc.

Printed in the United States of America

ISBN 0-387-07230-6   Springer-Verlag   New York Heidelberg Berlin

ISBN 3-540-07230-6   Springer-Verlag   Berlin Heidelberg New York

Preface

The control of cancer is at once a major public health problem and a problem of fundamental biologic interest. As a result of technologic developments and new insights in the realm of molecular biology, new and important approaches to an understanding of neoplasia are now possible. Several aspects of neoplasia are clearly of microbiologic interest, including the role of viruses in the etiology of cancer, control of the immune response to tumor cells, and the susceptibility of tumor-bearing hosts to overwhelming infection as a result of immuno-deficiency. Recent advances in these areas led us to organize this symposium, and, through this publication, to record some of the progress being made in laboratories around the world in understanding some of the basic aspects of the cancer problem.

This symposium was held as part of the commemoration of the twentieth anniversary of the Waksman Institute of Microbiology. Dr. Waksman's devotion to the study of the smallest forms of life and the commitment of the Waksman Institute to the free pursuit of knowledge are the underpinnings of the institute's research efforts in the broad area of microbiology, including the problem of neoplasia. It is of interest to note that actinomycin, one of the earliest antibiotics discovered in Waksman's laboratory, was also one of the first compounds found to be clinically useful in the treatment of certain types of cancer. In addition, the institute has been the training ground of several key figures in the National Cancer Program, including the current director. In recent years, the institute has developed several programs in virology and immunology that relate to the cancer problem, and several studies of the fundamental biochemical characteristics of tumor cells as well. The interests of the institute faculty in these areas led to the suggestion that it would be appropriate to devote this Twentieth Anniversary Symposium to the problem of neoplasia.

Three major themes emerge from the symposium.

1. The impossibility of planning scientific research in such areas as the biology of cancer, areas in which a high degree of uncertainty exists.
2. Several observations suggest that tumors are interesting biologic systems in themselves. Tumor cells can produce a variety of molecules; and some of these molecules may potentiate tumor cell growth and, thereby, be potential targets for chemotherapeutic drugs.
3. Although much has been learned about tumor viruses in animal systems, and although there is considerable indirect evidence that viral particles or

parts of viruses occur in human tumor tissue, the complex interactions of viruses and carcinogenic agents and the respective role that each play in the etiology of cancer remain to be determined.

We wish to express our appreciation for the financial support of the Charles and Johanna Busch Bequest, which made this symposium possible. We also wish to thank Dr. J. O. Lampen, Director of the Institute of Microbiology, Mr. E. R. Isaacs, Executive Secretary of the Institute, and Mr. Jack Faron, Division of Special Services of Rutgers University, who aided us in our planning and management of the symposium. We are especially indebted to Mrs. Jeanne Nied and other members of the Institute staff, who handled the heavy secretarial burdens, inherent in the preparation of the symposium, with efficiency and dispatch. Dr. Bruce Alberts, Dr. Sheldon Cohen, and Dr. Walter Schlesinger served as able chairmen of various sections of the symposium.

Finally, we are indebted to the speakers and their associates who through their efforts provided a valuable and memorable highlight to the institute's twentieth year.

A. Arthur Gottlieb
Otto J. Plescia
David L. Bishop

New Brunswick, N. J.

A. Arthur Gottlieb, M.D.
Professor and Chairman
Department of Microbiology and Immunology
Tulane University School of Medicine
New Orleans, Louisiana   70112

Formerly,
Professor of Microbiology
Institute of Microbiology
Rutgers University
New Brunswick, New Jersey   08903

Otto J. Plescia, Ph.D.
Professor of Immunochemistry
Institute of Microbiology
Rutgers University
New Brunswick, New Jersey   08903

David H. L. Bishop, Ph.D.
Professor of Microbiology
The Medical Center
University of Alabama
Birmingham, Alabama

Formerly,
Professor of Microbiology
Institute of Microbiology
Rutgers University
New Brunswick, New Jersey   08903

Prologue:
The National Cancer Plan
and its Relationship to Basic Research

Guy R. Newell

I thank you for inviting me to share with you this important occasion, which simultaneously commemorates the Twentieth Anniversary of the Institute of Microbiology of Rutgers University and honors the memory of the late Professor Selman A. Waksman. Professor Waksman's name is linked for all time with microbiology and Rutgers, and I was not surprised to learn that Dr. Waksman was associated with Rutgers University for more than half a century, as a student, faculty member, director of the Institute of Microbiology, and professor emeritus.

We of the National Cancer Institute are proud of the twelve professionals on its staff with degrees from Rutgers, including the director, Dr. Frank J. Rauscher. I suspect that the interest sparked while he was at Rutgers eventually led to Dr. Rauscher's discovery at the Institute, of the murine leukemia virus now known as the Rauscher virus. Dr. Rauscher immediately made his virus available to many investigators, and it is being widely used in studies of viral neoplasia in laboratories throughout the world. His discovery was one of a number of such advances in the 1950s and 1960s that led to an Institute decision to develop an expanded research program in viral oncology. During that time, the Institute was already conducting broad programs of research on chemotherapy and chemical carcinogenesis.

A mandate for a greatly intensified effort was given the Institute by the National Cancer Act of 1971, for a total mobilization of resources, people, and knowledge in a new national program to conquer cancer. At this time, knowledge and technology were believed sufficient to warrant the confidence that progress against cancer could be accelerated.

By the 1971 Act, the Institute was charged with developing and coordinating an overall national strategy for cancer research with many members of the scientific community collaborating to produce the National Cancer Program Plan. Now, what is the National Cancer Program Plan—and more importantly, what isn't it? The Plan provides the framework for coordinating, monitoring, updating, and reporting on the progress of the National Cancer Program. It is a progress report, to be updated annually, to reflect new scientific knowledge, new research leads, new opportunities for applying research findings to clinical medicine. The fact that the Plan will be updated points out its flexibility in reflecting the *state* of science, and not directing the *art* of science. The Plan does not measure the scientific merit of traditional investigator-initiated research; such research is currently and will continue to be, reviewed and measured by the peer review study section system. There is no built-in mechanism to allow the Plan to stifle new research initiatives.

I would now like to highlight briefly for you some scientific advances and opportunities, particularly in the clinical area of treatment, inasmuch as many advances in the more basic areas will be covered during the course of this symposium.

There are 44 drugs that produce remissions of clinical cancer. If analogues are subtracted, there remain 27 different chemical structures. Ten of these have been employed in regimens that produce cures or remissions (some quite impressive) in 11 different types of cancer.* Unfortunately, these are relatively uncommon tumors. Our question then is: Do these uncommon tumors share a process that is different from the processes in the more common tumors? Research has shown that they do: they are relatively fast growing tumors, with short doubling times. Successful chemotherapy of these uncommon tumors is pointing the way by which common tumors may be manipulated by other regimens to be more susceptible to this kind of chemotherapy.

Thus, direction for future research includes: (a) developing and screening new drugs that can act alone or in combination with other drugs. For example, adriamycin, an anticancer drug discovered in Italy, has shown a greater degree of activity against a broader range of tumors than any other single agent previously tested. Studies are under way to test the usefulness of the drug in combination with other treatments and to develop active analogues of adriamycin that are not cardiotoxic. (b) Applying new forms of radiation, such as the the laser beam, that spare normal tissue are not in themselves carcinogenic. (c) Certainly, developing new regimens for BCG and other forms of immunotherapy, both alone and in combinations. (d) Determining new combinations of known effective drugs to be administered at a time when a large majority of tumor cells are irretrievably committed to DNA replication and thus susceptible to differential kill by chemotherapeutic agents. Drugs may also be used as adjuvant therapy, given immediately following surgery for the removal of the primary tumor mass or irradiation and directed toward eradicating microscopic foci of metastases. This is a particularly exciting area with great

---

* *Drugs:* Cyclophosphamide, nitrogen mustard, thiotepa, 6-mercaptopurine, methotrexate, vincristine, actinomycin D, mithramycin, procarbazine, and prednisone.

Types of cancer: Wilms' tumor, choriocarcinoma, Burkitt's lymphoma, retinoblastoma, mycosis fungoides, acute lymphocytic leukemia, Ewing's sarcoma, Hodgkin's disease, rhabdomyosarcoma, histocytic lymphoma, and embryonal testicular cancer.

future promise. (e) Combining such modalities as surgery, irradiation, chemotherapy, and immunotherapy.

Results of research in the fields of cellular and molecular biology, and especially in immunology and virology, will be highlighted during this symposium, so, now, I would like to present in broader terms how the National Cancer Act affects basic research.

Several conditions following enactment of the National Cancer Act of 1971, and relating to the conduct of research, created sensitive issues for the Institute and for our colleagues in the scientific community. Because the Act *directed* the Institute to include within the National Cancer Program not only the programs of the Institute but related programs of other research institutes and federal and non-federal programs, we do have a responsibility to relate and respond to a much broader scope of activity than we previously had. This implies that the Institute is responsible for all cancer research done in the United States, in one way or another. Numerous departments, other than Health, Education, and Welfare, of which we are a part, and other federal government agencies fund or support cancer research and control. Many private voluntary organizations, such as the American Cancer Society, support cancer research and control. We are making every effort to establish meaningful liaisons with these other groups and agencies, and, at the very least, to try to assure that funds provided to the Institute are not used in research that duplicates other research.

Other sensitive issues related to budget, to ways of funding, and to our relationship to other institutes within the National Institutes of Health. These issues cannot be treated separately. The Act specifies that the director of the Institute prepare and submit an annual budget estimate for the National Cancer Program directly to the President; and that the Director receives from the President and the Office of Management and Budget directly all funds appropriated by Congress for obligation and expenditure by the Institute.

We have a legal and a moral responsibility to specify the amount of money we think the Institute can use to greatest effect. But the federal dollar is limited, and we recognize this. As a result, many people think cancer is being given such a high priority that other important areas of biomedical research are being neglected. No one, to my knowledge, has shown that this is, in fact, true. But the ordering of priorities is of great concern to us. We do not want resources for cancer to be increased at the expense of other disease-oriented and basic biomedical research. It seems to me that the key question to be asked is: If funds allocated to cancer research during the past few years had not been earmarked for cancer, would they have been provided to other areas of biomedical research? The fact is that the answer to this question will never be known. We sincerely hope that our advocacy of large sums of money for cancer research will help other research areas and that advocates for other diseases and research areas will be successful in obtaining their own funding. At the same time, we believe that information from cancer research will necessarily provide important leads in other disciplines and for categorical diseases and vice versa.

If we look at the numbers of grants awarded for both the Institute and the National Institutes of Health from 1962 through 1973, one readily sees that the trend was one of rapid decline. Since the National Cancer Act was passed, in late 1971, we have done considerably better, and funding for the National Institutes of Health has leveled off. We are hopeful, and even confident, that we shall both show further increases in grant-supported activities.

To assure that no promising research that may be related to the fundamental process of cell transformation goes unfunded, we have established a firm, dual-assignment policy. Thus, if projects related to cancer cannot be funded by other institutes, they are also assigned to the Institute. Their priorities as determined by NIH Study Sections or by other institutes, are considered along with the priorities of applications coming directly to the Institute. If their priorities are higher than the Institute's cut-off point, they are funded with cancer dollars. We currently support between 3.5 and 4.0 million dollars worth of research this way.

In fiscal year 1971, before the new National Cancer Program began, the Institute had a budget of $233 million. In 1972, the first year of the new Cancer Program, it was $378 million. In 1973, it was $432 million; and in 1974 our operating level was $589.2 million, including impounded funds released by the President.

I would like to further break down the allocation of these funds. Although most of the available money is in extramural programs, more than 15 percent is used in intramural research and direct operating costs, and, thus, it does not enter the competitive arena.

For fiscal year 1974, $39.0 million (6.6 percent) was used to support our intramural scientists, and $51.9 million (8.8 percent) paid for our own direct operating costs plus our share of the National Institutes of Health management fund. A small amount (2.4 percent) supported cancer research performed by other federal agencies; this is effected by an Interagency Agreement. But, clearly over 50 percent of extramural funds are expended in support of grants, and, if Interagency Agreements are excluded, the ratio is 58 percent grants and 42 percent contracts.

A comparison of research and research-supported activities by grant and by contract is of interest, as follows: Funds for total research grants, including traditional grants, cancer centers, and off-campus task forces, increased from 50 percent of grant and contract funds in 1972 to 55 percent in 1974, for an amount of $217.7 million. Of the $91 million for cancer centers, only $20 million was for core support; the remaining $71 million supported regular competitive research projects, which could just as well be shown in the category above. The figure of $217.7 million for research grants does not include *all* money funded through grants. Additional grant funds (amounting to about $70 million) are included with other activities, such as training, cancer control, and construction. I should also point out the sizable increases in funding for regular research grants from 1972 to 1974. On the contract side, about one-half of the research contract funds were for support activities, and these went to support grantees as well as other contractors. Research contracts and research support contracts decreased from 50 percent in 1972 to 45 percent in 1974, for an amount of $175.8 million. In addition, we managed to enhance our fellowship and training program to $25.6 million, surpassing the $20 million figure in 1972, which was our previous peak year for the support of training. You should be aware that Mr. Benno C. Schmidt, the chairman of the President's Cancer Panel, has championed the cause for the restoration and maintenance of training programs for the benefit of all of the National Institutes of Health.

A review of the history of the Institute grant support from 1964 through 1973 highlights the fact that the number of grants funded increased from 884 in 1970 to 1424 in 1973, from $63.8 million to $138.2 million. These figures also show that the rate of grant support has increased commensurate with the rate of contract support. Is this increase enough? Certainly not. Is good research going unfunded? Yes, it is. The point is that, along with the increase in funded grants, there has been a threefold increase in the number of applications submitted, which means a larger number of unfunded applicants. There is no doubt that some investigators, who would not have done so, are now gearing their work toward cancer. Balance is, of course, the key question. What is the appropriate cut-off level for funding approved applications to assure that the best research is done with the finite resources available? What is the best combination of grant and contract support to assure that knowledge is applied in clinical medicine, to be delivered to the American people? These are questions we grapple with every day, and we solicit your suggestions and and recommendations.

A final point is that substantial support is given by the Institute to research projects of young investigators. In fiscal year 1972, 52 percent of the applications of investigators 35 years of age and under were approved and funded: 32 percent of the applications of investigators over age 35 were approved and funded. For those under 35, only 35 percent of applications were disapproved, whereas 55 percent for those over 35 were disapproved. The average dollar amount was slightly more for the over 35 group ($47.6 thousand) than for the young group ($36.4 thousand). This seems reasonable, since the older investigator usually has attracted professionals and would be expected to maintain a somewhat larger laboratory.

Because of the scientific emphasis of this anniversary symposium on cancer virology, I would like to discuss the Virus Cancer Program briefly. As many of you in this audience know, the Institute, in 1964, received a special appropriation of $10 million from Congress to develop an intensified research program on cancer viruses and on leukemia and related diseases. An early task was to encourage investigators to apply for support through the Virus Cancer Program for studies that were deemed promising and important to the control of human leukemia. The Contracts were used to get the program going quickly. Contracts could be awarded to academic or commercial investigators within about three months. (It takes about nine months to process and award grants.) In addition, the Institute was encouraged to support research in private, commercial laboratories, where the contract is the only funding possible.

To a large extent, the work performed by investigators in this program taught us that approaches other than simple isolation of viruses must be used to determine whether viruses cause human cancers. We feel that the program has expanded the base of scientific information, so that additional advances can be made toward control of human cancer.

There were, however, growing criticisms of the virus program. Dr. Rauscher consulted with the National Cancer Advisory Board, which, in March 1973, appointed a committee headed by Dr. Norton Zinder of Rockefeller University to review the program. The committee's final report was submitted at the Board's meeting in March, 1974.

The committee unanimously felt that viral oncology was a high priority area and that area should be broadened and more virologists supported. The major criticism was on the management of the program. The report emphasized that contracts do not receive the same high quality peer review that grants receive, and that the program was too much an Institute in-house operation. The committee recommended a program with an appropriate mix of contract and grant-type work, all open to competition and decided upon by the collective wisdom of the working groups in coordination with a steering committee and the segment chairmen of the program. In response to the report, a board subcommittee, chaired by Dr. Harold Amos, was appointed to advise on the selective implementation of the recommendations. Recommendations endorsed by the subcommittee and approved by the Board are beginning to be implemented. I might add, the Institute has all this time been reviewing management and scientific aspects of the program and taking steps to make modifications, and, particularly, changes in the review process.

I do not want to close this discussion without mentioning another special mandate of the 1971 Act, and a major priority of the Institute—the Cancer Control Program. The main goal of cancer control is to mobilize all present research knowledge and technology to help people with cancer and at risk to cancer *now*. This program's high priority reflects a growing public, congressional, and scientific commitment to getting research results to the people.

Among the programs under way are:

- Some 30 breast cancer detection demonstration projects geographically distributed throughout the country to screen women at risk.
- Education programs to reduce lung cancer deaths due to cigarette smoking.
- Studies to detect early lung cancer through the use of sputum cytology and a flexible fiberoptic bronchoscope.
- Demonstration of the new treatments for acute lymphocytic leukemia, Hodgkin's disease, and other lymphomas.
- A national network of comprehensive cancer centers for a broad range of cancer-related research and demonstration activities, including outreach activities to local medical service communities.
- Specialized cancer centers for a wide variety of basic and clinical research activities; cooperative clinical trials under specified research protocols; and organ site task forces for study of cancer of particular body organs, such as the large bowel and bladder.

In closing then, I would like to state the two interrelated objectives of the National Cancer Program: to conduct research in promising areas and to assure the application of regimens derived from this research to all persons who can benefit from it. Thus, we support a vast array of fundamental research projects and many areas of clinical medicine.

The research of virologists and microbiologists is crucial to cancer research. I know the Institute of Microbiology will continue its excellent research record, and I am confident its future will be as bright as its past. Thank you again for inviting me to share this commemoration with you.

Contributors

P. Alexander
Chester Beatty Research Institute
Belmont, Sutton, Surrey
England

J. P. Bader
National Cancer Institute
Bethesda, Maryland

D. Baltimore
Department of Biology and Center for
    Cancer Research
Massachusetts Institute of Technology
Cambridge, Massachusetts

R. Baserga
Department of Pathology and Fels
    Research Institute
Temple University School of Medicine
Philadelphia, Pennsylvania

N. Battula
Institute for Cancer Research
Fox Chase Center for Cancer and
    Medical Sciences
Philadelphia, Pennsylvania

H. Bauer
Institut für Virologie
Gieben, West Germany

R. Benveniste
National Cancer Institute
Bethesda, Maryland

D. Berkoben
Waksman Institute of Microbiology
Rutgers University
New Brunswick, New Jersey

S. Bhaduri
Institute for Molecular Virology
St. Louis University School of Medicine
St. Louis, Missouri

J. M. Bishop
Department of Microbiology
University of California
San Francisco, California

S. Bowers
Waksman Institute of Microbiology
Rutgers University
New Brunswick, New Jersey

D. L. Bronson
Department of Urologic Surgery
University of Minnesota School of Medicine
Minneapolis, Minnesota

M. M. Burger
Department of Biochemistry
Universität Basel
Basel, Switzerland

V. S. Byers
Department of Medicine
University of California School of Medicine
San Francisco, California

R. Callahan
National Cancer Institute
Bethesda, Maryland

A. E. Castro
Department of Urologic Surgery
University of Minnesota School of Medicine
Minneapolis, Minnesota

P. H. Cleveland
Department of Urologic Surgery
University of Minnesota School of Medicine
Minneapolis, Minnesota

D. Colcher
Meloy Laboratories, Inc.
Springfield, Virginia

G. Delage
Institut Gustave-Roussy
Villejuif, France

I. Djerassi
Mercy Catholic Medical Center
Philadelphia, Pennsylvania

F. R. Eilber
Division of Oncology
Department of Surgery
UCLA School of Medicine
Los Angeles, California

Contributors

A. Y. Elliot
Department of Urologic Surgery
University of Minnesota School of Medicine
Minneapolis, Minnesota

C. Feit
Waksman Institute of Microbiology
Rutgers University
New Brunswick, New Jersey

S. Feldman
Institute for Cancer Research
Columbia University
New York, New York

E. Fenster
Institut Gustave-Roussy
Villejuif, France

S. Ferrone
Scripps Clinic and Research Foundation
La Jolla, California

J. Folkman
Department of Surgery
Children's Hospital Medical Center and the
Harvard Medical School
Boston, Massachusetts

E. E. Fraley
Department of Surgery
University of Minnesota School of Medicine
Minneapolis, Minnesota

H. H. Fudenberg
Department of Basic and Clinical Immunology
and Microbiology
Medical University of South Carolina
Charleston, South Carolina

R. E. Gallagher
National Cancer Institute
Bethesda, Maryland

R. C. Gallo
National Cancer Institute
Bethesda, Maryland

H. Gelderblom
Robert Koch-Institut
Berlin, West Germany

D. Gillespie
National Cancer Institute
Bethesda, Maryland

R. Glaser
Department of Microbiology
The Milton S. Hershey Medical Center of the
Pennsylvania State University
Hershey, Pennsylvania

S. H. Golub
Division of Oncology
Department of Surgery
UCLA School of Medicine
Los Angeles, California

A. A. Gottlieb
Waksman Institute of Microbiology
Rutgers University
New Brunswick, New Jersey
Present address:
Department of Microbiology and Immunology
Tulane University School of Medicine
New Orleans, Louisiana

M. Green
Institute for Molecular Virology
St. Louis University School of Medicine
St. Louis, Missouri

K. Grinwich
Waksman Institute of Microbiology
Rutgers University
New Brunswick, New Jersey

Y. Groner
Albert Einstein College of Medicine of
Yeshiva University
Bronx, New York

R. R. Guntaka
Department of Microbiology
University of California
San Francisco, California

R. K. Gupta
Surgical Services
Sepulveda Veterans Administration Hospital
Sepulveda, California

T. R. Hakala
Department of Urologic Surgery
University of Minnesota School of Medicine
Minneapolis, Minnesota

T. Harel
Institut Gustave-Roussy
Villejuif, France

C. Heidelberger
McArdle Laboratory for Cancer Research
University of Wisconsin
Madison, Wisconsin

xvi

I. Hellström
Department of Pathology
University of Washington
Seattle, Washington

K. E. Hellström
Department of Pathology
University of Washington
Seattle, Washington

E. C. Holmes
Surgical Services
Sepulveda Veterans Administration Hospital
Sepulveda, California

J. Hurwitz
Albert Einstein College of Medicine of
    Yeshiva University
Bronx, New York

M. Jacquet
Albert Einstein College of Medicine of
    Yeshiva University
Bronx, New York

M. Klagsbrun
Department of Surgery
Children's Hospital Medical Center and the
    Harvard Medical School
Boston, Massachusetts

R. Kurth
Robert Koch-Institut
Berlin, West Germany

F. Lacour
Institut Gustave-Roussy
Villejuif, France

J. Lacour
Institut Gustave-Roussy
Villejuif, France

A. S. Levin
Department of Medicine
University of California School of Medicine
San Francisco, California

A. J. Levine
Department of Biochemical Sciences
Princeton University
Princeton, New Jersey

M. M. Lieber
Meloy Laboratories, Inc.
Springfield, Virginia

L. A. Loeb
Institute for Cancer Research
Fox Chase Center for Cancer and
    Medical Sciences
Philadelphia, Pennsylvania

M. C. Loni
Institute for Molecular Virology
St. Louis University School of Medicine
St. Louis, Missouri

R. J. Mannino, Jr.
Department of Biochemistry
Universitat Basel
Basel, Switzerland

D. J. Marciani
National Cancer Institute
Bethesda, Maryland

A. M. Mauer
St. Jude Children's Research Hospital
Memphis, Tennessee

C. F. McKhann
Department of Surgery
University of Minnesota
Minneapolis, Minnesota

R. Michalides
Meloy Laboratories, Inc.
Springfield, Virginia

S. Mizutani
McArdle Laboratory for Cancer Research
University of Wisconsin
Madison, Wisconsin

G. Monroy
Albert Einstein College of Medicine of
    Yeshiva University
Bronx, New York

D. H. Moore
Institute for Medical Research
Camden, New Jersey

D. L. Morton
Division of Oncology
Department of Surgery
UCLA School of Medicine
Los Angeles, California

S. B. Murphy
St. Jude Children's Research Hospital
Memphis, Tennessee

G. R. Newell
National Cancer Institute
Bethesda, Maryland

D. E. Nicholson
Waksman Institute of Microbiology
Rutgers University
New Brunswick, New Jersey

A. M. Novi
Pathologishes Institut
Universität Düsseldorf
Dusseldorf, West Germany

S. Oh
Scripps Clinic and Research Foundation
La Jolla, California

A. Panet
Department of Biology and Center for
    Cancer Research
Massachusetts Institute of Technology
Cambridge, Massachusetts

E. Pankuch
Waksman Institute of Microbiology
Rutgers University
New Brunswick, New Jersey

M. A. Pellegrino
Scripps Clinic and Research Foundation
La Jolla, California

O. J. Plescia
Waksman Institute of Microbiology
Rutgers University
New Brunswick, New Jersey

E. H. Postel
Department of Biochemical Sciences
Princeton University
Princeton, New Jersey

F. Rapp
Department of Microbiology
The Milton S. Hershey Medical Center of the
    Pennsylvania State University
Hershey, Pennsylvania

R. A. Reisfeld
Scripps Clinic and Research Foundation
La Jolla, California

M. S. Robin
Institute for Molecular Virology
St. Louis University School of Medicine
St. Louis, Missouri

S. Salzberg
Institute for Molecular Virology
St. Louis University School of Medicine
St. Louis, Missouri

W. C. Saxinger
National Cancer Institute
Bethesda, Maryland

J. Schlom
National Cancer Institute
Bethesda, Maryland

G. Schochetman
Meloy Laboratories, Inc.
Springfield, Virginia

G. Seal
Institute for Cancer Research
Fox Chase Center for Cancer and
    Medical Sciences
Philadelphia, Pennsylvania

G. Shanmugam
Institute for Molecular Virology
St. Louis University School of Medicine
St. Louis, Missouri

C. T. Sherr
National Cancer Institute
Bethesda, Maryland

A. H. Smith
Waksman Institute of Microbiology
Rutgers University
New Brunswick, New Jersey

R. G. Smith
National Cancer Institute
Bethesda, Maryland

F. C. Sparks
Department of Surgery
Sepulveda Veterans Administration Hospital
Sepulveda, California

S. Spiegelman
Institute for Cancer Research
Columbia University
New York, New York

C. F. Springate
Institute for Cancer Research
Fox Chase Center for Cancer and
    Medical Sciences
Philadelphia, Pennsylvania

N. Stein
Department of Surgery
University of Minnesota School of Medicine
Minneapolis, Minnesota

H. L. Sulit
Division of Oncology
Department of Surgery
UCLA School of Medicine
Los Angeles, California

T. Sun Kim
Mercy Catholic Medical Center
Philadelphia, Pennsylvania

U. Suvansri
Mercy Catholic Medical Center
Philadelphia, Pennsylvania

H. M. Temin
McArdle Laboratory for Cancer Research
University of Wisconsin
Madison, Wisconsin

L. Thomas
Memorial Sloan-Kettering Cancer Center
New York, New York

G. J. Todaro
National Cancer Institute
Bethesda, Maryland

H. E. Varmus
Department of Microbiology
University of California
San Francisco, California

I. M. Verma
Department of Biology and Center for
    Cancer Research
Massachusetts, Institute of Technology
Cambridge, Massachusetts

T. Young
Meloy Laboratories, Inc.
Springfield, Virginia

Contents

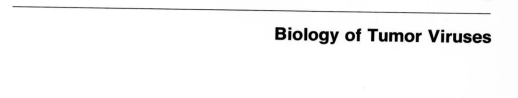

Biology of Tumor Viruses

1

On the Evidence for Type-C RNA Tumor Virus Information and Virus-Related Reverse Transcriptase in Animals and in Human Leukemia Cells

D. Gillespie, R. E. Gallagher, R. G. Smith, W. C. Saxinger, and R. C. Gallo

Introduction

RNA tumor viruses obtained from animals or from cultured animal cells can be divided into two categories, "endogenous" and "exogenous." Endogenous RNA tumor viruses can be obtained from ostensibly normal (uninfected) cells or animals, some have been shown to be vertically transmitted (parent to progeny *via* the germ line), and those viruses that have been tested contain RNA that is closely related in nucleotide sequence to the genes of normal animals of the species that generated the virus. It has not been convincingly demonstrated that endogenous viruses induce neoplasia in animals, nor that they transform cells in culture. Exogenous viruses, obtained from virus-producing tumor tissue, are not closely related in nucleotide sequence to the genes of normal host cells and do induce neoplasia in recipient animals.

It is important to determine whether *human* neoplasia is induced by endogenous or exogenous RNA tumor viruses. Neoplasia caused by an endogenous virus represent a physiologic disturbance, possibly trigged by an external factor (carcinogen), but, conceptually, it does not require invasion by a different biologic entity. Neoplasia caused by an exogenous virus might involve the introduction of foreign metabolites through infection. Our views on how best to detect, follow, and treat a given human cancer may depend on whether the etiologic agent originates within the patient or comes from an outside source.

It is useful to list in advance our conclusions, for they derive from several types of experiments. We believe that there exist in the genome of mammalian cells several different genes that normally govern special functions in differentiation but that can also induce RNA tumor viruses (9,12,15). These genes we call "class I" genes. They are equivalent, in some respects to the "virogenes" postulated by Huebner and Todaro, but in the context of our discussion,

Fundamental Aspects of Neoplasia,
edited by A. Arthur Gottlieb, Otto J. Plescia, and David H. L. Bishop.
© 1975 by Springer-Verlag New York Inc.

their physiologic role is in normal differentiation, not in virogenesis. We believe that an RNA tumor virus genome is created when a class I gene is improperly expressed, possibly, when the RNA transcript from a class I gene is processed by an unusual method (12,15). The class of viruses so generated are class I, or endogenous, viruses and, as such, have a slight pathologic effect on cells or none at all. From the evidence discussed below it is suggested that frankly tumorigenic RNA tumor viruses (exogenous or class II viruses) arise from a class I virus-cell interaction during infection (14,15) in a manner similar to that proposed by Temin (41). The two classes of viruses can often be distinguished by molecular hybridization and immunologic assays. With respect to human neoplasia, these assays reveal in peripheral blood white cells of some patients with leukemia, the presence of components of both virus classes, including reverse transcriptase and nucleic acid components genetically related to analogous components in tumorigenic, primate, type-C RNA tumor viruses. Normal human, dividing, peripheral blood white cells do contain some viral-related components, but they do not contain the primate, class II virus-related components mentioned above. The results leading to these conclusions are presented below. If we have interpreted them correctly, it means that experiments indicating infection as a cause for human leukemia will have to rule out the possibility that "foreign" virus components are endogenous virus elements that have been genetically modified. It also implies that a fruitful line of research will involve learning how an endogenous RNA tumor virus originates and how it becomes an exogenous virus.

Genetic Relationship between Endogenous (Class I) RNA Tumor Viruses and Cells

The simple fact that some apparently normal cells can be stimulated to produce RNA tumor viruses in the absence of any known biologic factor has prompted the conclusion that the genetic information of those viruses is identical to the genes in normal animals of the same species from which the progenitor cell was derived; that is, that the viruses are truly endogenous. The context in which these endogenous viruses are defined is one wherein particular genes of normal animals (virogenes) are derepressed, and the RNA transcripts of these genes are packaged into virus particles with the nucleotide sequence of the RNA unchanged (17). In practice, we cannot draw this conclusion from biologic experiments alone, for the experiments are concerned with the phenotype of the virus, not its genotype, and we cannot be absolutely sure that the progenitor cell is uninfected.

Reasonable presumptive evidence for this conclusion can be obtained by the use of molecular hybridization, in which the RNA of the virus is annealed to

DNA from normal animals. A positive result means that the nucleotide sequences in the animal DNA are similar to those in the viral RNA. If an excess of DNA is used, the fraction of viral RNA sequences shared by the animal genome can be determined. Table 1-1 describes the biologic origin of "endogenous" viruses tested by hybridization, and Table 1-2 presents the hybridization results (see also refs. 9,12,13,15,25,27,28). More than 70 per-

Table 1-1 Biologic Origin of RNA Tumor Viruses

A.	Endogenous (Class I) viruses	
	RAV_0 (Rous-associated virus)	Released spontaneously by normal embryos of line 7 chickens (cited in ref. 27)
	RD114	Cultured human rhabdomyosarcoma cells following passage in fetal kittens (cited in refs. 13 and 15).
	GPV (guinea pig virus)	Released following bromodeoxyuridine treatment of cultured normal or leukemic guinea pig cells (cited in ref. 25)
	$MMTV_{DW}$ (strain Dmochowski–Williams of mouse mammary tumor virus)	spontaneous mammary tumor in rIII mice (cited in ref. 28)
	BEV (baboon endogenous virus)	Released spontaneously by bat or canine cells following co-cultivation with baboon placental cells (cited in ref. 4)
B.	Exogenous (Class II) viruses	
	Rous sarcoma virus	Chicken sarcoma
	Avian myeloblastosis (leukemia) virus	Chicken leukemia
	Feline sarcoma virus, Gardner strain	Cat sarcoma
	Feline leukemia virus, Rickard strain	Cat leukemia
	Mouse leukemia virus, Rauscher strain	Plasma of a leukemic mouse
	Mouse leukemia virus, Moloney strain	Mouse sarcoma
	Mouse sarcoma virus, Moloney strain	Moloney leukemia virus, following maintenance in mouse fibroblast cells
	Gibbon ape leukemia virus	Cultured tumor cells from a gibbon ape with lymphosarcoma (cited in ref. 15). The virus produced by the gibbon ape tumor cells has also been grown in normal human lymphoid (NC37) cells
	Simian sarcoma virus	Marmoset cells, following culture with a cell-free extract from a woolly monkey fibrosarcoma (cited in ref. 15). The virus produced by the marmoset cells has also been grown in normal rat kidney (NRK) and human (NC37) cells

Table 1-2 Hybridization of 70 S RNA of Endogenous (Class I) Viruses to DNA from Normal Cells

In each case, ^{3}H-labeled 70 S RNA was isolated from isopycnically purified viruses. This RNA was annealed to an approximately 10^6-fold weight excess of sheared, denatured DNA purified from ostensibly normal animals under the conditions specified here. In the first two cases, with hybrids formed at 67°C, hybrids were detected by chromatography on hydroxyapatite columns; in the remaining three cases, hybrids were assayed by resistance to ribonuclease.

Source of 70 S RNA[a]	Source of Animal DNA	Hybridization conditions	Percent RNA hybridized	Reference
RAV$_0$	Chicken	0.4 M PO$_4$, 67°, $C_ot=10^4$	> 70	27
RD114	Cat	0.4 M PO$_4$, 67°, $C_ot=10^4$	> 60	13
		0.4 M PO$_4$, 67°, $C_ot=10^4$	> 60	14
GPV	Guinea pig	0.5 M PO$_4$, 70°, $C_ot=5\times10^4$	> 80	25
MMTV$_{DW}$	Mouse	0.4 M PO$_4$, 60°, $C_ot=10^4$	>100	14

[a] See Table 1-1 for abbreviations.

cent of the RNA of endogenous viruses hybridizes to DNA isolated from normal animals of the same species as the original host. It is not known whether the failure to hybridize all of the viral RNA is a technical problem, inherent in the hybridization assay, although this is suspected to be the case (see ref. 25).

Hybridization between the RNA of RNA tumor viruses and DNA of normal cells is a specific interaction. This is indicated by two parameters of the hybridization reaction: its specificity for DNA from the natural host cells and the thermal stability of the hybrid complex formed with that DNA. Table 1-3 presents data on the specificity of a hybridization reaction in which RNA from mouse mammary tumor virus and an endogenous cat virus RD114 were used. The RNA isolated from these viruses hybridizes preferentially to DNA from normal host cells; there is less hybridization to DNA from other mammals (see also refs. 12–15). Other work has shown that RNA from an endogenous chicken virus, RAV$_0$, and from an endogenous guinea pig virus also hybridize preferentially to DNA from natural host cells (25,27). Table 1-4 presents data from many sources concerning the thermal stability of hybrids formed between RNA from endogenous viruses and DNA from their natural host cells. All of the hybrids display a rather high t_m. The thermal stability of a hybrid complex is related to the number of hydrogen bonds per base pair; hence, poly (A):poly (dT) with two hydrogen bonds per base pair has a lower thermal stability (t_m) than poly (G):poly (C) with three hydrogen bonds per base pair. Mismatches, the presence of unpaired or non-Watson–Crick paired bases, reduces

6

Table 1-3 Hybridization of RNA from Class I Viruses to DNA from Different Animals

Hybridization was carried out in 0.4 M PO$_4$ buffer at 60°, under conditions described in the legend to Table 1-2. Hybrids were detected by resistance to ribonuclease. (The data are taken in part from Gillespie, et al., ref. 14.)

Source of RNA	Source of DNA	Percent RNA hybridized	
		$C_ot = 10^3$	$C_ot = 10^4$
Mouse mammary tumor virus, strain DW	Mouse	45	100
	Rat	0	24
	Cat	0	15
	Rabbit	1	—[a]
	Calf	0	—[a]
	Human	0	5
Cat virus, strain RD114	Cat	40	73
	Rat	0	10
	Mouse	3	9
	Calf	2	—[a]
	Human	0	9
Mouse rRNA	Mouse	76	—[a]
	Rat	74	—[a]
	Calf	77	—[a]
	Human	73	—[a]
Mouse poly (A)-containing RNA (cytoplasmic)	Mouse	—[a]	45
	Rat	—[a]	37
	Human	—[a]	15

[b] Not tested.

the t_m of a hybrid structure by reducing the number of hydrogen bonds per base pair in the hybrid. Table 1-4 shows that the thermal stability of the hybrid formed at the highest permissible temperature between RNA from RD114 virus and DNA from normal cat cells is the same as the thermal stability of a hybrid formed between ribosomal RNA and DNA under optimal hybridization conditions. (Ribosomal RNA:DNA was chosen as a standard because its (G+C) content is similar to that of RNA tumor virus RNA.) These data indicate that there is little difference in nucleotide sequences (0 to 2 percent) between certain genes in normal cats and the analyzed portion of RD114 virus RNA. The only other endogenous virus RNA analyzed with this precision is that from mouse mammary tumor virus. The t_m of the hybrid formed at the highest permissible temperature between this RNA and normal mouse DNA is

Table 1-4 Thermal Stability of Hybrids Formed between RNA from Endogenous (Class I) Viruses and DNA from Normal Cells

Hybrids were formed with each virus RNA–cell DNA pair as described in Table 1-2 and its legend. In the experiments utilizing RNA from MMTV and RD114 and assaying hybrids with ribonuclease, the t_m of hybrids formed at several temperatures was measured. The t_m was not influenced by the temperature of hybrid formation in these cases (12). The t_m of the rRNA:DNA hybrid was determined on hybrids formed at 75° and was the highest t_m observed with this RNA when hybrids formed at several temperatures was analyzed. DNA:DNA standard signifies reannealed cell DNA.

Virus RNA[a] Animal DNA	Hybrid assay conditions	t_m of hybrid	standard	t_m of standard	Reference
RAV₀	Hydroxyapetite, 0.18 M Na⁺	82.5°	DNA:DNA	85.7°	27
RD114	Hydroxyapetite, 0.18 M Na⁺	81°	DNA:DNA	85.5°	13
	Ribonuclease, 0.15 M Na⁺[b]	86.5°	rRNA:DNA	86.5°	14
GPV	Ribonuclease, 0.18 M Na⁺	90°[c]	None		25
MMTV_DW	Ribonuclease, 0.15 M Na⁺[b]	83°	rRNA:DNA	86.5°	14

[a] See Table 1-1 for abbreviations.

[b] Hybrids carried out to $C_0t = 10^3$; all others carried out to the C_0T value shown in Table 1-2.

[c] Incubation with ribonucleases A and Tl was carried out in 0.12 M PO₄. The effects of this inhibitory buffer on the specificity of ribonuclease is not known, at least to us.

83°, indicating about a 5 percent divergence in nucleotide sequence of the analyzed portion of this RNA from the mouse DNA. In neither of the above cases was the t_m influenced by the temperature of hybrid formation in the range 60° to 80°. Other hybrids formed between RNA from endogenous viruses and DNA from normal cells also have a high t_m (Table 1-4), but there is no appropriate standard, and the method of hybrid detection used precludes an estimate of the degree of RNA–DNA similarity in nucleotide sequence. It should be noted that the t_m are most readily interpreted if the hybrid is formed at the highest temperature that does not influence hybrid yield, for the genomes of higher animals are so complex that the t_m are strongly dependent on the temperature of hybrid formation.

In sum, these hybridization results show a genetic proximity between endogenous RNA tumor viruses and those animals from which the viruses are isolated. The results, however, also show that some viruses classified as endogenous on biologic criteria will be proved not to be truly endogenous by molecular hybridization criteria. Mouse mammary tumor virus (strain DW, from rIII mice) appears to carry nucleotide sequences that are slightly different from those in similar genes in the normal mouse, although it is classified as an endogenous virus. We prefer to call viruses that are genetically proximal to normal host cells—determined by molecular hybridization—class I viruses, as distinguished from the class II viruses. The utility of the class I–class II nomenclature is discussed later.

Although genes similar or identical to endogenous RNA tumor virus genomes have been found in the DNA of all normal progenitor cells examined, viral RNA or viral proteins have not. RD114-like RNA is found in several types of feline cells (30); mouse mammary tumor-like RNA is found in some normal mouse tissues but not all (34); RAV$_o$-like RNA is found in many "normal" chicken cells (16), and RNA similar to that of baboon placental virus is found in baboon placenta but not in baboon liver (4). Normal cells that produce viral-like RNA follow no discernible pattern, but apparently production of viral RNA by normal cells is not a universal process. At least one normal tissue produces RNA-dependent DNA polymerase (reverase transcriptase) that is immunologically similar to that found in the endogenous virus produced by that type of tissue: placentae of primates yield type-C viruses. Viruses from baboon placenta have been propagated in heterologous cells (4). Reverse transcriptase has been purified from the placenta of one primate, a rhesus monkey, and the purified enzyme was shown to be immunologically indistinguishable from that of a primate, placental, type-C virus particle (21); this is discussed later. But this is the only clear example of a normal tissue producing reverse transcriptase. When we consider the molecular hybridization results described earlier, it appears that all normal mammalian cells have the genetic mechanism required to produce endogenous RNA tumor viruses but only certain cells use this mechanism.

Genetic Relationship between Exogenous (Class II) RNA Tumor Viruses and Cells

Exogenous viruses are not a well-defined group of RNA tumor viruses. Biologically, exogenous viruses differ from endogenous viruses in that they are obtained from tumor tissue and cause neoplasia in recipient animals, whereas endogenous viruses may also be obtained from ostensibly normal cells and do not cause neoplasia in recipient animals. It is of some interest to determine the genetic relationship between exogenous viruses and normal host cells, for, although exogenous viruses have not yet been isolated from normal cells, this does not rule out the possibility that exogenous viruses, like endogenous viruses, represent escaped cell elements.

Molecular hybridization can be used to distinguish the two virus types. Only a small fraction of RNA from exogenous (class II) viruses can hybridize to DNA from normal animals (Table 1-5). Moreover, the thermal stability of

9

Table 1-5 Hybridization of 70 S RNA from Exogenous (Class II) Viruses to DNA from Normal Cells

In each case ^{3}H-labeled 70 S RNA was isolated from isopycnically purified viruses. This RNA was annealed to an approximately 10^6-fold weight excess of sheared, denatured DNA purified from ostensibly normal animals. Hybridization conditions were 0.4 M and 60°C, except in the case of Rous sarcoma virus where hybrids were formed in 0.4 M PO_4 at 67°C. The hybridization was carried out to $C_ot = 10^4$, although in every case except that of Rous sarcoma virus maximal hybridization was achieved by $C_ot = 10^3$. Hybrid formation was monitored by resistance to ribonuclease except in the case of Rous sarcoma virus where hybrids were detected by chromatography on hydroxyapatite columns.

Source of Virus 70 S RNA	Source of animal DNA	Percent RNA hybridized	Reference
Rous sarcoma virus	Chicken embryo	>30	26
Avian myeloblastosis (leukemia) virus	Chicken embryo	30	
Feline sarcoma virus, strain Gardner	Cat liver or spleen	18	14
Feline leukemia virus, strain Rickard	Cat liver or spleen	16	14
Mouse leukemia virus, strain Rauscher	Mouse liver, spleen, or cultured cells	20	14
Mouse sarcoma virus, strain Moloney	Mouse liver, spleen, or cultured cells	17	14
Simian sarcoma virus (produced by normal rat kidney cells)	Woolly monkey liver Normal human white blood cells Normal rat spleen	0[a,b] 2[a] 20[a]	
Simian sarcoma virus (produced by normal human lymphoid cells)	Normal human white blood cells	>40[a]	

[a] Unpublished results of W. C. Saxinger, S. Gillespie, W. Prensky, R. C. Gallo, and D. Gillespie.
[b] Hybrid formation is detectable at C_ots between 100 and 1,000, but the hybrid disappears with time. No hybrid is obtained at 70°C.

these hybrids is lower than that of similar hybrids involving RNA from endogenous viruses (12,14,26). It appears that the exogenous viruses are not as closely related to their hosts as are the endogenous viruses; it is clear, however, that the exogenous viruses are not totally unrelated to normal animals and that the percentage of the RNA that does hybridize varies with the conditions of hybrid formation and detection. In the case of Rauscher leukemia virus, some 30 percent of its RNA hybridizes to RNA from normal mice (e.g., NIH Swiss general-purpose mice) when the hybrid is formed at 60° C and detected by

RNase resistance. But, when hybrids are formed the same way are assayed by retention on nitrocellulose, over 70 percent of the RNA can be found complexed to mouse DNA (but not to human DNA) in a structure with a low t_m (F. Wong-Stall, unpublished work). A likely explanation of this is that the genome of the Rauscher leukemia virus originated from a cell gene and then evolved away from it. An examination of the interrelatedness of several leukemia viruses has lead to the same conclusion. Radioactive DNA copies of viral RNA have been made *in vitro* by reverse transcriptase and hybridized to RNA isolated from other RNA tumor viruses to determine the genetic relatedness among the viruses. When this analysis is restricted to leukemia viruses, it is found that leukemia viruses from different animals are related to one another; specifically, their relationship follows the pattern that relates their natural hosts (22). This finding has been interpreted to mean that exogenous and endogenous RNA tumor viruses both originate from host genes.

Some normal cells produce proteins that are antigenically similar to gs proteins of exogenous viruses, but, again, these proteins are not produced in all cells. Proteins like the gs antigen of Rauscher leukemia virus are produced in mouse embryo but not in mouse adult cells (cited in ref. 15). Embryos of some strains of chickens produce viral proteins; embryos from other strains do not (cited in ref. 15). Reverse transcriptase, related to the transcriptase of an exogenous virus, has never been detected in an uninfected cell. Antibody against viral reverse transcriptase does not inhibit DNA polymerases α, β, or γ of normal cells which, suggests that viral reverse transcriptase and the DNA polymerases of normal cells are not related genetically. This is not as sensitive a test for immunologic relatedness, however, as is a blocking antibody test, for example. In fact, it is likely that the viral gene coding for reverse transcriptase originated from information in the cell, at least in the case of the leukemia viruses. The interrelatedness of reverse transcriptases from leukemia viruses has been assessed immunologically by measuring the inhibition of activity of one reverse transcriptase by antibody prepared against another. As in the case of the virus genomes, the leukemia virus reverse transcriptases show an interrelatedness pattern similar to the pattern of genetic relatedness seen among the virus natural hosts (cited in refs. 9,12,15).

We note, in Table 1-5, that 70 S RNA from simian sarcoma virus produced by normal rat kidney cells does not form a stable hybrid with DNA from woolly monkeys or humans, but 20 percent of it will hybridize to rat DNA. On the other hand, 40 percent of the 70 S RNA from simian sarcoma virus grown in normal human lymphoid cells can form a hybrid structure with human DNA. Simian sarcoma virus was originally obtained from a woolly monkey and then propagated in marmoset cells (see ref. 9). The virus emanating from marmoset cells was introduced directly into the rat and human cells. It appears that the virus acquired nucleotide sequences from the genome of its rat and human host cells. This phenomenon may be similar to the acquisition of endogenous cat virus sequences, when the exogenous cat leukemia virus is cultured in feline embryo cells (5).

Class I and Class II RNA Tumor Viruses

Class I RNA tumor viruses are those viruses that are closely related genetically to genes in normal host cells; class II viruses are more distinctly related to cell genes (Tables 1-2 and 1-5). Classification is based solely on molecular hybridization assays, unlike the endogenous–exogenous classification that is based on biologic parameters. Evidence was presented in the previous two sections that the genomes of both classes of viruses obtained from cell DNA. We propose also that class II viruses evolve from class I viruses. Table 1-6 is a summary of our working hypothesis concerning the origin of avian, feline, murine, and primate RNA tumor viruses.

Table 1-6 Proposed Progenitor–Descendant Relationship among Normal Cells and RNA Tumor Viruses

See text for details.

Animal progenitor Cells	Class I viruses	Intermediate	Class II viruses
Chicken ⟶	RAV₀ ───────────	⟶	Rous sarcoma virus
		⟶	Avian myeloblastosis virus
Cat ⟶	? ───────────	⟶	Feline leukemia virus
		⟶	Feline sarcoma virus
Cat ⟶	RD114 ───────────	⟶	?
Mouse ⟶	?[a] ⟶	Mouse mammary tumor virus ⟶	?[a]
Mouse ⟶	Xenotropic type-C virus ⟶	AKR virus ⟶	Rauscher leukemia virus
		⟶	Moloney leukemia virua
		⟶	Moloney sarcoma virus
		⟶	
Primate ⟶	? ───────────	⟶	gibbon ape leukemia virus
		⟶	simian sarcoma virus virus
Primate ⟶	Placental type-C ───────────	⟶	?

[a] There may possibly be a spectrum of mammary tumor viruses. It would be interesting if the least tumorigenic were true class I and the most tumorigenic were Class II.

In the chicken virus group, RAV_0 is an endogenous class I virus with an RNA that hybridizes to DNA from normal chickens (27). Avian sarcoma virus, strain Rous, and avian myeloblastosis (leukemia) virus are class II viruses (26,38). But RAV_0 is closely related genetically to the class II viruses (29), and the DNA polymerases of these two classes of viruses appear to be immunologically identical (21). In the chicken system, it seems reasonable to conclude that the class II viruses evolved from RAV_0. In the cat viruses, RD114 is an endogenous class I virus, whereas the common strains of cat sarcoma and leukemia viruses are class II. Unlike the chicken system, however, RD114 is not genetically related to the class II cat viruses (5), nor is the RD114 reverse transcriptase immunologically related to the transcriptases of the class I cat viruses (20). The RD114 and the class II cat RNA tumor viruses appear to have different genetic origins. Mouse mammary tumor virus is an enigma. The RNA from this type-B virus hybridizes to DNA from normal mice, but the thermal stability of the hybrid complex is lower than that expected for a perfect hybrid, indicating that the virus has diverged slightly from its progenitor cell. It may represent an intermediate between a class I and class II virus. It is not genetically related to any other mammalian virus tested (22). Type-C mouse RNA tumor viruses are more easily categorized. Strains Rauscher and Moloney mouse leukemia viruses are class II viruses (14). The AKR virus is probably an intermediate between class I and class II (7), and the iododeoxyuridine-induced, xenotropic, type-C mouse viruses are probably class I. Genetically, AKR virus is related to Rauscher and Moloney virus, and all of the type-C mouse viruses share an antigenically common reverse transcriptase. These facts are consistent with the hypothesis that the xenotropic virus arises directly from cell components and that the AKR leukemia virus and the Rauscher and Moloney leukemia viruses evolved from the xenotropic virus. The classes of the primate RNA tumor viruses are similar to those of the cat viruses. The primate placental virus appears to be class I (4), and the simian sarcoma and gibbon ape leukemia viruses class II (36). The primate class I and class II viruses are not related genetically, nor are their reverse transcriptases related immunologically (37).

Virus Markers in Cells Producing RNA Tumor Viruses

Cells infected by and producing class II viruses contain viral nucleotide sequences in the DNA genome and viral RNA and viral proteins in the cytoplasm. One class II viral protein, in particular, viral reverse transcriptase, has never been convincingly demonstrated to occur in cells not producing RNA tumor viruses. At least some of the viral reverse transcriptase and RNA are associated in a particle obtained from the cytoplasmic fraction of disrupted cells. This association is a functional one in the sense that when the particulate fraction is fed deoxynucleoside triphosphates, DNA can be synthesized *in vitro*. The DNA synthesis ("endogenous" DNA synthesis) does not require added template or reverse transcriptase. The DNA contains viral sequences and is associated with RNA (presumably viral RNA) (35). It appears that the presence of class II virus reverse transcriptase and the endogenous synthesis of DNA sequences complementary to RNA from class II viruses indicates that the tested cells are producing RNA tumor viruses. In this section, we detail experiments that bear on the nature of viral reverse transcriptase in a cell that is obviously producing virus; in the next section, we correlate these results with similar data obtained from fresh human leukemic cells.

Reverse transcriptases isolated from several mammalian type-C RNA tumor viruses have been found to have molecular weights of 70,000 (cited in refs. 2,8). DNA polymerases isolated from a cytoplasmic particle (24) obtained from human lymphoid cells infected by and producing a type-C primate RNA tumor virus, the gibbon ape leukemia virus, are of two size classes, as judged by velocity sedimentation in sucrose density gradients. If we assume that both forms are globular proteins, the molecular weights of these forms are 70,000 (4.5 S) and 137,000 (6.5 S) (Fig. 1-1B). By several criteria, discussed below, both DNA polymerase forms have reverse transcriptase activity, which is not the activity seen in normal cell DNA polymerases.

There is now evidence that three distinct DNA polymerases exist in normal uninfected mammalian cells. These enzymes have been separated and partially characterized (Table 1-7). (Unless specifically mentioned, a selection of original articles are cited in refs. 12 and 15). The largest of these enzymes is called DNA polymerase alpha. It is a 7 S protein (MW$= 1.5 \times 10^5$) recovered preferentially from the cytoplasmic fraction of disrupted cells. It has also been called DNA polymerase I and "maxi-polymerase". *In vitro* it uses poly(dA) preferentially as a template, in the presence of a suitable primer, and it uses poly(rA) poorly and poly(rC) not at all. The DNA polymerase alpha fails to transcribe heteropolymeric regions of 70 S viral RNA. Its activity *in vitro* is not inhibited by antibody prepared against DNA polymerases isolated from any of several RNA tumor viruses, nor does antibody against it inhibit the activity of viral reverse transcriptase or the remaining two normal cell DNA polymerases (39). The smallest of the normal cell DNA polymerases is DNA polymerase beta. It is a 3.5 S protein (MW$= 0.4 \times 10^5$), which is recovered from both the nuclear and the cytoplasmic fractions of disrupted cells. It has also been called DNA polymerase II and "minipolymerase". *In vitro*, the template used most effectively by this enzyme is poly (dA), although poly (rA) can also be transcribed by DNA polymerase beta. Its activity *in vitro* is not inhibited by antibody prepared against viral reverse transcriptases or by

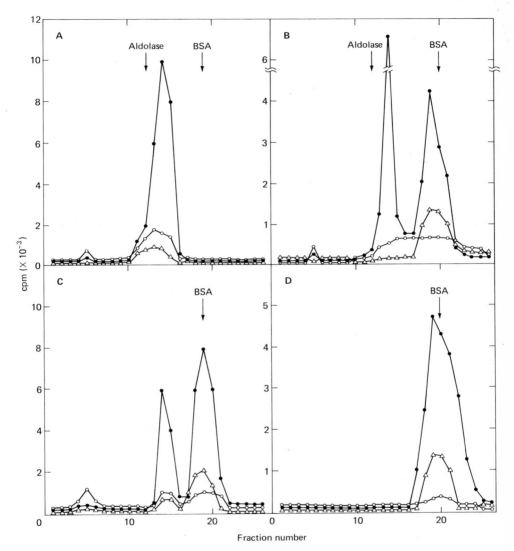

Figure 1-1. Effect of salt and detergent treatment on the sedimentation of RNA-directed DNA polymerases from human leukemic blood cells and gibbon ape virus-producing lymphosarcoma cells (10 to 60 percent glycerol gradients were prepared and run). Gradients were collected from below. DNA polymerase activities determined as described (24) and also with 40 μg/ml dG$_{12-18}$:C$_n$ (Collaborative Research, Waltham, Mass.), using 16 μm [^{3}H]dGTP (NEN, 4,628 cpm/pmole). (A) Human leukemic cell enzyme, 0.1 M KCl. (B) Gibbon ape lymphosarcoma cell enzyme, 0.1 M KCl. (C) Human leukemic cell enzyme, 0.5 M KCl, 0.5 percent Triton X-100. (D) Gibbon ape lymphosarcoma cell enzyme, 0.5 M KCl, 0.5 percent Triton X-100 (●), dT$_{12-18}$:A$_n$, (○), dT$_{12-18}$:dA$_n$, (△), dG$_{12-18}$:C$_n$. (Data taken from Mondal, et al., ref. 24.)

Table 1-7 Properties of Mammalian DNA Polymerases

Property	DNA Polymerase alpha	DNA polymerase beta	DNA polymerase gamma	Human leukemic reverse transcriptase
1. Cellular location	Cytoplasmic	Nuclear or cytoplasmic	Not known	Cytoplasmic
2. Molecular weight	1.3×10^5	0.4×10^5	About 10^5	1.3×10^{5b} 0.7×10^5
3. Utilization of oligo (dT):poly (rA) and oligo (dT):poly (dA)	Poly (dA)> poly (rA)	Poly (dA)> poly (rA)	Poly (rR)>poly (dA) (with Mn²⁺)	Poly (rA)>> poly (dA)
4. Utilization of oligo (dG):poly (rC)	None	None	None or very low	Yes
5. Utilization of polymeric regions of HMW viral RNA	None	None	Slight or none	Yes
6. Inhibition with antibody (IGG) prepared against purified DNA polymerases from				
SiSV or GaLV	None	None	None	Strong
MuLV	None	None	None	Weak
FeLV or AvLV	None	None	None	None
Mp-MV	None	None	None	None
Human cells (polymerase alpha)	Strong	None	None	None

ª Obtained specifically with human cells.

ᵇ The 1.3×10^5 is converted to a 0.7×10^5 form in high salt. (H. Mondal, R. E. Gallagher, and R. C. Gallo, unpublished observations.)

antibody prepared against DNA polymerase alpha (18). The remaining DNA polymerase activity found in normal cells is likely to be due to a separate enzyme, DNA polymerase gamma. This enzyme has also been called DNA polymerase III and "R"-DNA polymerase. It is a 6 to 6.5 S protein (MW~10^5). In vitro, DNA polymerase gamma uses poly (dA) and poly (rA) as a template. In the presence of M_n^{2+}, poly (rA) is the preferred template; in the presence of M_g^{2+}, DNA polymerase gamma uses poly (dA) preferentially. The enzyme uses poly (rC) poorly, if at all. Like the other two normal cell DNA polymerases, DNA polymerase gamma is not inhibited in vitro by antibodies prepared against viral reverse transcriptase or by antibodies prepared against DNA polymerase alpha (18).

The DNA polymerases detected in the cytoplasmic particle of cells producing gibbon ape leukemia virus have properties unlike any of the three normal cell DNA polymerases, but similar to the properties of reverse transcriptases purified from extracellular viral reverse transcriptase (Table 1-8). The enzyme with 70,000 MW activity uses poly (rC) as a template and is effectively inhibited by antibodies prepared against reverse transcriptase isolated from extracellular gibbon ape leukemia virus. The 137,000 MW form does not use poly (rC) as efficiently, nor is it as easily inhibited by anti-reverse transcriptase antibodies, but, unlike the normal cell DNA polymerases, it can effectively transcribe viral 70 S RNA.

The 137,000 MW form of DNA polymerase detected in the cytoplasmic particle of the virus-producing cell is probably an alternate state of the 70,000 MW form. When the cytoplasmic particle is exposed to 0.5M NaCl and 0.5 percent Triton X-100, only the 70.000 MW form is detectable (Fig. 1-1D). When the 137,000 MW form is collected after velocity centrifugation, it can be converted to a 70,000 MW form by exposure to high salt and Triton X-100. But, removal of salt and Triton from the 70,000 MW form thus generated results in a transition back to the 137,000 MW form. Finally, the 70,000 and 137,000 MW forms derived by changing salt and Triton concentrations have the same template and immunologic properties as their analogues obtained directly from the cytoplasmic particle. Enzyme activities having properties characteristic of viral reverse transcriptase have not been detected in uninfected control cells, although attempts have been made to find them. The particles purified from the cytoplasm of gibbon ape leukemia virus-producing cells can carry out endogenous DNA synthesis. The DNA product synthesized hybridizes to 70 S RNA isolated from extracellular gibbon ape leukemia virus particles (H. Mondal, unpublished results). From the results presented above, we suggest that the presence of particulate reverse transcriptase immunologically related to class II type-C RNA tumor viruses is indicative of a cell producing a class II RNA tumor virus. Transformed mouse cells not producing virus particles have so far not yielded true reverse transcriptase (cited in ref. 9).

In the primates, the reverse transcriptases of the class II viruses (simian sarcoma virus and gibbon ape leukemia virus) are immunologically distinct from those enzymes of the known endogenous virus (e.g., the type-C particles seen in monkey placentae and propagated in the case of the baboon placental virus particle). It was of some interest to purify the DNA polymerases from monkey placentae and determine (a) whether intracellular reverse transcriptase could be detected and (b) if it could, whether the placental reverse transcriptase was immunologically related to that of class I or class II primate, type-C RNA tumor viruses. The techniques used to purify the DNA polymerases from rhesus monkey placenta are detailed elsewhere (19); Tables 1-9

Table 1-8   Primer–Template Responses of the High and Low Molecular
Weight Forms of RNA-Directed DNA Polymerase Isolated from
Human Leukemic Blood Cells, from Gibbon Ape Lymphosarcoma
Cultured Cells Producing Gibbon Ape Leukemia Virus (GAL
Cells), and from Extracellular Gibbon Ape Leukemia
Virus (GALV)

The enzymes used in these studies were the pooled activities shown and described earlier
(24), which were adjusted to a final glycerol concentration of 50 percent stored at $-20°C$.
Reactions with the oligomeric-homopolymeric hybrids were performed as described in
Figure 1-1. For the experiments with AMV 70 S RNA, 25 μg/ml of RNA was used with
or without 20 μg/ml of dT_{12-18}. The 70 S RNA was heated to 90°C for 1 min and slowly
cooled to room temperature to permit reannealing. Reactions with AMV 70 S RNA were
performed under the same conditions as described in Figure 1-1 except that 3 mM DDT,
0.1 M APT, and all four deoxyribonucleoside trisphosphates (16 μM each) were used.
Sources and specific activities of deoxyribonucleoside were as follows: [³H]dTTP; 6,200
cpm/pmole; [³H]dGTP, 4,000 cpm/pmole; [³H]dATP, 4,600 cpm/pmole; [³H]dCTP,
4,300 cpm/pmole; all were obtained from New England Nuclear Corp., Boston, Mass.
No significant stimulation of deoxyribonucleoside monophosphate incorporation was
observed with AMV 70 S in the presence of dG_{12-18}, dC_{12-18}, or dA_{12-18} over values with
AMV 70 S RNA alone. Protein determinations were by the method of Lowry et al. (23).
Values are reported as picomoles of deoxyribonucleoside monophosphate incorporated
per 10 μg of enzyme protein per hour reaction time. With AMV 70 S RNA, values were
calculated by determining the average specific activity of the deoxyribonucleoside
triphosphate precursors, and equimolar incorporation of all four substrates is assumed.
(Data taken from Mondal et al., ref. 24.)

---

and 1-10 describe the biochemical and immunologic properties of the one DNA
polymerase found that resembled viral reverse transcriptase. This enzyme uses
poly (rA) in preference to poly (dA) in the presence of M_n^{2+} or M_g^{2+} and
effectively transcribes poly (rC). It is recovered as a 70,000 MW form, but
an initial step in the purification procedure is exposure of the cell extract to
high concentrations of salt and detergent. No attempt has yet been made to
convert it to a 137,000 MW form. As described in Table 1-9, the activity of
this enzyme is inhibited by antibodies prepared against reverse transcriptase of
the endogenous, baboon placental type-C virus particle but is not inhibited by
antibodies prepared against reverse transcriptase from the simian sarcoma virus
or the gibbon ape leukemia virus. This result is useful from two points of
view. First, it is the first DNA polymerase isolated from a normal tissue that
meets the rigid biochemical and immunologic criteria defining a reverse transcriptase. Since the enzyme was isolated from fresh tissue, there is not the

	DNA polymerase activity (pmoles/10 μg/hr)				
	Human leukemic cell enzyme		"GAL cell" enzyme		
Primer–template	137,000 form	70,000 form	137,000 form	70,000 form	"GALV" enzyme[a]
$dT_{12-18}:A_n$	2.05	10.41	11.51	63.42	56.21
$dT_{12-18}:dA_n$	0.60	2.12	2.17	2.5	2.32
dT_{12-18}	0.01	0.01	0.01	< 0.05	0.05
$dG_{12-18}:C_n$	0.70	3.41	0.56	12.32	26.52
dG_{12-18}	<0.01	<0.01	0.01	0.02	<0.01
AMV 70 S RNA					
Complete	1.20[b]	0.64[b]	2.88[b]	2.52[b]	0.48[b]
	1.20[c]	0.72[c]	3.44[c]	2.04[c]	—[d]
Complete+dT_{12-18}	1.08[b]	1.16[b]	2.60[b]	8.72[b]	18.44[b]
	1.16[c]	1.44[c]	3.00[c]	5.24[c]	—[d]
Complete−dGTP	0.04	0.04	0.04	0.10	—[d]
Complete−dTTP	0.04	0.04	0.12	0.04	—[d]

[a] Only one enzyme form with an approximate molecular weight of 70,000 was detected.

[b] Activity using [³H]TTP, [³H]dATP, and [³H]dCTP with cold dGTP.

[c] Activity using [³H]dGTP, [³H]dATP, and [³H]dCTP with cold dTTP.

[d] Not tested.

nagging doubt that somehow the cells became inadvertently infected by a laboratory RNA tumor virus, unless the animal itself had become infected. Second, it comes from normal tissue known by electron-microscope studies to be capable of producing type-C viruses (33) but not suspected of being a malignant tissue. We would predict, based on the results presented in the preceding discussions, that this tissue would not produce reverse transcriptase immunologically related to the transcriptases of class II, primate, type-C RNA tumor viruses. A single study of the placental reverse transcriptase verifies this prediction.

Virus Markers in Human Leukemic Cells

We describe below two markers in some human leukemic cells, which we feel are characteristic of class II RNA tumor viruses. The first marker is a

Table 1-9   Reverse Transcriptase from Rhesus Monkey Placenta: Effect of Template–Primer and Divalent Cations on Enzyme Activity

Assay mixtures contained 10 μl of enzyme and were initiated by adding 40 μl of a mixture to give a final concentration of 0.05 M Tris HCl (pH 7.5): 0.001 M dithiothreitol; either 0.1 M MgCl$_2$ or 0.0008 M MnCl$_2$; 80 μM each of unlabeled deoxynucleoside triphosphate [dATP for assays containing $(A)_n:(dT)_{12-18}$ and $(dA)_n:(dT)_{12-18}$, and $(dG)_{12-18}$]; 14.5 μM [^{3}H]TTP (28,000 cpm/pmole); and template–primer (31 μg/ml). All reactions were performed at 37°C for 30 min. Acid-insoluble precipitates were collected on nitrocellulose filters, and the radioactivity was counted in a liquid scintillation counter. Enzyme activity is expressed as picomoles of ^{3}H-labeled deoxynucleoside monophosphate incorporated per milliliter of reaction mixture. (Data taken from Mayer et al., ref. 21.)

Template–primer	Tritium-labeled substrate	Divalent cation	Enzyme activity
$(A)_n:(dT)_{12-18}$	TTP	Mn^{2+}	3.140
$(A)_n:(dT)_{12-18}$	TTP	Mg^{2+}	<0.500
$(C)_n:(dG)_{12-18}$	dGTP	Mn^{2+}	4.980
$(C)_n:(dG)_{12-18}$	dGTP	Mg^{2+}	2.600
$(dA)_n:(dT)_{12-18}$	TTP	Mn^{2+} or Mg^{2+}	<0.500
Primer alone			
[$(dT)_{12-18}$ or $(dG)_{12-18}$]	TTP or dGTP	Mn^{2+} or Mg^{2+}	<0.500

reverse transcriptase isolated from a cytoplasmic particle that is biochemically and immunologically related to reverse transcriptase purified from class II, but not class I, primate, type-C RNA tumor viruses. The second is a DNA product synthesized endogenously *in vitro* in a reverse transcriptase-like reaction, to yield a DNA population of which at least one fraction is associated with RNA through a heat-sensitive linkage; another large fraction is capable of hybridizing specifically to RNA isolated from a primate, class II RNA tumor virus (simian sarcoma virus). The results detailed below suggest that some human leukemic cells have properties comparable to properties of cultured cells that produce class II RNA tumor viruses.

Reverse transcriptase has been detected in and partially purified from the cytoplasm of human leukemic cells but not the cytoplasm of proliferating white blood cells from normal donors (6,11,32,40). The enzyme has template preferences that resemble those of viral reverse transcriptase (32) and is immunologically related to reverse transcriptase purified from class II, primate, type-C RNA tumor viruses (8,24,42). But three properties of the human leukemic enzyme appeared to differ from the properties of the reverse tran-

Table 1-10   Effect of Antibody (IgG) to Primate Viral Reverse
Transcriptases on Enzyme Activity of the Reverse Transcriptase

Variable amounts of IgG were mixed with 10 μl of enzyme. Each sample was brought
to a volume of 20 μl by the addition of buffer (0.1 M Tris HCl, pH 8.0) or a sufficient
amount of nonimmune (control) IgG to bring the total IgG input to 100 μg (except in
the reactions containing IgG to M7 polymerase, where the total IgG was 20 μg), and the
mixture was kept at 0°C for 10 min. Reverse transcriptase assay mixtures were processed
as described in Table 1-9, except that the incubation period was 120 min at 30°C. The
template–primer was $(A)_n:(dT)_{12-18}$ and the divalent cation was Mn^{2+}, except in the
reactions containing the Mason–Pfizer viral enzyme, where Mg^{2+} was substituted. Antibody
to woolly monkey sarcoma virus reverse transcriptase was prepared in a rat; antibodies
to Mason–Pfizer and M7 virus reverse transcriptase were prepared in rabbits. Control IgG
was purified from serums of unimmunized rats and rabbits, respectively. IgG against
woolly monkey and Mason–Pfizer virus reverse transcriptase was isolated from serums by
Sephadex G-200 chromatography (29), concentrated by precipitation in 50 percent
ammonium sulfate, and dialyzed against 0.1 M Tris HCl. The IgG against M7 virus
reverse transcriptase was purified as described (37). (Data taken from Mayer et al., ref. 21.)

		Micrograms of purified immune IGG required to inhibit reverse transcriptase activity by 25 or 50 percent						
		Woolly monkey virus		Mason–Pfizer virus		Baboon placental virus		
	Control							
Source of reverse transcriptase	25%	25%	50%	25%	50%	25%	50%	
Woolly monkey virus	>100	10	45	>100	>100	—	—	
Mason–Pfizer	>100	>100	>100	39	74			
Rhesus monkey placenta	>100	>100	>100	>100	>100	3	9	
Baboon placental (M7) virus	> 20	—	—			3	9	

scriptase purified from extracellular mammalian RNA tumor viruses. First, the
human enzyme exhibited a molecular weight of 137,000 compared to the
70,000 MW consistently obtained with reverse transcriptase from extracellular
type-C mammalian cells. Second, the human enzyme utilized viral 70 S RNA
more efficiently than the mammalian virus enzymes assayed under similar conditions. Third, although the human leukemic enzyme could be neutralized by
antibodies prepared against viral reverse transcriptase, the inhibition was often
incomplete and sometimes required an unusually large amount of antibody.
Our experience with the cytoplasmic particles of human lymphoid cells
producing gibbon ape leukemia virus provided a possible solution to this
apparent contradiction, for the properties of the human leukemic enzyme were

strikingly similar to those of the 137,000 MW intracellular form of reverse transcriptase from the gibbon ape leukemia virus-producing cells. Graph A in Figure 1-1 shows that the DNA polymerase activity fraction extracted from a particle isolated from the cytoplasm of peripheral leukocytes from a patient with acute myelogenous leukemia sediments in a glycerol gradient as would a globular protein with a molecular weight of 137,000. Upon exposure to 0.5M NaCl and 0.5 percent Triton X-100, most of the activity is reduced to a 70,000 MW for m(Figure 1-1C), paralleling the behaivor of the enzyme activity of the gibbon ape leukemia virus-producing cells (Fig. 1-1B, and D). Table 1-8 and Figure 1-2 show that the biochemical and immunologic properties of the high and low molecular weight forms of the intracellular human leukemic enzyme are the same as those of the analogous forms detected in virus-producing cells. Specifically, the human leukemic DNA polymerase activity acquires the capacity to transcribe poly (rC) and loses some of its ability to transcribe viral 70 S RNA upon conversion from the high to low molecular weight form (Table 1-8) and, at the same time, becomes more sensitive to antibodies prepared against reverse transcriptase purified from simian sarcoma virus (Figure 1-2). Human leukemic enzymes sensitive to these antibodies have not been observed in every leukemic patient studied, but they have been observed in the majority of cases of acute myelogenous leukemia (five out of seven cases studied). In no case has an enzyme been detected in human leukemic cells that is sensitive to antibodies that inhibit reverse transcriptase from the class I primate virus from baboon placenta. These results suggest the presence in some human leukemic cells of a reverse transcriptase that is specifically related to reverse transcriptase isolated from primate, class II RNA tumor viruses. No enzyme with these properties has been found in proliferating white blood cells from normal donors.

A preparation of particles obtained from the cytoplam of human leukemic cells can carry out the endogenous synthesis of DNA *in vitro* (13,27). In several cases it has been shown that over 50 percent of this DNA population is capable of hybridizing to RNA isolated from class II RNA tumor viruses (9,42). One such case is illustrated in Table 1-11 and is compared to a population of DNA synthesized endogenously by particles prepared from the cytoplasm of proliferating white blood cells from normal donors. A note is appropriate here, concerning the characteristics of endogenous DNA synthesis by particles of normal cells contrasted to those of DNA synthesis by particles of leukemic cells. Normal cell synthesis is carried out on a DNA template as judged by its sensitivity to actinomycin D anl from a physical analysis of the DNA product–template complex (31). The same analyses show that endogenous DNA synthesis carried out by particles in leukemic cells is effected, at least in part, by an RNA template (1,10). Both DNA populations contain

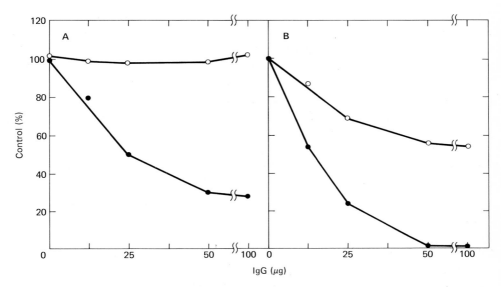

Figure 1-2. Effect of antisera (IgG) to RNA-directed DNA polymerase from woolly monkey type-C virus on RNA-directed DNA polymerase from human leukemic blood cells and from gibbon ape virus-infected lymphosarcoma cells. Antisera were prepared in rats, and IgG was purified as described elsewhere (39). The enzymes used in these studies were the pooled activities from the glycerol fractions shown in Figure 1-2. The respective enzymes were preincubated at 4°C for 30 min with an equal volume of mimune or nonimmune rat IgG. The IgG was diluted with 0.1 M Tris HCl (pH 8.0) to give the indicated quantity. Assays for the incorporation of [^{3}H]TMP on dT$_{12-18}$:A$_n$, using the enzyme preincubated with IgG, were performed as described in Figure 1-1. In the absence of immune IgG, cpm of [^{3}H]TMP were incorporated 10,000 to 25,000. The values are expressed as percent of activity in the presence of an equal amount of nonimmune IgG, which had a negligible effect on all enzymes. (A) Human leukemic cell enzymes, (B) Gibbon ape lymphosarcoma enzymes; (○) 137,000 dalton enzyme, (●) 70,000 dalton enzyme. (Data taken from Mondal et al., ref. 24.)

sequences that hybridize to 70 S RNA isolated from RNA tumor viruses; only the DNA product synthesized by the particle from leukemic cells, however, hybridizes to DNA known to be from a class II, RNA tumor virus–simian sarcoma virus grown in normal rat kidney cells. The DNA synthesized by particles from both leukemic and normal human white blood cells hybridizes to RNA from simian sarcoma virus grown in normal human lymphoid cells. As described earlier, 70 S RNA isolated from this virus contains a major component capable of hybridizing to DNA from normal human cells. It is possible

Table 1-11 Hybridization of DNA Synthesized Endogenously by Cytoplasmic Particles from Normal and Leukemic Cells to 70 S RNA from RNA Tumor Viruses

The results are expressed as percentage of input [³H]DNA hybridized to the indicated RNA [0=less than 1 percent hybridized after background was subtracted]. The [³H]DNA was synthesized from material in the 1.17 g/ml density regions of a sucrose isopycnic gradient centrifugation of the 100,000×*g* cytoplasmic pellet, which was obtained from homogenized cells after removal of mitochondria, nuclei, and other large structures (10). The [³H]DNA synthesis was carried out in the presence of all four ³H-labeled nucleotide triphosphates, 50 mM Tris (pH 7.4), 1 mM MnCl₂, 5 DDT, 20 mM KCl and (where indicated) 50 μg/ml actinomycin D (Act. D) and 0.03 percent Triton X-100. There was no exogenous template nucleic acid added. The viral 70 S RNA was purified and immobilized on filter discs as described (10,22). The hybridizations, with the DNA in solution (1,000 to 3,000 cpm), were carried out in 100 μl of 50 percent formamide, 3×SSC (0.45 M NaCl–0.045 M Na citrate), 0.01 M Tris HCl (pH 7.4), at 37°. After 1 week, the filters were removed from the hybridization solutions, washed with 0.01×SSC, 0.5 percent SDS, dried, and the amount of radioactivity remaining on each filter was determined. (Details on DNA synthesized by particles from several patients and hybridized to other viral RNAs can be found in ref. 9.)

	Percent DNA hybridized, using DNA synthesized endogenously by cytoplasmic particles from	
Source of viral RNA	Patient (MT) with acute myelogenous leukemia	Normal donors (pooled)
Simian sarcoma virus grown in normal rat kidney cells	34	0
Simian sarcoma virus grown in normal human lymphoid cells	26	25
Mouse leukemia virus (AKR)	0	3
Feline sarcoma virus, strain Gardner	0	—ᵃ
Poly (A)	0	0

ᵃ Not tested.

that this isolate of simian sarcoma virus contains some type of endogenous human viral information, and it is our working hypothesis that normal human white blood cells express this information or that they, at least, have the capacity to express it. The hybridization of DNA products synthesized by particles from normal cells and several cases of leukemic cells to RNA from RNA tumor viruses, other than those listed in Table 1-10, provides additional information (9,10) and, as far as we know, does not change the conclusions drawn here.

In summary, some human leukemic white blood cells have viral reverse transcriptase and viral endogenously synthesized DNA similar to markers found in human lymphoid cells infected by, and actively producing, class II, primate, type-C, RNA tumor viruses. As described earlier, class II viruses are categorized by molecular hybridization but, also, as a group, they represent those viruses isolated from malignant tissues; they are also capable of inducing neoplasia in recipient animals. This is in contrast to class I viruses, which can be isolated from normal cells and which, for the most part, do not induce neoplasia in recipient animals. Our interpretation of the results presented here, in concert with the experiments of Baxt and Spiegelman (2,3), is that they constitute indirect evidence that class II, RNA tumor viruses are etiologic agents in at least some cases of human leukemia.

REFERENCES

1. Baxt, W., Hehlman, R., and Spiegelman, S. Human leukemic cells contain reverse transcriptase associated with a high molecular weight virus-related RNA. Nature [New Biol.], 244:72, 1972.

2. Baxt, W. G. and Spiegelman, S. Nuclear DNA sequences present in human leukemic cells and absent in normal leukocytes. Proc. Natl. Acad. Sci. USA, 69:3737, 1972.

3. Baxt, W. G. and Spiegelman, S. Leukemia-specific DNA sequences in leukocytes of the leukemic member of identical twins. Proc. Natl. Acad. Sci. USA, 70:2629, 1973.

4. Benveniste, R. E., Heinemann, R., Wilson, G. L., Callahan, R., and Todaro, G. J. Detection of baboon type-C viral sequences in various primate tissues by molecular hybridization. J. Virol., 14:56, 1974.

5. Benveniste, R. E. and Todaro, G. J. Homology between type-C viruses of various species determined by molecular hybridization. Proc. Natl. Acad. Sci USA, 70:3316, 1973.

6. Bobrow, S. N., Smith, R. G., Reitz, M. S., and Gallo, R. C. Stimulated normal human lymphocytes contain a ribonuclease-sensitive DNA polymerase which is distinct from viral RNA-directed DNA polymerase. Proc. Natl. Acad. Sci. USA, 69:3228, 1972.

7. Chattopadhyay, S. K., Lowy, D. R., Teich, N. M., Levine, A. S., and Rowe, W. P. Evidence that the AKR murine-leukemia-virus Genomes is complete in DNA of the high-virus AKR mouse and incomplete in the DNA of the "virus-negative" NIH mouse. Proc. Natl. Acad. Sci. USA, 71:167, 1974.

8. Gallagher, R. E., Todaro, G. J., Smith, R. G., Livingston, D. M., and Gallo, R. C. Relationship between reverse transcriptase from human acute leukemic blood cells and primate type-C viruses. Proc. Natl. Acad. Sci. USA, 71:1309, 1974.

9. Gallo, R. C., Gallagher, R. E., Miller, N. R., Mondal, H., Saxinger, W. C., Mayer, R. J., Smith, R. G., and Gillespie, D. H. Relationships between components in primate RNA

tumor viruses and in the cytoplasm of human leukemic cells: Implications to leukemogenesis. Cold Spring Harbor Sypm. Quant. Biol., 39:933, 1974.

10. Gallo, R. C., Miller, N. R., Saxinger, W. C., and Gillespie, D. Primate RNA tumor virus-like DNA synthesized endogenously by RNA-dependent DNA polymerase in virus-like particles from fresh human acute leukemic blood cells. Proc. Natl. Acad. Sci. USA, 70:3219, 1973.

11. Gallo, R. C., Yang, S. S., and Ting, R. C. RNA dependent DNA polymerase of human acute leukemic cells. Nature, 228:927, 1970.

12. Gillespie, D. and Gallo, R. C. RNA processing and the origin and evolution of RNA tumor viruses. Science, 188:802, 1975.

13. Gillespie, D., Gillespie, S., Gallo, R. C., East, J. L., and Dmochowski L. Genetic origin of RD114 and other RNA tumor viruses assayed by molecular hybridization. Nature [New Biol.], 244:51, 1973.

14. Gillespie, D., Gillespie, S., and Wong-Steal, F. RNA-DNA hybridization applied to cancer research: Special reference to RNA tumor viruses. *In* Methods in Cancer Research (H. Busch, ed.), vol. 11, in press.

15. Gillespie, D., Saxinger, W. C., and Gallo R. C. Information transfer in cells infected by RNA tumor viruses and extension to human neoplasia. *In* Progress in Nucleic Acid Research and Molecular Biology (Academic Press, New York, W. Cohn, ed.) 15:1 (1975).

16. Hayward, W. S. and Hanafusa, H. Detection of avian tumor virus RNA in uninfected chicken embryo cells. J. Virol., 11:157, 1973.

17. Huebner, R. and Todaro, G. J. Oncogenes of RNA tumor viruses as determinants of cancer. Proc. Natl. Acad. Sci. USA, 64:1087, 1969.

18. Lewis, B. J., Abrell, J. W., Smith, R. G., and Gallo, R. C. Human DNA polymerase III (R-DNA polymerase): Distinction from DNA polymerase I and reverse transcriptase. Science, 183:867, 1974.

19. Lewis, B. J., Abrell, J. W., Smith, R. G., and Gallo, R. C. DNA polymerases in human lymphoblastoid cells infected with simian sarcoma virus. Biochim. Biophys. Acta, 349:148, 1974.

20. Long, C., Sachs, R., Norvell, J., Huebner, V., Hatanaka, M., and Gilden, R. Specificity of antibody to RD114 viral polymerase. Nature [New Biol.] 241:147, 1973.

21. Mayer, R. J., Smith, R. G., and Gallo, R. C. Reverse transcriptase in normal rhesus monkey placenta. Science, 185:864, 1974.

22. Miller, N. R., Saxinger, W. C., Reitz, M. S., Gallagher, R. E., Wu, A. M., Gallo, R. C., and Gillespie, D. Systematics of RNA tumor viruses and virus-like particles of human origin. Proc. Natl. Acad. Sci. USA, 71:3177, 1974.

23. Mizutani, S. and Temin, H. M. Specific serological relationships among partially purified DNA polymerases of avian leukosis–sarcoma viruses, reticuleondoliosis viruses, and avian cells. J. Virol., 13:1020, 1973.

24. Mondal, R., Gallagher, R. E., and Gallo, R. C. RNA-directed DNA polymerase from human leukemic blood cellsan d from primate type-C virus-producing cells: High and low molecular weight forms with variant biochemical and immunological properties. Proc. Natl. Acad. Sci. USA, 71:1194, 1974.

25. Nayak, D. P. Endogenous guinea pig virus: Equability of virus-specific DNA in normal, leukemic, and virus-producing cells. Proc. Natl. Acad. Sci. USA, 71:1164, 1974.

26. Neiman, P. Rous sarcoma virus nucleotide sequences in cellular DNA. Science, 179: 750, 1972.

27. Neiman, P. E. Measurement of endogenous leukosis virus nucleotide sequences in the DNA of Normal Avian Embryos by RNA–DNA hybridization. J. Virol., 53:196, 1973.

28. Neiman, P. E. Measurement of RD114 virus nucleotide sequences in feline cellular DNA. Nature [New Biol], 244:62, 1973.

29. Neiman, P., Wright, E. E., McMillin, C., and MacDonnell, D. Nucleotide sequence relationships of avian RNA tumor viruses. J. Virol., 13:837, 1974.

30. Okabe, H., Gilden, R. V., and Hatanaka, M. Extensive homology of RD114 virus DNA with RNA of feline origin. Nature [New Biol.], 244:54, 1973.

31. Reitz, M. S., Smith, R. G., Roseberry, E. A., and Gallo, R. C. DNA-Directed and RNA-primed DNA synthesis in microsomal and mitochondrial fractions of normal human lymphocytes. Biochem. Biophys. Res. Commun., 57:934, 1974.

32. Sarngadharan, M. G., Sarin, P. S., Reitz, M. S., and Gallo, R. C. Reverse transcriptase activity of human acute leukemic cells: Purification of the enzyme, response to AMV 70 S RNA, and characterization of the DNA product. Nature [New Biol.] 240:67, 1972.

33. Schidlovsky, G. and Ahmed, M. C-Type virus particles in placentas and fetal tissues of rhesus monkeys. J. Natl. Cancer Inst., 51:225, 1973.

34. Schlom, J., Michalides, R., Kufe, D., H. Hehlmann, Spiegelman, S., Bentvelzen, P., and Hageman, P. A comparative study of the biologic and molecular basis of murine mammary carcinoma. J. Natl. Canc. Inst., 51:541, 1973.

35. Schlom, J. and Spiegelman, S. Simultaneous detection of reverse transcriptase and high molecular weight RNA unique to oncogenic RNA viruses. Science, 174:840, 1971.

36. Scolnick, E. M., Parks, W., Kawakami, T., Kohne, D., Okabe, H., Gilden, R., and Hatanaka, M. Primate and murine type-C viral nucleic acid association kinetics. J. Virol., 13:363, 1974.

37. Scolnick, E. M., Parks, W. P., and Todaro, G. J. Reverse transcriptases of primate viruses as immunological markers. Science, 177:1119, 1972.

38. Shoyab, M., Baluda, M. A., and Evans, R. Acquisition of new DNA sequences after infection of chicken cells with avian myeloblastosis virus. J. Virol., 13:331, 1974.

39. Smith, R. G., Abrell, J. W., Lewis, B. J., and Gallo, R. C. Serologic analysis of human DNA polymerases. Preparation and properties of antiserum to DNA polymerase α from human lymphoid cells. J. Biol. Chem., 250:1702, 1975.

40. Smith, R. C. and Gallo, R. C. DNA-Dependent DNA polymerases I and II from normal human-blood lymphocytes. Proc. Natl. Acad. Sci. USA, 69,2879, 1972.

41. Temin, H. M. The protovirus hypothesis: Speculations on the significance of RNA-directed DNA synthesis for normal development and for carcinogenesis. J. Nat. Cancer Inst., 46:III, 1971.

42. Todaro, G. J. and Gallo, R. C. Immunological relationship of DNA polymerase from human acute leukemia cells and primate and mouse leukemia virus reverse transcriptase. Nature, 244:206, 1973.

2

Evolution of Primate Type-C Viral Genes

R. E. Benveniste, C. J. Sherr, M. M. Lieber, R. Callahan, and G. J. Todaro

Introduction

The spontaneous appearance of complete, infectious type-C viruses in the animals of certain mammalian species and in cultured cells derived from these animals led to the hypothesis that the information for the production of such viruses might be transmitted genetically from parent to progeny along with the other cellular genes (15,33). DNA sequences (type-C virogenes) homologous to the RNA genomes of known type-C viruses have been detected in the somatic cell DNA of normal tissues from chickens (2) and from a variety of mammalian species (reviewed in ref. 18) and, when fully expressed, can lead to the production of complete, infectious virus particles.

Type-C virogene sequences offer several distinct advantages for the study of evolutionary relationships. As cellular genes, type-C virogenes are subject to the pressures of mutation and selection; thus, closely related animal species would be expected to have closely related, but not identical, endogenous type-C virogenes. The complete expression of virogenes, with concomitant production of type-C viruses containing specific viral proteins, a reverse transcriptase, and a high molecular weight RNA, offers a unique possibility for the isolation of a discrete set of cellular genes and their products. Because these viruses can be propagated in heterologous hosts the isolation of cellular genes with species specific properties is possible. Single-stranded [³H]DNA transcripts that represent the majority of the viral RNA sequences, synthesized *in vitro* by the viral reverse transcriptase, can be used to detect information in the cellular DNA of related species. Mammalian type-C viruses are present in cellular DNA in multiple copies (five to fifteen per haploid genome) as a family of related, but not identical, gene sequences. These sets of type-C virogene sequences appear to evolve faster than the unique sequence cellular genes. It is thus possible to establish taxonomic relationships among closely related species that are not revealed by previously described methods involving the annealing of entire unique sequence DNA.

In this chapter, we present evidence that shows that DNA sequences related

Fundamental Aspects of Neoplasia,
edited by A. Arthur Gottlieb, Otto J. Plescia, and David H. L. Bishop.
© 1975 by Springer-Verlag New York Inc.

to the sequences of endogenous baboon type-C virogenes can be identified in the genomes of all Old World monkey and ape species so far studied and that the degree of relatedness of the virogene sequences closely correlates with the taxonomic relatedness of the monkey species based upon anatomic criteria and the fossil record. DNA sequences partially homologous to the endogenous baboon type-C virogenes can also be detected in the genome of domestic cats, and baboon type-C viral RNA is shown to be partially homologous to the viral RNA of the RD114/CCC group of endogenous domestic cat viruses. Antigenic studies of the viral proteins and biologic studies *in vitro* also demonstrate such partial relatedness. Further, studies with other feline species suggest that domestic cat viruses of the RD114/CCC group originated from an exogenous infection of progenitors of domestic cats by a type-C virus that also gave rise to the present-day, endogenous type-C viruses of Old World monkeys.

Endogenous Baboon Type-C Virus

Isolation and Characterization

Six separate isolates of infectious baboon type-C virus have been obtained in this laboratory by co-cultivation of kidney, lung, testes, and placenta from several different animals of the baboon species *Papio cynocephalus* (5,34). These isolates are all morphologically and biochemically typical of mammalian type-C viruses (27,34) and have been shown to be infectious for cells of human, rhesus monkey, dog, and bat origin. Although the six isolates are all closely related by host range, viral neutralization and interference, and by immunologic and nucleic acid hybridization criteria, they are distinctly different by these same criteria from all previously studied type-C viruses (5,34) except for the viruses of the RD114/CCC group (see below).

Evolution of Primate Type-C Viral Genes

[³H]DNA transcripts prepared from three of the baboon type-C virus isolates hybridize completely to DNA extracted from tissues of various baboons of the species *P. cynocephalus* (4,5). This suggests that these type-C viruses are endogenous viruses of the baboon. If the baboon viruses were transmitted from parent to offspring as cellular genes, they would be expected to have evolved as the monkey species had evolved. It would be reasonable to suspect that other Old World monkeys that are close relatives of the baboon would have related, but not identical, gene sequences in their cellular DNA. And primates at a greater taxonomic distance from baboons would be expected to have a much more extensive mismatching of their virogene sequences.

The evolutionary relationships among the primates is the subject of much controversy. Primate ancestors are believed to have evolved from primitive mammalian insectivores during the lower Eocene and Paleocene (60 to 70 million years ago). The exact origin of the higher primates, the anthropoids (New World monkeys, Old World monkeys, apes, and man) from prosimians is not clear (29). It is believed, however, that the New World monkeys diverged from both the apes and the Old World monkeys approximately 50 to 60 million years ago. The Old World monkeys (Cercopithecoidea), which include the baboon species, are thought to have been separated from the great apes and man (Hominoidea) for 30 to 40 million years. The exact evolutionary relationship among the various genera within the Old World monkey and ape families is also uncertain. For example, estimates of divergence time between two Old World monkey genera, baboons and macaques, varies from 4 to 15 million years (17,24).

Figure 2-1,A shows a DNA reassociation experiment performed using a [³H]DNA transcript of baboon type-C virus grown in a dog thymus cell line (5) and DNA extracted from various primate species. The extent of DNA–DNA hybridization was monitored with the single-strand specific nuclease, S_1. The greatest homology is found between the baboon viral probe and *P. cyno-cephalus* tissue, as expected. At the maximal extent of the reaction approximately 80 percent of the [³H]DNA is resistant to digestion by S_1 nuclease. The DNA from another species of baboon, *P. hamadryas*, hybridizes to a lesser extent (60 percent) to the [³H]DNA probe. In order of decreasing extent of hybridization, DNA from the following genera of the Old World monkey subfamily Cercopithecinae contain nucleic acid sequences that are partially homologous to the baboon viral [³H]DNA probe: *Cercocebus* (mangabeys), *Erythrocebus* (patas monkey), *Cercopithecus* (African green monkey), and *Macaca* (stump-tailed macaque). An ape (chimpanzee) DNA hybridizes to a much smaller extent to the baboon viral probe than the DNA from any of the Old World monkey species examined, whereas New World monkey and prosimian DNA exhibit essentially background values (i.e., not significantly higher than hybridization to the DNA of various nonprimates) under the hybridization conditions employed. Thus, the baboon type-C viral DNA probe detects homologous nucleic acid sequences in all the Old World monkeys examined and shows less homology to the ape virogene sequences; no homology can be detected by these techniques in various New World monkey DNAs.

That such species as the baboon and rhesus monkey, which have diverged genetically and have been geographically separated for several million years, still retain related virogene sequences demonstrates that these sequences have been highly conserved during the course of evolution. The virogenes of Old World monkeys have thus evolved as cellular entities diverging from one another in the different genera and species in a manner consistent with a common ancestry and their presence in the ancestral primate germ line. The low, but consistently observed hybridization to ape (chimpanzee) DNA with the baboon viral probe demonstrates that this virogene information has been in the primate stock for at least 30 to 40 million years.

The presence of baboon type-C viral-specific information in tissues from various Old World primates suggests that a virus related to the baboon type-C viruses is present in the genomes of these other Old World monkeys, even though infectious virus has yet to be isolated from them. Expression of viral-specific RNA and p30 antigen has been found in normal stumptail spleen tissue and in a rhesus ovarian carcinoma (26). Thus, virogene information is not only present in various other Old World primates but is also expressed as viral-specific RNA and as p30 antigen. These genes, then, are not silent but are normally expressed; the level of expression varies from animal to animal and from tissue to tissue in a given animal.

The eucaryotic genome consists of redundant and unique (non-repeated) DNA sequences. The non-repeated DNA sequences comprise a large fraction of mammalian DNA; each sequence is believed to occur only once per haploid

---

Figure 2-1. Hybridization of baboon type-C viral [³H]DNA probe and baboon unique sequence cellular [³H]DNA to various primate cellular DNAs. The [³H]thymidine-labeled DNA probes were synthesized from detergent disrupted type-C virus in the presence of actinomycin D as described (6). The specific activity of the [³H]DNA was 1.5×10⁷ cpm/ug. The [³H]DNA probes used in these experiments contained 50 to 75 percent of their respective 70 S viral RNA sequences at a [³H]DNA [³²P]viral RNA molar ratio of 1.5 (4), thus, they contain most of the sequences present in viral RNA; and these sequences are in proportions similar to their content in 70 S RNA. Cellular

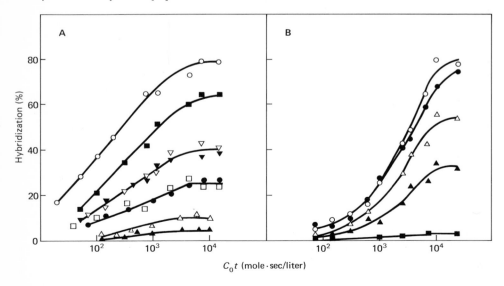

C_0t (mole·sec/liter)

genome (11). Non-repeated DNA sequences held in common between species must be the direct descendants of the same sequence present in the most recent common ancestor. Unique sequence DNA is, therefore, a suitable probe for determining the extent of nucleotide diversity acquired since two species diverged. The extent of cross-hybridization or the thermal stability measurements of the heterologous duplexes reflect interspecies evolutionary divergence. Radioactive, unique-sequence, baboon *cellular* DNA was obtained by annealing labeled cellular DNA for a sufficient time ($C_0t = 100$) to reassociate the repeated DNA sequences. This DNA was then fractionated on hydroxylapatite, and the single-stranded non-repeated fraction was isolated. The data obtained when labeled, baboon cellular DNA is hybridized to Old World monkey, ape, New World monkey, and nonprimate DNA are shown in Figure 2-1,B. The extent of reassociation between these various primate DNAs agrees with the classic paleontologic view of the relationships among the primates tested. As expected, for example, stump-tailed macaque cellular DNA is most closely related to baboon unique-sequence cellular DNA, followed by an ape (chim-

---

DNA was extracted from tissues and cell lines as described (4). All DNAs were sonically treated so as to yield a mean size of 6 to 8 S (the size of the [³H]DNA probes) as determined by centrifugation on alkaline sucrose gradients (4). The DNA: DNA hybridizations were incubated at 65°C in reaction mixtures containing 0.01 M Tris (pH 7.4), 0.75 M NaCl, 2×10^{-3} M EDTA, 0.05 percent SDS, 10,000 to 20,000 cpm/ml [³H]DNA, and 1 to 3 mg of cellular DNA/ml. Hybridizations were started by heating the mixtures to 98°C for 10 min, cooling on ice to 4°C, and incubating at 65°C. At varying times (ranging from 15 min to 96 hr), 0.05-ml aliquots were removed and frozen at −80°C until digested with the single-strand specific nuclease, S_1, as described (6). The C_0t values (C_0 is the concentration of cellular DNA in moles of nucleotide per liter, and t is the time in seconds) were calculated as suggested by Britten and Kohne (11), as $A_{260}/ml/2 \times h$ and corrected to a monovalent cation concentration of 0.18 M (12).

(A) Annealing of [³H]DNA probe prepared from the baboon type-C virus (M7) (5) grown in a canine thymus cell line (FCf2Th) to DNA extracted from

(○) baboon (*Papio cynocephalus*) lung,
(■) baboon (*Papio hamadryas*) liver,
(▽) sooty mangabey (*Cercocebus atys*) liver,
(▼) patas (*Erythrocebus patas*) liver,
(□) African green monkey (*Cercopithecus sabaeus*) liver,
(●) stump-tailed macaque (*Macaca arctoides*) spleen,
(△) chimpanzee (*Pan troglodytes*) brain,
(▲) capuchin monkey(*Cebus sp.*) or rat liver.

(B) Annealing of unique sequence baboon cellular [³H]DNA to the cellular DNA of various primates. Baboon cell line DNA was labeled with [³H]thymidine and extracted (4). Unique sequence cellular DNA was isolated by removing the highly reiterated DNA sequences that anneal by a C_0t of 100 by fractionation on hydroxylapatite (4). This [³H]thymidine-labeled unique sequence DNA was then hybridized to
(○) baboon lung DNA,
(●) stump-tailed macaque liver DNA,
(△) chimpanzee spleen DNA,
(▲) capuchin liver DNA,
(□) cat liver DNA,
(■) mouse liver DNA.

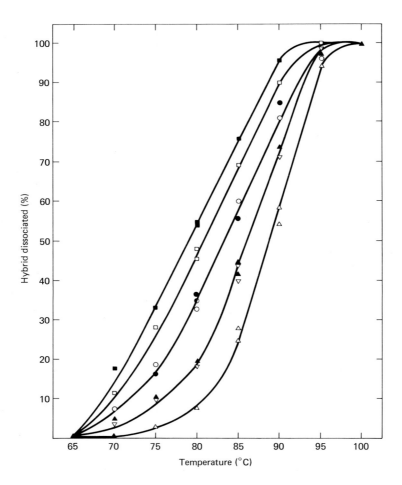

Figure 2-2. Thermal stability of hybrids formed between baboon viral [³H]DNA probe and various Old World monkey cell DNAs. The baboon [³H]DNA probe was hybridized to DNA extracted from tissues of three baboon species: ($\triangle$) (*P. cynocephalus*), ($\blacktriangle$), (*P. hamadryas*), and ($\triangledown$) (*P. papio*), and to DNA from the following primates: ($\bigcirc$) mangabey, ($\bullet$) patas, ($\square$) African green monkey, and ($\blacksquare$) rhesus. After being hybridized to $C_0t = 10^4$, aliquots containing 600 to 1,000 cpm were heated for 5 min in 0.75 M NaCl at the indicated temperatures. The amount of hybrid remaining was determined with the single-strand specific nuclease, S_1.

panzee) and a New World monkey (capuchin). The relative final extent of hybridization agrees well with the data previously obtained by Kohne (17), using hydroxylapatite to establish the relationships among the non-repetitive DNA of primates.

The thermal stability of nucleic acid hybrids can be used as an index of the degree of base-pair mismatching between the strands of a double-strand DNA molecule. Base-pair mismatching results in the formation of hybrids that melt at a lower temperature; the overall effect of mismatched base pairs on the thermal stability is reported to be between 0.7 and 1.6°C/1 percent altered base pairs (10,20). Figure 2-2 shows the melting curves obtained when a single-stranded, [³H]DNA transcript of baboon, type-C viral RNA is hybridized to the DNA from various Old World primates. The family of curves obtained exhibits a decrease in thermal stability (and, therefore, a greater degree of base-pair mismatching) that correlates well with the extent of hybridization between [³H]viral DNA and the DNA of the primates shown in Figure 2-1,A. The highest thermal stability ($T_m = 88°C$) is obtained when the baboon viral probe is hybridized to DNA from *P. cynocephalus*, the baboon species from which the virus was isolated. When DNA from two other baboon species are examined (*P. hamadryas* and *P. papio*), the T_m is slightly reduced (1.5 to 2.0°C lower than in the homologous system). The other Old World monkeys studied are more distantly related to *P. cynocephalus* by taxonomic criteria, and their DNA contain sequences that are less closely related by T_m criteria to the baboon viral probe. The lower thermal melting points obtained with the other Old World monkey DNAs further indicates that the partial homology detected between the baboon type-C viral probe and DNA from the various Old World monkey species is not the result of a strict preservation of discrete continuous segments of the viral genome in these various species, but, rather, the result of a more general base-pair substitution involving the entire viral genome.

Table 2-1 summarizes the thermal stability data obtained among the various primates using either labeled, non-repeated, baboon *cellular* DNA or ³H-labeled, baboon type-C *viral* DNA as a probe. It is evident that the baboon viral probe permits a finer discrimination among the Old World monkey species (even with different species of baboons) than would be possible by using the total, unique sequence, baboon cellular DNA. Stump-tailed macaques and baboons are believed to have diverged 4 to 15 million years ago (17,24); their unique sequence DNA exhibits a 1.5°C reduction in T_m compared to the homologous baboon hybrid. When the baboon viral DNA is used as a probe, however, T_m values obtained with the DNA from four different species of the *Macaca* genus, i.e., *M. arctoides* (stump-tailed monkey). *M. nemestrina* (pig-tailed monkey), *M. fascicularis* (crab-eating monkey), and *M. mulatta* (rhesus monkey) are all 8.5 to 9.0°C lower. Mangabey, patas, and African green

Table 2-1 Thermal Stability of Hybrids Formed between Baboon unique Sequence Cellular DNA and Type-C Viral DNA and the DNA from Various Primate Species

Species[a]	Unique sequence baboon cellular [^{3}H]DNA[b]		Baboon type-C viral [^{3}H]DNA[c]	
	Hybrid (%)	ΔT_m	Hybrid (%)	ΔT_m
Old World monkeys				
Baboon				
(P. cynocephalus)	100	<0.5	100	<0.5
(P. papio)			81	1.5
(P. hamadryas)	100	<0.5	74	2.0
Mangabey			48	5.5
Patas			38	6.0
African green			30	7.0
Macaque				
stump-tailed	91	1.5	25	8.5
pig-tailed			27	9.0
crab-eating			22	9.0
rhesus			23	9.0
Apes and man				
Chimpanzee	61	4.5	9	—[d]
Gorilla	66	4.5	8	—[d]
Gibbon	66	4.0	4	—[d]
Man	63	4.3	5	—[d]
New World monkeys				
Capuchin	31	7.5	2	>15
Howler	29	8.0	2	>15
Nonprimates				
Mouse	<2	>15	<2	>15
Dog	<2	>15	<2	>15
Domestic cat	<2	>15	19	11.0

[a] Cellular DNA was extracted from various tissues of the species listed as described (4). The scientific names of the primate species are listed in Figure 2-1, with the exception of pig-tailed macaque (*Macaca nemestrina*), crab-eating macaque (*M. fascicularis*), rhesus monkey (*M. mulatta*), gibbon ape (*Hylobates lar*), gorilla (*Gorilla gorilla*), and howler (*Alouatta spp.*).

[b] The [^{3}H]thymidine-labeled unique sequence baboon cellular DNA (4) was hybridized to the various species as described in Figure 2-1. The percent hybrid is the normalized value obtained after digestion of the hybrids with S$_1$ nuclease. The temperature at which 50 percent of the hybrids are dissociated (T_m) was 83°C for the homologous baboon:baboon hybrid; the ΔT_m is the difference in T_m between the other DNA:DNA hybrids and the T_m of the homologous hybrid.

[c] The [^{3}H]DNA probe was prepared from the baboon virus (M7) grown in the canine thymus cell line (FCf2Th) (5). The T_m of the homologous baboon:baboon hybrid was 88°C.

[d] Not tested.

monkey DNA form hybrids that are somewhat more stable. The most stable hybrids are formed with the DNA from the three baboon species, although it is clear that the viral [³H]DNA probe can even distinguish between different species of the same genus in which the *overall* unique sequence DNA is not distinguishable by these methods. Thus, it is possible (see Figure 2-3), based on the thermal stability of DNA hybrids and the final extent of reassociation, to identify Old World monkeys as belonging to one genus (*Papio*), to any of four other genera (*Cercocebus, Erythrocebus, Cercopithecus,* or *Macaca*), or to the subfamily Cercopithecinae. Members of the more primitive Old World monkey subfamily Colobinae, including the leaf-eating colobus and langur monkeys, have not been examined. A low but significant level of homology is also obtained with DNA extracted from various ape (chimpanzee, gorilla, and gibbon) and human tissues. This low level of homology can be amplified by lowering the stringency of the annealing conditions (8).

The reduction in T_m among the various primate species for the type-C viral genes and for the unique sequence cellular DNA is plotted in Figure 2-4. The primate type-C viral genes, although evolving in a fashion that correlates well with the classic paleontologic view of primate evolution, are doing so at approximately six times the rate of overall, unique sequence, primate cellular DNA. What is the basis for this apparently faster rate of evolution among primate type-C viral genes, relative to the average unique sequence cellular genes? Baboons, cats, pig, rats, and mice have all been shown to contain five to fifteen related, but not identical copies of endogenous type-C viruses (9). Specific repeated DNA sequences have been shown to diverge more rapidly than overall unique sequence DNA; examples are mouse satellite DNA (23) and the "spacer" regions of 5 S RNA (13). The presence of multiple, related virogene sequences, *each* of which presumably evolve independently of the others, may well explain why virogene sequences of primates appear to have diverged more than other cellular genes. It is this apparent faster evolutionary divergence of the primate type-C viral genes that allows one to discriminate to such a fine degree among the various Old World monkey species.

Since all mammalian species tested to date contain multiple, partially related copies of these endogenous type-C virogene sequences, one would expect the apparent faster rate of evolution demonstrated here for the primate type-C viral genes to be a general property of type-C viruses. In Table 2-2, it can be seen that pig, cat, and rat endogenous type-C viruses have also diverged faster than the unique sequence DNA of the related species. For example, among the rodents, mouse, hamster, and rat unique sequence cellular DNA was shown to be partially related, when examined in detail by other investigators (21). As can be seen, however, [³H]DNA probes prepared from rat type-C viruses do not hybridize to murine or hamster cell DNA. Moreover, various rat and

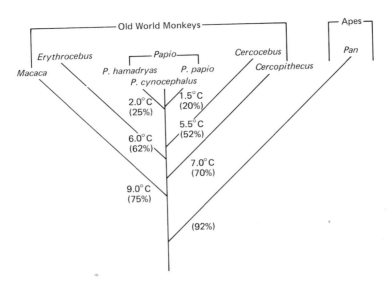

Figure 2-3. Schematic tree depicting relationships among the primates obtained with the baboon type-C viral probe. The thermal stability difference compared to the homologous (*P. cynocephalus*) hybrid, and the percent nucleic acid dissimilarity as determined with S_1 nuclease are shown.

mouse type-C isolates have previously been shown to be unrelated by viral RNA: [³H]DNA (viral) hybridization (7). Rats and mice are believed to have diverged approximately 10 million years ago, and the unique sequence cellular DNA hybrid formed between these two species melts at a temperature 9°C lower than the homologous rat:rat DNA hybrid. An equivalent reduction in T_m among unique sequence primate DNA corresponds to 70 million years of evolution. When the generation time of rodents (approximately 0.3 years) is taken into account, however, the rate of nucleotide divergence among rodents and primates is more nearly equal (17). Using the data plotted in Figure 2-4, one would expect that the nucleic acid sequences of the endogenous viruses of two species whose unique sequence *cellular* DNA melts with a T_m more than 4°C below that of the homologous T_m would not hybridize to each other to any appreciable extent under the conditions used. Therefore, as also shown in Table 2-2 for the artiodactyls (pig and cow) and the carnivores (cat, dog, mink), one would not expect the type-C viruses of those species to be sufficiently related to one another to be detected by nucleic acid hybridization. The inability to detect viral-related sequences in more distantly related species, then, reflects the more extensive changes in base sequence that have accumulated in the virogenes since divergence.

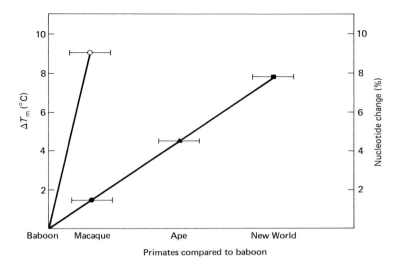

Figure 2-4. Comparison of the rate of divergence of unique sequence primate cellular DNA to that of endogenous primate type-C viral DNA. The [³H]Thymidine-labeled unique sequence baboon cellular DNA was hybridized to the following primate DNA: (●) Old World monkey (rhesus), (▲) ape (chimpanzee), and (■) New World monkey (howler). A baboon type-C viral [³H]DNA probe was annealed to (○) rhesus DNA. The scale along the abscissa is arbitrary; the T_m plotted for each hybridization is that obtained compared to the homologous (baboon:baboon) hybrid T_m. The data plotted were obtained from that given in Table 2-1.

Figure 2-5 summarizes the data for the relationship between the percent hybridization detected with nuclease S₁ and the ΔT_m for the hybridization of both unique sequence DNAs and viral type-C [³H]DNA to the cellular DNA of related species. As can be seen, the lower the percent hybridization detected between two heterologous species, the lower the thermal stability for the hybrids. The relationship is not linear, especially with hybrids that exhibit a very low homology. This curve, which is applicable only to S₁ nuclease under the hybridization conditions employed, is shown to be the same for virogenes and for unique sequence cellular genes and would be the expected curve for any diverging set of nucleic acid sequences. It should not be possible to generate data points that lie in the region above the curve (no fully homologous hybrid detected with S₁ nuclease could have a low T_m), but points lying significantly below the curve would be found if a portion of the viral gene sequence remained constant in different species (while other regions were deleted), or if a virus arose as a recombinant and contained portions of virogene sequence from two heterologous species. The data for divergence of the type-C virogene

39

Table 2-2   Thermal Stability of Hybrids Formed between Baboon, Rat, Pig, and Cat Unique Sequence Cellular DNA and Type-C Viral DNA and the DNA of Various Related Species

Cell DNA:Cell DNA[a]			Viral DNA:Cell DNA[b]		
Hybrid	T_m	$\triangle T_m$	Hybrid	T_m	$\triangle T_m$
Baboon: baboon	83	<0.5	Baboon (M7): baboon	88	< 0.5
: rhesus		1.5	: rhesus		9.0
: chimpanzee		4.5	: chimpanzee		—[c]
: capuchin		7.5	:capuchin		>15
Rat: rat	84	<0.5	Rat (RT21c): rat	89	< 0.5
: mouse		9.0	: mouse		>15
: hamster		10.0	: hamster		>15
Pig: pig	85	<0.5	Pig (PK15): pig	87	< 0.5
: cow		11.0	: cow		>15
Cat: cat	85	<0.5	Cat (CCC): cat	88	< 0.5
: mink		10.0	: mink		>15
: dog		11.0	: dog		>15

[a] The [³H]Thymidine-labeled unique sequence baboon, rat, pig, and domestic cat cellular DNA were hybridized to the cellular DNA of the species listed. The T_m was determined as described in Figure 2-2.

[b] The [³H]DNA probes were prepared from the endogenous baboon (M7) (5), rat (RT21c) (30), pig (PK15) (32), and domestic cat (RD114/CCC) (19) type-C viruses and hybridized to the cellular DNA of the species listed.

[c] Not tested.

sequences in the various primates fit this curve and thus, as mentioned above, these sequences have evolved with the primate species.

Homology between Primate and Feline Endogenous Type-C Viruses

Evidence for Partial Homology between RD114 and Baboon Type-C Viruses

The data shown in Table 2-1 demonstrate that domestic cat DNA contains sequences partially related to endogenous baboon type-C viral sequences, even though unique sequence baboon and cat *cellular* DNA show no homology. Since other primates (i.e., New World monkeys and prosimians) as well as other mammals (mouse, rat, hamster, pig, sheep, cow, dog, and mink) do not contain those related sequences, the finding of baboon type-C viral sequences in the distantly related domestic cat *(Felis catus)* clearly cannot be explained strictly on evolutionary grounds.

Domestic cat DNA is known to contain type-C virogenes, which can lead

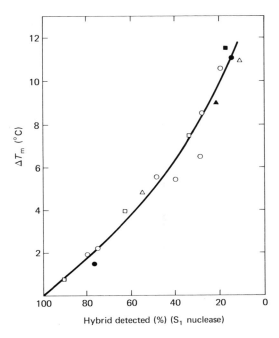

Figure 2-5. The relationship between percent hybrid detected with S_1 nuclease and the thermal melting point of DNA:DNA hybrids for various diverging nucleic acid sequences. Shown are data obtained for the hybridization of the baboon type-C [³H]DNA probe to (○) the cellular DNA of various primates, for the hybridization of an endogenous feline type C-virus probe (RD114) to (●) various cats and primates, for the hybridization of unique sequence cow cellular DNA to (△) sheep and pig DNA, (▲) unique sequence rat celular DNA to mouse cellular DNA, unique sequence baboon cellular DNA to (□) rhesus, chimpanzee and capuchin DNA, and for the hybridization of (■) cat unique cellular DNA to dog DNA. The data plotted were obtained from that shown in Tables 2-1 through 2-3.

y-axis: ΔT_m (°C)

x-axis: Hybrid detected (%) (S_1 nuclease)

to the production of endogenous type-C viruses of the RD114/CCC group (3,22). Several lines of evidence demonstrate that it is the RD114/CCC virogene information in the domestic cat that is partially homologous to the endogenous baboon type-C viral sequences. Of all the known mammalian type-C viruses (including another cat virus [FeLV]), only RD114/CCC viral RNA hybridizes to the baboon viral [³H]DNA probe (5). In reciprocal experiments, [³H]DNA probes prepared from either RD114 or CCC viruses hybridize to baboon viral RNA, to the DNA of all the Old World monkey species tested (4), and, as expected, to domestic cat cell DNA. Figure 2-6 shows the results of these reciprocal hybridization studies: There are nucleic acid sequences in baboon tissue DNA that are partially homologous to RD114, and there are nucleic acid sequences in domestic cat tissue DNA that are partially homologous to the baboon type-C virus.

Figure 2-7 shows the results of a competitive radioimmunoassay using ^{125}I-labeled purified p30 protein from the baboon virus and an antiserum developed against this antigen (28). There is a substantial cross-reaction with the p30 antigen of the RD114 virus but not with several other mammalian type-C viruses tested. The decreased slope of the RD114 competition curve indicates that the antigenic determinants of the RD114 p30 antigen are related but not identical to those of the p30 antigen of the baboon type-C virus. Also, in a radioimmunoassay developed against the purified p30 protein of the RD114

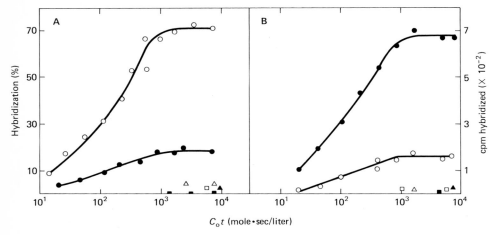

Figure 2-6. Hybridization of endogenous feline and baboon viral [³H]DNA products to DNA extracted from various mammals. Details of the hybridization are described in the legend to Figure 2-1. (A) The [³H]DNA product was prepared from baboon type-C virus grown in a canine thymus cell line (FCf2Th) and hybridized to cellular DNA extracted from (○) baboon lung, (●) domestic cat liver, (△) dog liver, (▲) mouse liver, (□) calf thymus, (■) salmon sperm. (B) The [³H]DNA product was prepared from CCC virus grown in FCf2Th. Symbols are the same as in (A). (Appeared originally in Benveniste et al., 1974, ref. 4.)

virus, the baboon virus p30 antigen shows a similar pattern of partial, but not identical cross-reaction (28).

The antigenic determinants of the reverse transcriptase of both the baboon and domestic cat endogenous viruses are also partially related (34). Figure 2-8 shows a polymerase inhibition study in which reverse transcriptase from mouse, woolly monkey, baboon, and RD114 viruses and antisera developed against partially purified RD114 reverse transcriptase were used. Enzymes from three different baboon virus isolates show marked inhibition, but not as marked as that observed with the homologous RD114 enzyme. Further, preinfection with either RD114 or baboon virus of a cell line permissive for both of these viruses (the mink cell line, CCL64) results in an interference of focus formation by murine sarcoma virus pseudotypes by either the RD114 or baboon virus but not by any of several other mammalian type-C viruses (14). Thus, by many different criteria, these viruses are related but distinct from one another.

Detection of Nucleic Acid Sequences Related to RD114 in Various Species of the Cat Family

It seems unlikely that the close relationship between the endogenous baboon type-C viruses and the endogenous cat viruses could be fortuitous. One is,

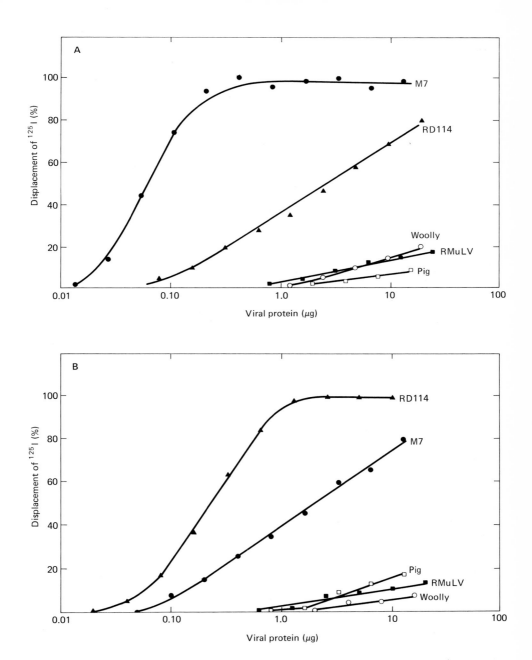

Figure 2-7. Competitive radioimmunoassays for the p30 antigens of the baboon (M7) virus (A) and feline RD114 virus (B). Detergent-disrupted virions were used as sources of competing antigens (28). The endogenous pig virus, PK15 (32), the woolly monkey type-C virus (31), and the Rauscher strain of murine leukemia virus (7) are shown.

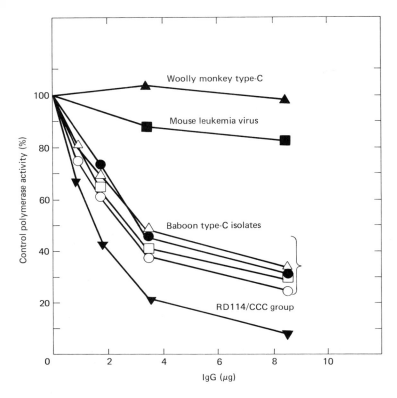

Figure 2-8. Inhibition of reverse transcriptases of different type-C viruses with antiserum raised against the polymerase from the RD114 virus (34). (Appeared originally in Todaro et al., *Cell*, 2:57, 1974.)

therefore, compelled to conclude that the viruses have a common ancestor type-C virus, even though they now behave as the endogenous viruses of two evolutionarily distant mammalian species. The progenitor virus may have been derived from virogenes of one of the species or from an infectious virus from still a third source. Further clarification of the origin of the endogenous cat viruses can be obtained by examining the DNA from other cat species of the family Felidae.

Relatively little is known about cat phylogeny; all carnivores seem to have had a common ancestor approximately 35 million years ago. The data obtained when radioactive unique sequence domestic cat DNA is hybridized to the DNA of various Felidae are shown in Figure 2-9,B. All cats DNA examined, including that from the more distantly related lion and tiger, could not be readily distinguished from domestic cat cellular DNA in these hybridization studies. The

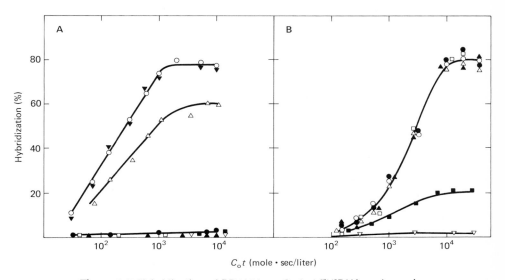

Figure 2-9. Hybridization of RD114 type-C viral [³H]DNA probe and domestic cat unique sequence cellular [³H]DNA to various feline cellular DNAs. (A) Annealing of [³H]DNA probe prepared from RD114 grown in RD cells (19) to DNA extracted from (○) domestic cat (*F. catus*) kidney, (▼) European wildcat (*F. sylvestris*) liver, (△) jungle cat (*F. chaus*) liver, (●) leopard cat (*F. bengalensis*) spleen, (□) tiger (*Panthera tigris*) liver, (▲) lion (*P. leo*) spleen, (■) dog liver, (▽) human spleen. (B) Annealing of unique sequence, domestic cat cellular [³H]DNA to the cellular DNA of various cats. A domestic cat cell line DNA was labeled with [³H]thymidine and extracted (4). Unique sequence cellular DNA was isolated by removing the highly reiterated sequences that anneal at $C_o t = 100$ by fractionation on hydroxylapatite (4). This [³H]thymidine-labeled unique sequence DNA was then hybridized to the DNA listed above. Symbols are the same as in (A). (Reprinted from *Nature*, 252:456, 1974).

DNA of another carnivore (dog) demonstrates much less sequence homology, whereas human and mouse cell DNA share no detectable sequences in common with domestic cat cell DNA. The cellular DNA of the cats of the family Felidae examined thus contain nucleic acid sequences that are as closely related to each other as are those of the Old World monkey subfamily Cercopithecinae (see Fig. 2-1 and Table 2-1).

The hybridization of the cat cellular DNAs to a [³H]DNA transcript prepared from RD114 type-C virus is shown in Figure 2-9,A. The greatest extent of homology is observed with domestic cat DNA; at the maximal extent of the reaction approximately 80 percent of the [³H]DNA is resistant to digestion with nuclease S₁. The cell DNA from two other species of cats, European wildcat (*F. sylvestris*) and jungle cat (*F. chaus*), also contains nucleic acid

45

R. E. Benveniste et al.

sequences that are partially homologous to the RD114 viral [³H]DNA probe. Under the hybridization conditions employed, however, no other cat belonging to the genus *Felis* or to other feline genera possesses DNA base sequences that are related to RD114. This result is in striking contrast to that obtained with the baboon type-C virus: The DNA of all primate species in which the unique sequence *cellular* DNA is homologous (on nearly so) to baboon cellular DNA hybridizes extensively to the baboon type-C virus probe. The seemingly total lack of RD114-related information in the other cats is most consistent with an acquisition of this virus relatively recently in feline evolution.

Table 2-3 summarizes the thermal stability data obtained with 13 feline species (representing five genera) using either labeled, non-repeated, domestic cat *cellular* DNA or ³H-labeled, RD114, type-C *viral* DNA as a probe. Although the overall unique sequence *cellular* DNA of all 13 cat species are highly homologous (the difference in thermal stability is less than 1°C), only three species of the genus *Felis* contain RD114 related sequences. There are no sequences related to RD114 [³H]DNA in two carnivore species (mink and dog) or in mouse DNA. But it is apparent from the data that there is information related to RD114 that can readily be detected in six species of Old World monkeys (two baboon species; patas; African green; and two macaques, rhesus and stump-tail).

Models for the Transmission of Type-C Viruses among Species

The unexpected homology between the type-C viruses of domestic cat, European wildcat, and jungle cat, and those of the Old World monkeys suggests the possibility of transmission of viruses from one species to another with the subsequent integration of that information into the DNA and its perpetuation through the germ line. Figure 2-10 shows three possible interpretations of the data. In model A, a common ancestor type-C virus of unknown origin infects the ancestors of domestic cats and of Old World monkeys. In model B, a cat virus ancestral to the three species of cats discussed above infects an ancestor of Old World monkeys. In model C, the converse occurs: A primate virus, which is ancestral to the Old World monkeys, infects a recent ancestor of the domestic cat. The fact that RD114-related nucleic acid sequences can only be found in three species of cats, even though the overall unique sequence DNA of all feline species is highly homologous, favors model C as the most likely explanation of the data. Since RD114 type-C–related information can be found essentially in *all* the Old World monkeys to the same extent, arrow III in model C is the least likely to be correct. The approximate time of infection of cats with the primate virus thus probably occurred before the Old World monkeys had diverged significantly [about 5 to 15 million years ago (17,24)].

46

Table 2-3 Thermal Stability of Hybrids Formed between Domestic Cat Cellular DNA and RD114 Type-C Viral DNA and the DNA from Various Feline Species

Species[a]	Unique sequence domestic cat cellular [³H]DNA[b]		RD114 viral [³H]DNA[c]	
	Hybrid (%)	ΔT_m	Hybrid (%)	ΔT_m
Cats				
Domestic cat	100	<0.5	100	<0.5
European wildcat			95	
Jungle cat			72	1.5
Leopard cat	95	<0.5	<2	>15
Golden cat	96	<0.5	<2	>15
Geoffroy's cat			<2	>15
Caracal cat			<2	>15
Bobcat			<2	>15
Lion	91	<1.0	<2	>15
Leopard			<2	>15
Tiger	92	1.0	<2	>15
Snow leopard			<2	>15
Cheetah			<2	>15
Other mammals				
Mink	23	10.0	<2	>15
Dog	19	11.0	<2	>15
Mouse	2	>15	<2	>15
Primates				
Capuchin	2	>15	<2	>15
Human	1	>15	<2	>15
Baboon				
(*P. cynocephalus*)	2	>15	16	10.5
(*P. hamadryas*)			18	11.0
Patas			17	11.0
African green			19	11.0
Macaque				
rhesus	2	>15	20	11.0
stump-tailed			17	11.5

[a] Cellular DNA was extracted from various tissues of the species listed. The scientific names of the feline species are listed in Table 2-4.

[b] The [³H]Thymidine-labeled unique sequence domestic cat cellular DNA was hybridized to the various species as described in Figure 2-1. The percent hybrid is the normalized value obtained after digestion of the hybrids with S_1 nuclease. The temperature at which 50 percent of the hybrids are dissociated (T_m) was 87°C for the homologous domestic cat:domestic cat hybrid; the ΔT_m is the difference in T_m between the other DNA:DNA hybrids and the T_m of the homologous hybrid.

[c] The [³H]DNA probe was prepared from RD114 virus grown in a human cell line. The T_m of the homologous RD114:domestic cat DNA hybrid was 88.5°C.

A

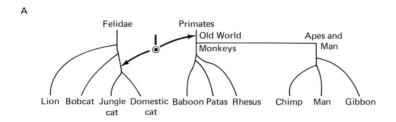

B

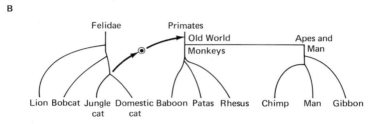

C

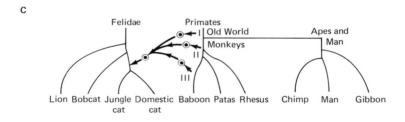

Figure 2-10. Schematic representation of various models that could account for the presence of related virogene information in Old World monkeys and domestic cats. (A) Common foreign virus infection of ancestors of both Old World monkeys and domestic cats. (B) Infection of the ancestors of Old World monkeys and apes by a feline virus. (C) Infection of the ancestors of domestic cats and jungle cats by an Old World monkey (primate) virus. Three possible times for the infection are shown and discussed in the text: (I) before the Old World monkeys and apes diverged, (II) before the Old World monkeys diverged, and (III) recently by a baboon type-C virus. (Reprinted from *Nature*, 252:458, 1974.)

All hypotheses shown in Figure 2-10 require the horizontal transpecies transmission of type-C viral information. Since RD114 now exhibits all of the properties of an endogenous feline type-C virus (see Table 2-4), this virus information had to become incorporated into the germ line of the newly infected species.

Table 2-5 lists the geographic habitat of the various cat species examined.

26. Sherr, C. J., Benveniste, R. E., and Todaro, G. J. Type-C viral expression in primate tissues. Proc. Natl. Acad. Sci. USA, 71:3721, 1974.

27. Sherr, C. J., Lieber, M. M., Benveniste, R. E., and Todaro, G. J. Endogenous baboon type-C virus (M7):Biochemical and immunologic characterization. Virology, 58:492, 1974.

28. Sherr, C. J. and Todaro, G. J. Radioimmunoassay of the major group specific protein of endogenous baboon type-C viruses: Relation to the RD-114/CCC group and detection of antigen in normal baboon tissues. Virology, 61:168, 1974.

29. Simons, E. L. The deployment and history of Old World monkeys. *In* Napier, J. R. and Napier, P. H., eds. Old World Monkeys: Evolution, Systematics, and Behavior. New York, Academic Press, 1970, pp. 97–138.

30. Teitz, Y., Lennette, E. H., Oshiro, L. S., and Cremer, N. Release of C-type particles from normal rat thymus cultures and those infected with Moloney leukemia virus. J. Natl. Cancer Inst., 46:11, 1971.

31. Theilen, G. H., Gould, D., Fowler, M., and Dungworth, D. C. C-Type virus in tumor tissue of a woolly monkey (*Lagothrix spp.*) with fibrosarcoma. J. Natl. Cancer Inst., 47:881, 1971.

32. Todaro, G. J., Benveniste, R. E., Lieber, M. M., and Sherr, C. J. Characterization of a type-C virus released from the porcine cell line PK(15). Virology, 58:65, 1974.

33. Todaro, G. J. and Huebner, R. J. The viral oncogene hypothesis: New evidence. Proc. Natl. Acad. Sci. USA, 69:1009, 1972.

34. Todaro, G. J., Sherr, C. J., Benveniste, R. E., Lieber, M. M., and Melnick, J. L. Type-C viruses of baboons: Isolation from normal cell cultures. Cell, 2:55, 1974.

3

The Mammary Tumor Viruses

D. H. Moore

Introduction

In the mouse, the mammary tumor viruses represent a group of closely related RNA viruses (type-B particles), which are functionally distinct, so far as is known, from type-C particles. Some mouse strains have milk-transmitted infectious mammary tumor viruses with an infectivity depending upon the recipient strain. In addition, there are endogenous viruses that remain after the milk-transmitted virus is removed by foster-nursing, which may or may not be expressed. Molecular hybridization experiments have shown that multiple copies of the mouse mammary tumor virus genomes are present in DNA of all strains of mice tested (17). These viral genomes have not yet been found in the DNA of any other species (17,18). Viral RNA and antigens related to these viruses, however, have been found in humans.

In 1971 it was reported (8,9), that virus-like particles morphologically indistinguishable from those responsible for mammary tumors in mice were found in human milk. Since that time much additional evidence has accumulated, indicating that there is indeed a human virus with properties that parallel those of the type-B particles of the murine mammary tumor virus (MuMTV).

Compared with milk from high mammary-tumor strains of mice, human milk contains a relatively low number of type-B particles. The virions in most human milks represent only a minute fraction (less than one-millionth) of those found in mice. Furthermore, these virions are unstable in human milk (6,12).

Antiviral Factors in Human Milk

In the process of trying to improve the procedure for isolating virus-like particles, mouse type-B particles were added to samples of human milk; different methods were then used to recover them. Destructive effects were readily observed; type-B particles were found in various stages of degradation, and bioactivity was greatly reduced (12). Despite this, RNA-directed DNA polymerase (RDDP) was found in some human milk, and a procedure was devised for the simultaneous detection of RDDP and its association with high

Fundamental Aspects of Neoplasia,
edited by A. Arthur Gottlieb, Otto J. Plescia, and David H. L. Bishop.
© 1975 by Springer-Verlag New York Inc.

molecular weight RNA (60 to 70 or 35 S) (13,14). By the end of 1972, there was general agreement on the occurrence of the oncornavirus specific RDDP and 35 S and/or 70 S RNA in many human milks (15).

Despite the fact that there was no correlation between the detection of type-B particles in density gradient isolates and the presence of 35 S and/or 70 S RNA and associated RDDP, the location of human milk RDDP in density gradients corresponded to the density of the type-B particles of mouse leukemia. Why did the buoyant density at which the RDDP was found correspond to that of type-B particles, while the virus particles could not consistently be found? The explanation might be that the "needle in the haystack" approach inherent in electron microscopy did not provide significant particle incidence data when the concentration of the particles was at the limit of detectability. Out of the milk specimens examined from more than 1,000 women, only three women had milk with a significant number of type-B particles or what appeared to be injured type-B particles; the RDDP in these milks was of a different (and higher) order or magnitude from the other milks. The high mammary tumor strains of mice, such as RIII, have 10^{12} particles/ml, whereas most human milks have a concentration of less than 10^6/ml, which, even after virion concentration, is at the limit of detectability with the electron microscope.

The fact that human milk rapidly destroys the virions (6,12) is another reason for the poor correlation of the detection of intact type-B particles with RDDP activity and 70 S RNA concentration. It was shown that "hind" milk, taken as it was synthesized, had much more of these biochemical markers (RDDP and 70 S RNA) than "fore" milk, which had been stored in the breast for some time (Moore et al., unpublished data).

Type-B Particles in Human Milk

Evidence that RDDP and 70 S RNA was associated with type-B rather than type-C particles came from two different findings. In gradient centrifugation, type-C particles band at a buoyant density of 1.16 g/ml in sucrose, whereas type-B particles band at 1.18 g/ml (11). In human milk, the RDDP activity and the 70 S RNA are associated with particles that band at 1.18 g/ml. Moreover, the same cation (Mg^{2+}) that activates the RDDP of MuMTV also activates that from the particles of human milk (5). The RDDP from type-C particles found in the mouse (Rauscher leukemia virus; Moloney sarcoma virus), cat (feline leukemia virus), rat (R35 virus), and certain primate (gibbon ape and woolly monkey) all can use Mn^{2+} for activation. Thus, these two findings, the buoyant density of the particles and the cation that best activates their associated RDDP, indicate that these human milk particles are type-B rather than type-C.

Cross-Species Nucleic Acid Hybridization

The results from a number of nucleic acid hybridization experiments indicate a close relationship between the RNA of MuMTV and the RNA found in some human breast cancer or precancerous tissues. Axel et al. prepared radioactive DNA probes using RDDP and 70 S RNA extracted from particles isolated from human breast carcinoma tissues. There was some hybridization of MuMTV RNA with the labeled DNA probes made from 30 out of 38 human mammary adenocarcinomas tested.

Das et al. (4) made DNA probes by using RDDP and 70 S RNA extracted from particles isolated from human milk. The polysomal RNA from one of three breast adenocarcinomas, an undifferentiated carcinoma, showed homology with these DNA probes.

In cross-species molecular hybridization experiments, Vaidya et al. (16) employed single-strand specific nuclease S_1 for digesting any unhybridized nucleotide sequences. DNA probes were made utilizing 70 S RNA and RDDP from Mason–Pfizer monkey virus and from MuMTV. Out of twenty-two human tumors tested (one adenocarcinoma, colon; one carcinoma, cecum; twenty carcinomas, breast) eight of the breast cancers had RNA that hybridized from 18 to 77 percent of the MuMTV DNA probes; no breast cancer or breast cancer human tissue RNA hybridized with the Mason–Pfizer monkey virus probes. The mean number of MuMTV-related RNA molecules per cell, based on the total RNA concentration and time of reaction, was 1.5 to 8.0 molecules/cell. Thermal stability studies indicated less than 5 percent mismatching for the molecules of the two species. These hybridization studies support and help explain the immunologic cross-reactivities that have been observed.

Immunology

There are now a number of indications of immunologic cross-reactivities between human and mouse products. One of the strongest is the evidence provided by Black et al. (3) showing the similarity of antigens of MuMTV and human mammary carcinomas. Black et al. employed a leukocyte migration procedure to demonstrate cellular hypersensitivity responses to human breast cancer tissue, since breast cancer tissue antigens can inhibit the migration of leukocytes (2). Responses (leukocyte migration inhibition) from breast cancer patients were found in 70 percent of tests against autologous *in situ* breast tumor tissue, in 35 percent of tests against autologous invasive breast tumor tissue, and in 15 percent of tests against homologous invasive breast tumor tissue. When leukocytes from unselected breast patients were tested against mouse milk (RIII) containing MuMTV, positive responses were obtained in

9 of 34 tests (27 percent). Leukocytes responsive to *in situ* breast cancer tissues cross-reacted with MuMTV-containing RIII milk in 6 of 11 tests; they did not react to MuMTV-free RIIIf or C57BL milk. When leukocytes responsive to MuMTV were tested against homologous *in situ* breast cancer, positive responses occurred in 36 (55 percent) of 66 tests. Leukocytes that failed to respond to MuMTV rarely (2/61) responded to human *in situ* breast cancer tissue. Thus, a large proportion of human *in situ* tumors appears to contain antigen(s) similar to those of MuMTV (3).

Experiments that indicate that some human sera contain antibodies that affect MuMTV include neutralization, immunofluorescence of virus-rich mouse mammary tumor tissue, and immunoprecipitation of human serum component(s) on budding MuMTV virions.

More than 100 human sera have been tested for neutralization of RIII MuMTV (Charney et al., unpublished data). One-fourth of these showed various degrees of neutralization whether or not the sera came from breast cancer patients. Some sera completely neutralized the mouse virus. Activity was eliminated by absorption by RIII milk but was not affected by absorption of the serum with MTV-free C57BL milk.

From immunofluorescence tests, Müller et al. (10) found that sera from some women with breast cancer or fibrocystic mastopathy reacted with slices of MuMTV-rich tumors. These results were confirmed with peroxidase-labeled anti-human IgG. Hoshino and Dmochowski (7), also using peroxidase-coupled anti-human globulin, showed that sera from human breast cancer patients formed a specific precipitate on budding virions in thin sections of mouse mammary tumor when examined with the electron microscope.

The results of many different experiments indicate that human milks and breast tumors contain virus closely related to the mouse mammary tumor virus, but the route of infection or means of transfer is unknown. Although there is much evidence for the presence in humans of RNA sequences and of antigens closely related to those of the mouse mammary tumor virus, no related DNA sequences have yet been found; detection of such sequences would indicate that the virus is endogenous in man.

REFERENCES

1. Axel, R., Gulati, S. C., and Spiegelman, S. Particles containing RNA-instructed DNA polymerase and virus-related RNA in human breast cancers. Proc. Natl. Sci. USA, 69:3133, 1972.

2. Black, M. M., Leis, H. P. Jr., Shore, B., and Zachrau, R. E. Cellular hypersensitivity to breast cancer: Assessment by a leukocyte migration procedure. Cancer, 33:952, 1974.

3. Black, M. M., Moore, D. H., Shore, B., Zachrau, R. E., and Leis, H. P., Jr. Effect of

murine milk samples and human breast tissues on human leukocyte migration indices. Cancer Res., 34:1054, 1974.

4. Das, M. R., Sadasivan, E., Koshy, R., Vaidya, A. B., and Sirsat, S. M. Homology between RNA from human malignant breast tissue and DNA synthesized by milk particles. Nature [New Biol.], 239:92, 1972.

5. Dion, A. S., Vaidya, A. B., and Fout, G. S. Cation preferences for poly(rC):oligo (dG)-directed DNA synthesis by RNA tumor viruses and human milk particulates. Cancer Res., 34:3509, 1974.

6. Fieldsteel, A. H. Nonspecific antiviral substances in human milk active against arbovirus and murine leukemia virus. Cancer Res., 34:712, 1974.

7. Hoshino, M. and Dmochowski, L. Electron microscope study of antigens in cells of mouse mammary tumor cell lines by peroxidase-labeled antibodies in sera of mammary tumor-bearing mice and of patients with breast cancer. Cancer Res., 33:2551, 1973.

8. Moore, D. H. Evidence for a human breast cancer virus. Indian J. Cancer, 8:80, 1971.

9. Moore, D. H., Charney, J., Kramarsky, B., Lasfargues, E. Y., Sarkar, N. H., Brennan, M. J., Burrows, J. H., Sirsat, S. M., Paymaster, J. C., and Vaidya, A. B. Search for a human breast cancer virus. Nature, 229:611, 1971.

10. Müller, M., Kemmer, C., Zotter, St., Grossmann, J., and Michell, B. Cross-reaction between human breast cancer and mastopathy and murine mammary carcinoma: Localization of the antigens in type-A particle virus. Arch. Geschwulstforsch., 41:100, 1973.

11. Sarkar, N. H. and Moore, D. H. Separation of B and C type virons by centrifugation in gentle density gradients. J. Virol. 13:1143, 1974.

12. Sarkar, N. H., Charney, J., Dion, A. S., and Moore, D. H. Effect of human milk on the mouse mammary tumor virus. Cancer Res., 33:626, 1973.

13. Schlom, J. and Spiegelman, S. Simultaneous detection of the reverse transcriptase and high molecular weight RNA unique to the oncogenic RNA viruses. Science, 174:840, 1971.

14. Schlom, J., Spiegelmen, S., and Moore, D. H. Reverse transcriptase and high molecular weight RNA in particles from mouse and human milk. J. Natl. Cancer Inst., 48:1197, 1972.

15. Vaidya, A. B. Molecular biology of human milk. Science, 180:776, 1973.

16. Vaidya, A. B., Black, M. M., Dion, A. S., and Moore, D. H. Homology between human breast tumour RNA and mouse mammary tumour virus genome. Nature, 249:565, 1974.

17. Varmus, H. E., Quintrell, N., Medeiros, E., Bishop, J. M., Nowinski, R. C., and Sarkar, N. H. Transcription of mouse mammary tumor virus genes in tissues from high and low tumor incidence mouse strains. J. Mol. Biol., 79:663, 1973.

18. Varmus, H. E., Stavnezer, J., Medeiros, E., and Bishop, J. M. Detection and characterization of RNA tumor virus-specific DNA in cells. Proc. VIth Intl. Symp. on Comparative Leuk. Res. (in press), 1974.

Biochemical Evidence for Viral Involvement in Human Breast Cancer

J. Schlom, D. Colcher, R. Michalides,
G. Schochetman, J. Young, S. Spiegelman, and
S. Feldman

Introduction

Definitive proof of a viral etiology in many animal cancers has been obtained in experiments that satisfy Koch's criteria for the identification of the causative agent. In 1936, J. J. Bittner (5) revealed that breast cancer in mice is due, in part, to the presence in milk of a factor since identified as the mouse mammary tumor virus (MMTV). Genetic constitution, hormonal stimulation, immune response, diet, nursing, and cocarcinogens may also be involved in the genesis of murine breast cancer. Whether MMTV is the common denominator in the etiology of this disease is not yet known.

In 1970, Temin and Mizutani (23) and Baltimore (3) reported the detection of an RNA-instructed DNA polymerase (reverse transcriptase) in two RNA tumor viruses. This discovery was to make possible a new approach in the study of cancer by providing previously unavailable molecular probes for the presence of viral agents. We describe here the utilization of these probes in the study of human breast cancer.

Biochemical Evidence for a Putative RNA Tumor Virus in Human Milk

It has been shown (21) that certain human milks contain particles, with a density of 1.16 to 1.19 g/ml, that contain an RNA-dependent DNA polymerase (reverse transcriptase). The demonstration of the viral origin of this reverse transcriptase activity is of obvious importance, since mouse milk has been shown to be a primary site of expression of the mouse mammary tumor virus. Numerous human milk preparations have been examined for the presence of "virus" particles by the simultaneous detection assay (20,22). This assay demonstrates the presence of particles that contain a 60 to 70 S RNA in association with a reverse transcriptase. The [^{3}H]DNA complexes generated in an endo-

Fundamental Aspects of Neoplasia,
edited by A. Arthur Gottlieb, Otto J. Plescia, and David H. L. Bishop.
© 1975 by Springer-Verlag New York Inc.

genous reaction with human milk particles sediment in the 60 to 70 S region of a glycerol velocity gradient and band at the density of RNA in a cesium sulfate gradient. These complexes are eliminated from the 60 to 70 S region if they are incubated with RNase before sedimentation analysis. Similar results have recently been reported by other researchers (10,12,13). We have observed that different women differ in their content of particles with 60 to 70 S RNA and reverse transcriptase and, furthermore, that different samples from an individual woman taken several days apart may also differ. This may be due to an actual variation of the number of particles in the milk or to the presence of inhibitors in milk that may obscure the outcome of these assays (22).

Numerous investigators have found that the 60 to 70 S RNA of the known RNA tumor viruses contains polyadenylic acid (poly A) regions approximately 200 nucleotides long, comprising about 1.5 percent of the viral genome. It was found (17) that the 60 to 70 S RNA of human milk particles also contain poly A sequences of the same length as those found in the mouse mammary tumor virus, Mason–Pfizer monkey virus, and in other known RNA tumor viruses. Thus, this technique is a useful method for the quantitation of a putative RNA tumor virus in human milk. We have thus far observed that certain human milks contain from 5×10^5 to 10^7 particles/ml.

Synthetic templates have been used to detect the presence of RNA tumor viruses. Extensive use has been made of oligo dT:poly rA as a template for demonstrating the presence of a reverse transcriptase associated with these viruses. This template, however, can also be used by other DNA polymerases. Several investigators have shown that oligo dG:poly rC can be used to differentiate a reverse transcriptase from other DNA polymerases, since the known DNA polymerases utilize it poorly as a template (16,4). No dG:rC-templated activity was found in NIH Swiss mouse milk, devoid of MMTV. On the other hand, RIII mouse milk containing MMTV, and certain human milks, contained large amounts of dG:rC-templated activity. This activity was confined to the 1.15 to 1.20 g/ml density regions of sucrose equilibrium gradients.

Cores from avian tumor viruses and from murine leukemia and murine mammary tumor viruses have been produced by the use of surfactants and ether. These cores contain the viral 60 to 70 S RNA and demonstrate a DNA polymerase activity. Recently, we reported (11) that phospholipase C can be used to prepare cores from the mouse mammary tumor virus and from human milk particles. These "subviral" particulates band at a density of approximately 1.26 g/ml in sucrose and contain a 60 to 70 S RNA in association with a reverse transcriptase. In addition to offering further evidence of similarity between the human milk particles and the known RNA tumor viruses, core isolation obviates certain technical difficulties. Because of their uniquely higher densities, cores, unlike complete virions, band in a region comparatively free of cellular contaminants. This minimizes the problems generated by enzyme inhibitors and the presence of cellular debris found in human milk. Under these conditions, the assays for particles become more sensitive and reliable.

Nucleic Acid Sequence Homology between cDNA of Particles from Human Milk and RNA of Human Mammary Adenocarcinomas

Using cDNA synthesized from MTV from mouse milk as a probe, a homology in nucleic acid sequence between the RNA in virus particles from mouse milk and RNA from the mouse mammary tumors can be demonstrated (18,24). A homology can also be shown in nucleic acid sequences between the particles of human milk and the RNA from human mammary adenocarcinomas (9). In the experiments undertaken in our laboratory, the ^{3}H-labeled DNA probe complementary to the RNA of the human milk particles is synthesized via an endogenous reaction using "cores" from these human particles. When 1000 cpm of this probe was hybridized to 350 μg of polysomal RNA of human mammary adenocarcinomas to $C_rt=2,500$, positive hybridization results were obtained upon analysis by cesium sulfate equilibrium gradient centrifugation (18). When the same probe was annealed to polysomal RNA from human benign breast tumors, the results were negative. The polysomal RNA of seven out of fourteen malignant human breast tumors hybridized significantly with the [^{3}H]DNA probe synthesized from the RNA of human milk cores with standard deviation values ranging from 3.0 to 11.0. An arbitrary cut-off of three standard deviations of the background value was used (18), thus providing a 99.9 percent confidence that those hybrids scored as positive are significant. No significant hybridization could be detected if the same probe was hybridized to the polysomal RNA of human benign breast tumors, normal human breast tissue, human sarcoma and leukemic cells, or normal human spleen.

To increase the sensitivity of the hybridization assay, [^{3}H]DNA probe, synthesized from the human milk "core," was hybridized to the RNA isolated from the 1.15 to 1.20 g/ml density regions of sucrose gradients of extracts of human malignant breast tumors. The hybridizations were carried out to a C_rt value of 7,000. Increased hybridization was observed when human milk cDNA was hybridized to RNA isolated from material banding between densities 1.15 to 1.20 (Fig. 4-1,A). The hybridizations between this same [^{3}H]DNA probe and the RNA extracted from analogous fractions of human benign breast tumors (Fig. 4-1,B), leukemias, or sarcomas were negative, with standard deviation values of 0 to 1.2.

These data show that this [^{3}H]DNA probe synthesized from the RNA of human milk "cores" detects sequences in the RNA specific for malignant breast tumors. We did not estimate the extent of transcription of the RNA of the

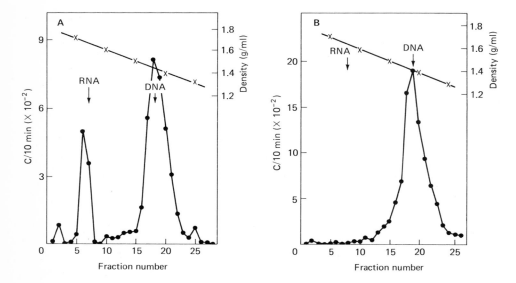

Figure 4-1. Hybridization of [³H]cDNA synthesized from human milk cores and RNA extracted from the 1.15 to 1.20 g/ml density region of (A) human malignant breast tumor (carcinoma) and (B) human benign breast tumor (fibroadenoma). See Schlom et al. (20) for methods.

human milk particles into a [³H]DNA probe, nor did we estimate the extent of homology of this probe with the RNA from human malignant breast tumors, so we can only indicate that there is a degree of homology in the nucleic acid sequences of both.

Sequence Homology between the RNA of Mason–Pfizer Monkey Virus and the RNA of Human Malignant Breast Tumors

The Mason–Pfizer monkey virus (MPMV) was isolated from a mammary carcinoma of a female rhesus monkey. The virus has been successfully propagated by co-cultivation of the original mammary tumor with monkey embryo cells and by cell-free infection of monkey, chimpanzee, and human cells. A virus (X-381) with all the properties of MPMV has also been isolated from a rhesus lactating mammary gland biopsy. (1). MPMV has the biochemical and biophysical properties that characterize the known RNA tumor viruses. It has a buoyant density of 1.16 g/ml in sucrose, an RNA-instructed DNA polymerase, and a 60 to 70 S RNA (19). This high molecular weight RNA contains polyadenylic acid approximately 200 nucleotides in length and consists of subunits of 2 to 3×10^6 daltons. The RNA-instructed DNA polymerase has been partially purified and is immunologically distinct from that of other oncornaviruses, but it cross-reacts with X-381. Morphologically, MPMV is similar but not identical to the type-B mouse mammary tumor virus (8).

It was of obvious interest to determine if any nucleotide sequence homology existed between this putative primate mammary tumor virus and the RNA of human mammary adenocarcinomas.

Synthesis of MPMV [³H]cDNA

The MPMV cDNA probe was synthesized from endogenous reverse transcriptase reactions using purified Mason–Pfizer virions and from reactions using AMV reverse transcriptase and MPMV 60 to 70 S RNA as template. Both types of ³H-labeled cDNA were analyzed to determine their efficacy in hybridization to MPMV 60 to 70 S RNA. The two probes synthesized by the endogenous virus reactions hybridized only 15 and 25 percent to MPMV RNA, whereas the cDNA synthesized with purified 60 to 70 S RNA and AMV reverse transcriptase gave as high as 70 percent hybridization, as measured by cesium sulfate analysis. Further studies were conducted to determine the degree of copying, if any copying occurred, of poly A stretches known to be present in MPMV RNA. A cDNA containing poly T stretches would be of limited value, since this would result in hybridization to normal messenger RNAs. Three of the seven probes analyzed showed significant hybridization to poly rA when analyzed by hydroxylapatite.

The [³H]DNA probes that exhibited the most hybridization to MPMV 60 to 70 S RNA and had no poly T stretches were further characterized on hydroxylapatite. They were shown to consist solely of a single-stranded DNA and hybridized 98 percent to MPMV 60 to 70 S RNA under formamide hybridization conditions, and were used in all subsequent experiments. These results illustrate the variation that is often seen in the synthesis of these cDNA probes and emphasizes the importance of monitoring the efficacy of each preparation before use.

Analysis of MPMV [³H]cDNA

Experiments were performed to determine how much of the MPMV 60 to 70 S RNA was copied into cDNA by the purified reverse transcriptase, and if any regions were selectively copied. Thus, ^{32}P-labeled MPMV 60 to 70 S RNA was prepared, and the specific activity determined to be 5×10^5 cpm/μg. Then 5,000 cpm was annealed to 2×10^5 cpm of [³H]cDNA to give a DNA:RNA molar ratio of 1.0. Hybrids were analyzed for RNase A resistance of the ^{32}P-label. The percent of the RNA that is resistant to the RNase digestion represents the fraction of the RNA that was copied by the reverse transcriptase when the [³H]cDNA was synthesized. The [³H]cDNA probes were shown to protect

56 percent of the 60 to 70 S [^{32}P]RNA when equimolar amounts of the DNA and RNA were used. Therefore, the probes used in these studies represent at least 56 percent of the viral genome.

The MPMV [^{3}H]cDNA probes were then analyzed for use in hybridization experiments by equilibrium density analysis in cesium sulfate. As expected, the [^{3}H]cDNA bands sharply at a density of 1.45 g/ml (Fig. 4-2,A). When this probe is annealed to purified MPMV 60 to 70 S RNA, approximately 70 percent of the [^{3}H]cDNA hybridizes and is shifted into the DNA/RNA hybrid regions of the density gradient (Fig. 4-2,B). If the [^{3}H]cDNA probe is annealed to AMV 60 to 70 S RNA, no hybrids are observed (Fig. 4-2,C).

Additional evidence for the specificity of the [^{3}H]cDNA probes was obtained by C_rt analysis by hydroxylapatite chromatography. The [^{3}H]cDNA probes were annealed to MPMV 60 to 70 S RNA from virus grown in CMMT (a cell line consisting of rhesus mammary tumor cells co-cultivated with rhesus embryo cells) and NC37 cells and to AMV 60 to 70 S RNA. The hybridization reactions, containing 1,000 cpm MPMV cDNA and 0.05 µg viral RNA, were incubated in 0.63 M Na$^+$ at 65°C for various times to obtain the desired C_rt values. The MPMV [^{3}H]cDNA specifically annealed to the viral RNA from

Figure 4-2. Characterization of MPMV cDNA probe. (A) Cesium sulfate equilibrium gradient centrifugation of the MPMV [^{3}H]cDNA alone, (B) after annealing in 50 percent formamide to 0.1 µg of 60 to 70 S RNA of MPMV, and (C) 0.1 µg of 60 to 70 S RNA of AMV (C).

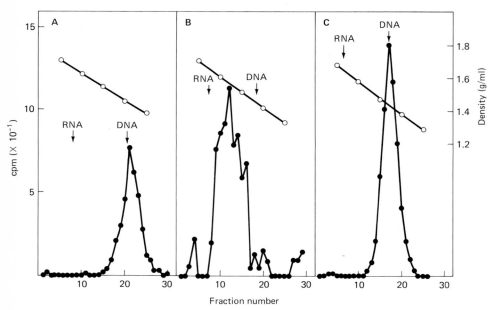

which it was synthesized with a $C_r t_{\frac{1}{2}} = 4 \times 10^{-2}$ (Fig. 4-3). The shape of the hybridization curve indicates little or no redundancy in the [³H]cDNA (7). There were no hybrids formed with AMV 60 to 70 S RNA even at 100-fold greater $C_r t$ values (Fig. 4-3).

The MPMV [³H]cDNA probe was also annealed to RNA of cells producing the virus. Annealing reactions were incubated for various times with 300 μg cellular RNA. There was no difference in the amount of viral-related RNA found in the two infected cell lines (NC37 and CMMT) examined. Both had a $C_r t_{\frac{1}{2}} = 2 \times 10^2$, indicating that approximately 0.02 percent of the cellular RNA is viral related. There was no hybridization of the [³H]cDNA probe to RNA of the uninfected NC37 cells, even to $C_r t$ values of 10^5 (Fig. 4-3), or to the DNA of the uninfected cells. This demonstrates that no RNA sequences expressed in normal cells were copied in the reverse transcriptase reaction.

Hybridization to Human Breast Tumor RNA, Cesium Sulfate Analysis

The MPMV [³H]cDNA synthesized from MPMV 60 to 70 S RNA, was used in annealing reactions with 300 μg of polysomal RNA (pRNA) from human adenocarcinomas of the breast. The reactions, containing 50 percent

Figure 4-3. A $C_r t$ analysis of the MPMV cDNA probe: analysis of annealing reactions with MPMV [³H]cDNA by hydroxylapatite analysis. The [³H]cDNA probe was annealed to 0.05 μg of MPMV 60 to 70 S RNA isolated from virions grown in (●) NC37-infected cells, (▲) CMMT cells, and (■) to 0.05 μg AMV 60 to 70 S RNA. The probe was also annealed to 300 μg of cytoplasmic RNA of (○) MPMV-infected NC37 cells, (△) MPMV-infected CMMT cells, and uninfected NC37 cells (□).

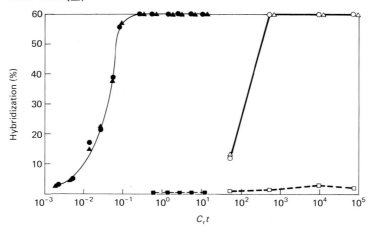

formamide and 0.4M NaCl, were incubated at 37°C for 18 to 24 hr, added to half-saturated Cs₂SO₄ in 0.001 M EDTA, and centrifuged to equilibrium. The results of one such reaction are shown in Figure 4-4,A. Approximately 25 percent of the MPMV [³H]cDNA hybridized to the pRNA and is, therefore, found in the DNA/RNA hybrid region of the gradient. This profile contrasts with the negative results obtained in similar reactions using pRNA isolated from benign fibroadenomas of the breast (Fig. 4-4,B) and normal breast tissue (Fig. 4-4,C). Figure 4-4 shows a tabulation of the results of tissues tested. An arbitrary cut-off of three standard deviations of the background value was used (18); this provided a 99.9 percent confidence that those hybrids scored as positive are significant. Twenty of the twenty-nine individual human breast adenocarcinomas were positive when the three standard deviations (S.D.) cut-off was used; these ranged from 3 to 30 S.D. (Fig. 4-5). None of the pRNA samples from normal human breast, fibrocystic tissue, and the fibroadenomas yielded positive reactions when tested in the same way with the MPMV [³H]cDNA. RNA from normal human spleens, livers, and kidneys also yielded negative results as did pRNA isolated from mouse tissues, including RIII

Figure 4-4. Hybridization of MPMV [³H]cDNA probe to human breast RNA: A cesium sulfate equilibrium gradient analysis of MPMV [³H]cDNA after annealing to 300 μg of polysomal RNA from (A) human breast adenocarcinoma, (B) benign breast tumor, and (C) normal breast tissue.

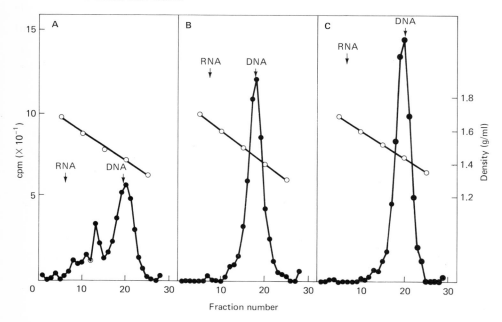

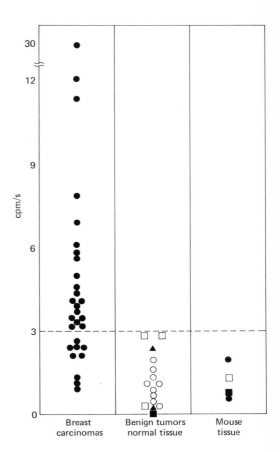

Figure 4-5. Results of annealing reactions with MPMV [³H]cDNA and pRNA from human breast tumors and other tissue. The DNA probe was hybridized to 300 μg of polysomal RNA of tissues and analyzed by cesium sulfate equilibrium gradient centrifugation. The results are plotted against the number of standard deviations of the operational background. The [³H]cDNA probe was hybridized to the following human tissue: (●) breast adenocarcinomas, (○) benign breast tumors, (▲) normal breast tissue, (□) normal liver, and (■) normal spleen. It was also hybridized to the following mouse tissue: (●)Rill breast tumors, (■) spleens of Rauscher-infected Balb/c, and (□) NIH Swiss livers.

breast tumors, Rauscher leukemia virus-infected spleens, and normal livers (Fig. 4-5).

Hybridization to Human Breast Tumor RNA, Hydroxylapatite Analysis

Analysis of annealing reactions between MPMV [³H]cDNA and human breast adenocarcinoma RNA was also conducted by hydroxylapatite chromatography. Total cytoplasmic RNA from individual adenocarcinomas were incubated with the MPMV cDNA at 65°C for various times to obtain $C_r t$ values up to 10^5. Figure 4-6 shows a compilation of the tissues tested. Each bar represents the percent hybridization of MPMV [³H]cDNA to the cytoplasmic RNA from an individual tumor annealed to $C_r t = 10^5$. Seven of the ten mammary carcinomas tested by hydroxylapatite analysis showed hybridization greater than the 5 percent operational background. None of the benign breast tissues, i.e., fibrocystic and fibroadenomas tested (Fig. 4-6), or normal human

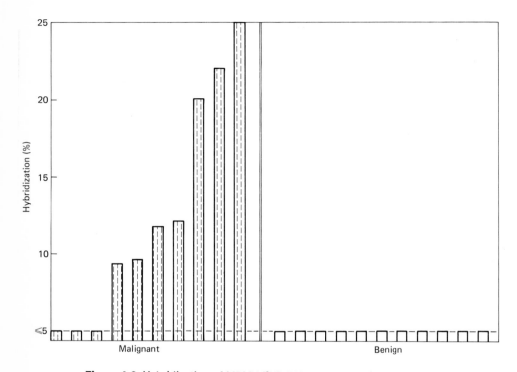

Figure 4-6. Hybridization of MPMV [³H]cDNA to human breast tumor RNA as analyzed by hydroxylapatite chromatography. The [³H]cDNA probe was hybridized to 300 μg of cytoplasmic RNA of human malignant adenocarcinomas and benign breast tumors and incubated at 65°C to achieve a $C_r t = 10^5$. Each bar represents an individual tumor.

breast, spleen, liver, or kidney showed hybridization above background levels.

The $C_r t$ curves made for several of the breast adenocarcinomas demonstrated $C_r t_{1/2}$ values of between 1 and 5×10^4 (Fig. 4-7), even though they reached different final percentages. There may be more MPMV-related RNA present in these tumors than was detected by this analysis because of the possibility of RNA degradation during the prolonged incubations at high temperatures. But $C_r t$ analysis of benign breast tumors to values of 10^5 showed no significant hybridization (Fig. 4-7).

Thermal Analysis of the MPMV-Breast Tumor Hybrids

Cytoplasmic RNA of human breast adenocarcinomas was annealed to MPMV [³H]cDNA to a $C_r t$ value of 5×10^4. The annealing reactions were then subjected to thermal analysis on hydroxylapatite. The hybrids were denatured by increasing temperature and eluted with 0.12 M PB with 0.4 percent SDS.

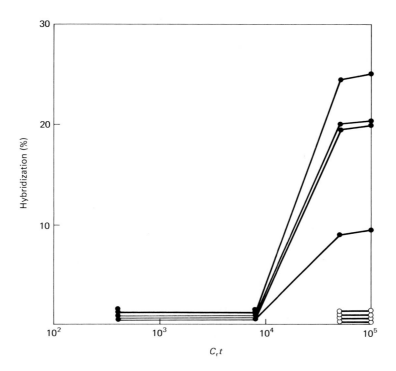

Figure 4-7. Analysis of hybridization of MPMV [^{3}H]cDNA to human breast tumor RNA. The probe was hybridized to 300 μg of cytoplasmic RNA of individual breast tumors and incubated for 10, 20, 100, and 200 hr at 65°C to achieve the desired $C_r t$ values; ($\bullet$) malignant breast adenocarcinomas, ($\bigcirc$) benign breast tumors.

Figure 4-8 compares the elution profile of the hybrids formed between MPMV cDNA and malignant breast tumor RNA, RNA from MPMV-infected NC37 cells, and purified MPMV 60 to 70 S RNA. The midpoint of the thermal elution profile (T_e) from hydroxylapatite of the hybrids formed with breast tumor RNA and the NC37-infected cellular RNA was 80.5°C, whereas the T_e of the MPMV [^{3}H]cDNA–MPMV RNA duplex was 81.5°C. This indicates that there is approximately 1.5 percent mismatching in the hybrids between the viral-related RNA in the human breast adenocarcinomas and the MPMV cDNA (15). The difference in the slopes of the temperature elution is most likely due to different sizes and base composition of the viral related RNA (7,14).

These studies demonstrate sequence homology between Mason–Pfizer monkey virus RNA and RNA isolated from human breast adenocarcinomas. The hybrids formed between the MPMV [^{3}H]cDNA probe and the malignant breast tumors were analyzed by both equilibrium density centrifugation in

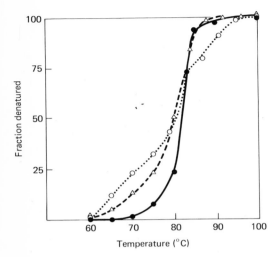

Figure 4-8. Thermal analysis of MPMV [^{3}H]cDNA hybrids. The MPMV [^{3}H]cDNA was hybridized as follows: (●) to 0.05 μg of 60 to 70 S MPMV RNA, (△) to 300 μg of cytoplasmic RNA isolated from infected NC37 cells, and to (○) 300 μg of cytoplasmic RNA isolated from a human breast adenocarcinoma. The annealing reaction were run to $C_r t = 0.5$ for the viral RNA and $' \times 10^4$ for the cytoplasmic RNA and loaded at 60°C onto hydroxylapatite. The single strands were eluted with 0.12 M PB with 0.4 percent SDS at various temperatures.

Cs_2SO_4 and by hydroxylapatite chromatography. Both methods gave positive results in more than two-thirds (27 of 39) of the breast adenocarcinomas tested, whereas no RNA from 20 human benign breast tumors, or normal tissue from human breast, spleen, liver, or kidney showed any homology to MPMV. The studies reported here provide further evidence that a virus may be involved in human breast cancer and that a putative human breast cancer virus may be related to MPMV.

Biochemical Characterization of Subviral Particulates (SVP) from Murine and Human Breast Tumors

Biochemical studies have indicated the presence of a putative oncornavirus in certain human milks. Recently, a technique using phospholipase C was employed (11) to isolate and characterize the particulates from human milk that have the biochemical properties characteristic of cores and ribonucleoproteins of RNA tumor viruses. We have used a modification of the method of BOLOGNESI et al. (6), using sterox-SL, to isolate particulates from murine and human malignant breast tumors. These "subviral particulates" (SVP) have the biochemical properties associated with RNA tumor viruses, i.e., a density of 1.23 g/ml and higher in sucrose, a 60 to 70 S RNA, and an RNA-instructed DNA polymerase. The isolation of SVP minimizes certain technical difficulties of nucleic acid and enzyme assays; because of their uniquely higher densities, SVPs band at regions comparatively free of cellular contaminants. Under these circumstances, assays become more sensitive and reliable than those previously reported (2).

Subviral Particulates from Mouse Breast Tumors

Here RIII mouse mammary tumors, containing MMTV, were minced, homogenized, and extracts were subjected to velocity and sucrose equilibrium gradient centrifugation. Fractions with densities ranging from 1.15 to 1.30 g/ml were divided into five distinct density regions. Material from each region was diluted and centrifuged at 90,000×g for 1 hr. The pellets that were obtained were assayed for endogenous RNA-directed DNA polymerase and 60 to 70 S RNA by the simultaneous detection test (20). As seen in Figure 4-9,A-E, there were several density regions with evidence of *de novo* DNA synthesis. Although some of the DNA synthesized was in the 60 to 70 S region (Fig. 4-9,C-E), the results were not conclusive. The biochemical demonstration of MMTV in these tumor preparations can be made more reliable, however, by the generation of MMTV SVP, i.e., cores, ribonucleoproteins, or transitional forms with some of the core membrane removed. One-half of the original material banding between 1.15 to 1.20 g/ml (the density of MMTV in sucrose is approximately 1.18 g/ml) was pelleted, treated with sterox-SL, and subjected to sucrose equilibrium gradient centrifugation. Resultant fractions were pooled into the same five distinct density regions described above, and each fraction was diluted, pelleted at 90,000×g, and assayed by the simultaneous detection test. As can be seen in Figure 4-9(I) no DNA synthesis on a high molecular weight template in the "viral" (1.15 to 1.20 g/ml) region of the gradient remains. This activity has now shifted to the 1.28 to 1.30 g/ml SVP density region of the gradient (Fig. 9,F). To demonstrate that the distinct DNA peak observed in the 60 to 70 S region (Fig. 4-9,F) is due to an RNA-directed DNA synthesis, parallel reactions were carried out in the absence of one deoxyribonucleoside triphosphate (dGTP) and in the presence of ribonuclease. Both of these reactions were negative.

Extracts from lactating mammary glands of NIH Swiss mice, shown to be free of mouse mammary tumor virion expression, were prepared and tested in an identical manner to the RIII tumors. Both the "viral" and "SVP" regions, before and after sterox-SL treatment, were negative.

"Putative Subviral Particulates" from Human Breast Tumors

The techniques developed for the preparation of subviral particulates of MMTV from murine breast tumors was applied to human malignant adenocarcinoma tissue. Human breast tumors were treated in an identical manner as the murine breast tumors had been. After mincing, homogenization, velocity sedimentation and sucrose equilibrium gradient centrifugation, the individual density regions from 1.15 to 1.30 g/ml were tested by the simultaneous detection assay. Contrary to previous reports (2), none of nine human tumor

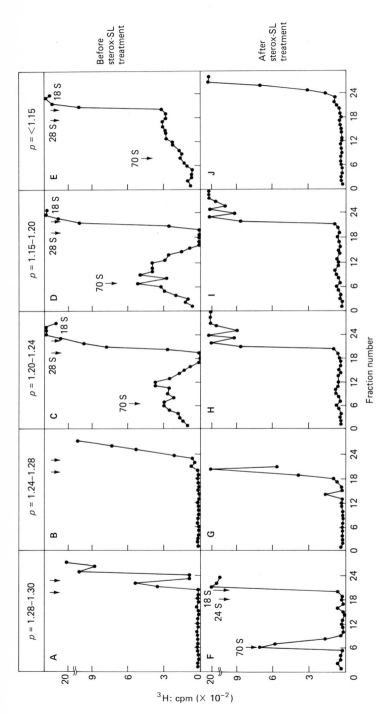

Figure 4-9. Conversion of simultaneous detection activity in mouse mammary tumor (RIII) from "viral" to "core" density region. Eight grams of mouse mammary tumor (RIII) was minced, homogenized, and centrifuged at 8,000×g for 10 min. The supernatant was layered over a 20 to 70 percent linear sucrose gradient and centrifuged for 3 hr at 98,000×g at 4°C. Fractions with the indicated densities were collected, diluted to 10 percent sucrose, and pelleted at 98,000×g for 1 hr at 4°C. The resulting pellets were dissolved in 0.01 M Tris (pH 8.3), and half of each sample was used in a simultaneous detection test (20) (A-E). Sterox-SL was added to the other half of fraction D (1.15 to 1.20 g/ml). This then was layered over a 20 to 70 percent sucrose gradient in TNE, 0.1 M DTT, and centrifuged at 98,000×g for 4 hr at 4°C. The indicated density regions (F-J) were diluted with 0.01 M Tris HCl, pelleted at 98,000×g for 1 hr, and assayed by the simultaneous detection test. The TCA-precipitable [³H]TTP of the 10 to 30 percent glycerol gradient is given.

extracts gave a distinct peak of DNA in the 60 to 70 S region in any of the density fractions tested. Positive results were obtained, however, when the material banding between the densities of 1.15 to 1.20 g/ml in the sucrose equilibrium gradient was treated with sterox-SL, and centrifuged to equilibrium in a 20 to 50 percent sucrose gradient. The resulting regions were concentrated and assayed by the simultaneous detection test. Putative subviral particulates,

Figure 4-10. Conversion of simultaneous detection activity in human malignant breast tumor from "viral" to "subviral particulate" density region. As described in the legend of Figure 4-9, 25 g of human malignant breast tumor was processed. Sterox-SL was added to the other half of fraction (C) (1.15 to 1.20 g/ml) and then layered over a 20 to 70 percent sucrose gradient in TNE, 0.1 M DTT, and centrifuged at 98,000×g for 4 hr at 4°C. The indicated density regions (D-F) were pelleted and assayed by the simultaneous detection test (20). Fractions heavier than 1.24 g/ml were also tested and found negative. The TCA-precipitable [³H]TTP of the 10 to 30 percent glycerol gradient is given.

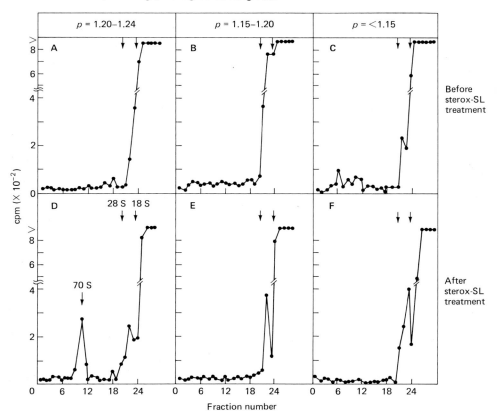

75

i.e., particles with a density of 1.23 g/ml and greater, which contain a 60 to 70 S RNA and a reverse transcriptase, were observed. Figure 4-10 exemplifies the results from one such experiment. The TCA-precipitable [^{3}H]TTP in the 60 to 70 S RNA region of these glycerol gradients was eliminated when RNase was added to the reaction mixtures. The omission of one of the deoxyribonucleoside triphosphates (dGTP) also significantly decreased these peaks, thus demonstrating that the synthesis represented a proper heteropolymer and not simply an end addition. No RNA-directed DNA polymerase activity was observed in normal breast tissue or benign breast tumors when they were tested before or after sterox-SL treatment.

Concluding Comments

The presence of particulates having the biochemical properties of RNA tumor viruses that appear in the milk of some normal women, and in malignant breast tumors, is strikingly similar to the murine model; the mouse mammary tumor virus appears in the milk of many normal mice and later appears in the breast tumors. This situation exists in the mouse, moreover, regardless of the mode of transmission of the virus. Further immunologic and biologic studies are of course needed before one can make more definitive statements about a human breast cancer virus. The data presented here, however, do provide new biochemical evidence to implicate a viral involvement in human breast cancer.

ACKNOWLEDGMENTS

These studies were conducted under National Cancer Institute Contracts NIH-NCI-43223 and NIH-NCI-E70-2049 with the Virus Cancer Program. We thank O. Posen, J. Greenfield, C. Metz, J. Castrop, and P. Uhric for their assistance.

REFERENCES

1. Ahmed, M., Korol, W., Schidlovsky, G., Vidrine, J., and Mayyasi, S. Detection of Mason–Pfizer monkey virus in normal monkey mammary tissue and embryonic cultures. Proc. Am. Assoc. Cancer Res., 14:34, 1973.

2. Axel, R., Gulati, S. C., and Spiegelman, S. Particles containing RNA-instructed DNA polymerase and virus-related RNA in human breast cancers. Proc. Natl. Acad. Sci. USA, 69:3133, 1972.

3. Baltimore, D. Viral RNA-dependent DNA polymerase. Nature, 226:1209, 1970.

4. Baltimore, D., McCaffrey, R., and Smoler, D. F. Virus Research, 1st ed. New York, Academic Press, 1973, pp. 51–59.

5. Bittner, J. J. Some possible effects of nursing on the mammary gland tumor incidence in mice. Science, 84:162, 1936.

6. Bolognesi, D. P., Gelderblom, H., Bauer, H., Molling, E., and Huper, G. Polypeptides of avian RNA tumor viruses. Virology, 47:567, 1972.

7. Britten, R. J. and Kohne, D. E. Repeated sequences in DNA. Science, 161:529, 1968.

8. Chopra, H. C. and Mason, M. M. A new virus in a spontaneous mammary tumor of a rhesus monkey. Cancer Res., 30:2081, 1970.

9. Das, M. R., Sadavisan, E., Koshy, R., Vaidya, A. B., and Sirsat, S. M. Homology between RNA from human malignant breast tissue and DNA synthesized by milk particles. Nature [New Biol.], 239:92, 1972.

10. Das, M. R., Vaidya, A. B., Sirsat, S. M., and Moore, D. H. Polymerase and RNA studies on milk virions from women of the Parsi community. J. Natl. Cancer Inst., 48:1191, 1972.

11. Feldman, S. P., Schlom, J., and Spiegelman, S. Further evidence for oncornaviruses in human milk: The production of cores. Proc. Natl. Acad. Sci. USA, 70:1976, 1973.

12. Feller, W. F. and Kantor, J. The clinical status of women whose milk contains reverse transcriptase and 70 S RNA. Colloque, Recherches Fondamentales Sur les Tumeurs Mammaires, 1972, pp. 279–86.

13. Gerwin, B., Ebert, P., Chopra, H., Smith, S., Kvedar, J., Albert, S., and Brennan, M. DNA polymerase activities of human milk. Science, 180:198, 1973.

14. Kohne, D. E. and Britten, R. J. Hydroxylapatite techniques for nucleic acid reassociation. Proc. Nucleic Acid Research, 2:500, 1972.

15. Kohne, D. E., Chiscon, J. A., and Hoyer, D. H. Nucleotide sequence change in non-repeated DNA during evolution. Carnegie Inst. Washington Ybk., 69:488, 1972.

16. Sarngadharan, M. G., Sarin, P. S., Reitz, M. S., and Gallo, R. C. Reverse transcriptase activity of human acute leukaemic cells: purification of the enzyme, response to AMV 70 S RNA, and characterization of the DNA product. Nature [New Biol.], 240:67, 1972.

17. Schlom, J., Colcher, D., Spiegelman, S., Gillespie, S., and Gillespie, D. Quantitation of RNA tumor viruses and virus-like particles in human milk by hybridization to poly A sequences. Science, 179:696, 1973.

18. Schlom, J., Michalides, R., Kufe, D., Hehlman, K., Spiegelman, S., Bentvelzen, P., and Hageman, P. A comparative study of the biologic and molecular basis of murine mammary carcinoma: A model for human breast cancer. J. Natl. Cancer Inst., 51:541, 1973.

19. Schlom, J. and Spiegelman, S. DNA polymerase activities and nucleic acid components of virions isolated from a spontaneous mammary carcinoma of a rhesus monkey. Proc. Natl. Acad. Sci. USA, 68:1613, 1971.

20. Schlom, J. and Spiegelman, S. Simultaneous detection of reverse transcriptase and high molecular weight RNA unique to oncogenic RNA viruses. Science, 174:840, 1971.

21. Schlom, J., Spiegelman, S., and Moore, D. RNA-dependent DNA polymerase activity in virus-like particles isolated from human milk. Nature, 231:97, 1971.

22. Schlom, J., Spiegelman, S., and Moore, D. H. Detection of high molecular weight RNA in particles from human milk. Science, 175:542, 1972.

23. Temin, H. M. and Mizutani, S. RNA-dependent DNA polymerase in virions of Rous sarcoma virus. Nature, 226:1211, 1970.

24. Varmus, H. Quintrell, N., Medeiros, E., Bishop, J. M., Nowinski, R. C., and Sarkar, N. H. Transcription of mouse mammary tumor virus genes in tissues from high and low tumor incidence mouse strains. J. Mol. Biol., 79:663, 1973.

Tumor Immunology

5

Immunologic Properties of Cell Surface Antigens Induced by RNA Tumor Viruses

H. Bauer, R. Kurth, and H. Gelderblom

Introduction

Since it is now recognized that surface interactions strongly influence the social behavior of cells, the expression of new macromolecules on the tumor cell surface, which can be detected by immunologic means, may be a key phenomenon in the process of malignant transformation of a cell. Also, further studies of the immunologic, biochemical, and biosynthetic reactions of tumor-specific, cell surface antigens (TSSA) could lead to a better understanding of this transformation and, hence, carcinogenesis. On the other hand, TSSA that are foreign to the tumor-bearing host and that can generally provoke an immunologic defense reaction could lead to techniques useful in the prevention or cure of cancer by immunologic means.

For the above reasons, we have undertaken an investigation of TSSA. As a model, we have chosen the avian tumor virus (ATV) system because it offers a variety of technical advantages for study. As in other tumor virus systems, but in contrast to chemically induced tumors, ATV-directed TSSA are virus specific in the sense that all tumors with the same virus etiology contain immunologically cross-reacting TSSA. The special advantages of the ATV system over other systems include (a) the existence of a variety of well-defined, clone-derived virus strains, which are closely related with respect to structure and mode of replication, but otherwise biologically distinct, (b) the existence of temperature-sensitive mutants, which are defective at a restrictive temperature for either replication or transformation or both (for review, see ref. 3); and (c) the occurrence of different interactions between a given virus strain and different host cells. Thus, there exist a variety of virus-host cell interactions for an investigation of cellular modifications related to the transformation process.

Viruses and Methods

Chick embryo fibroblasts (CEF) are transformed by infection with avian sarcoma viruses (ASV), but they can replicate avian leukosis viruses (ALV)

Fundamental Aspects of Neoplasia,
edited by A. Arthur Gottlieb, Otto J. Plescia, and David H. L. Bishop.
© 1975 by Springer-Verlag New York Inc.

without any change in their cell morphology or growth behavior. This makes it possible to distinguish between antigens that are expressed concomitant to virus replication and antigens that are specific for transformed cells. The fact that mammalian cells are non-permissive for replication of most strains of ASV, although they can be transformed, is experimentally useful here. The use of ASV strains from different subgroups (A through D) that vary with respect to the host range and virus envelope (Ve) antigen has made possible the definition of type, subgroup, or group specificity for any new antigen detected at the cell surface.

Since *in vivo* methods are necessarily very limited in any study of TSSA, we have performed studies *in vitro* only. The methods for assaying cell surface antigens have been described in detail in the literature: immunoelectron microscopy (4); immunofluorescence tests and humoral and cellular microcytotoxicity assays (8,9), and radio-immune assays (13).

Results

Distinction between Virion and Non-virion Cell Surface Antigen

RNA tumor viruses mature by budding through the cell membrane to expose Ve antigen at the cell surface. Therefore, it was long thought, and it still is a matter of intense discussion, that Ve antigen is the only antigen expressed at the surface of RNA tumor virus-transformed cells. Such an expression contrasts with the expression of non-virion antigens on the cell surface, which occurs with DNA tumor viruses (6). By comparative studies with ALV strains and non-defective ASV strains of the same and different subgroups, i.e., with related and unrelated Ve antigens we were able to obtain a clear answer to that question in the ATV system.

When ALV-infected (nontransformed) and ASV-infected (transformed) CEF were labeled with ferritin-bound chicken IgG, two kinds of antibody arrangements could be observed under the electron microscope. Antibody obtained from ALV-injected chicken appeared on the virus envelope as well as in certain distinct surface regions of cells infected or transformed by ALV or ASV of the homologous subgroup (Fig. 5-1,A). Antibody obtained from ASV-injected chicken, however, also appeared on the surface but not in the virus particles of cells transformed by an ASV strain of a heterologous subgroup (Fig. 5-1,C and D; Table 5-1) (4).

These results indicate that transformed cells express, in addition to Ve antigen, a further virus-directed antigen at the cell surface (Fig. 5-1,D), which is therefore, tumor specific and can be called tumor-specific cell surface antigen (TSSA). These results further indicate that TSSA are group specific, i.e., that they cross-react among all ASV strains tested.

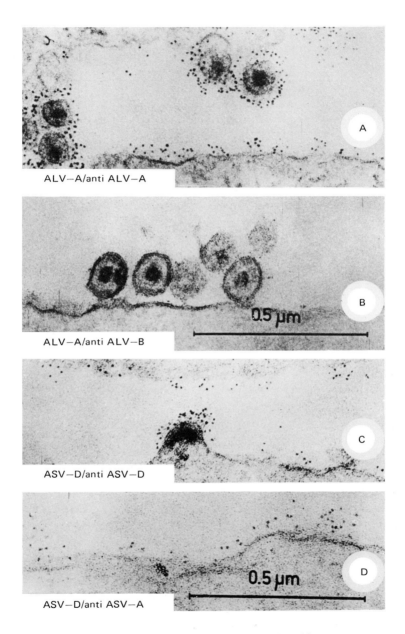

Figure 5-1. Immunoferritin labeling of transformed and/or productively infected chicken embryo cells. (A) Untransformed cells: The antigen detected represents virus envelope antigen.
(B) Untransformed cells: negative control in that heterologous ALV antibody do not react with ALV-B virus or cell surface.
(C) Transformed cells stained with homologous ASV antiserum.
(D) Transformed cells revealing TSSA, as labeled by heterologous ASV antiserum.

Table 5-1   Reaction of Chicken Immune Sera against ASV-Infected (Transformed) and ALV-Infected (Nontransformed) CEF, Respectively

CEF infected with		Immune sera against			
		Subgroup A		Subgroup D	
		ALV	ASV	ALV	ASV
Subgroup A	ALV	+ (Ve–Ag)	+ (Ve–Ag)	0	0
	ASV	+ (Ve–Ag)	+ + (Ve–Ag+TSSA)	0	+ (TSSA)
Subgroup D	ALV	0	0	+ (Ve–Ag)	+ (Ve–Ag)
	ASV	0	+ (TSSA)	+ (Ve–Ag)	+ + (Ve–Ag+TSSA)

a The type of antigen detected in the respective reaction is indicated in parentheses.

When immune lymphocytes, taken from chickens injected with several different viruses, were tested for their cytotoxic activity against a similar set of CEF as in the experiment described above, a cytotoxic pattern similar to that described in Table 5-1 was observed (9). Thus, TSSA, as well as Ve antigen, appears to be able to induce a cytotoxic immune reaction in the host. The one discrepancy between the cytotoxic data and the ferritin-labeled antibody data will be discussed below.

Cross-Reaction between ALV- and ASV-Induced TSSA

Immune lymphyocytes obtained after repeated injections of ALV into the chicken revealed a group-specific cytotoxic effect but only when tested against transformed cells (8). This was in contrast to the observations with humoral antibodies (Table 5-1) made 4 weeks after a single virus injection and interpreted to mean that, during the longer incubation period, the ALV had transformed hemopoietic target cells with a concomitant expression of TSSA, which then cross-reacted with the TSSA in sarcoma cells. A cross-reaction of leukemia and sarcoma cell TSSA was also suggested by *in vivo* experiments in mice and chicken, in which a protective effect of injected ALV against sarcoma development was demonstrated; according to experimental design, this effect could not have been due to Ve antigen (1,14).

This phenomenon was directly investigated in an experiment designed to show that TSSA-specific antisera prepared in mice against sarcoma cells exert a cytotoxic effect against chicken leukemic cells. Confirmation was also obtained

6

Studies on the Mechanisms of Tumor Immunity: Some Recent Data on Cellular Immunity to Common, Possibly Embryonic Antigens in Mouse Sarcomas

K. E. Hellström and I. Hellström

Introduction

Studies performed during the last decade have shown that lmphocyte-mediated cytotoxic reactions can be detected *in vitro* against many autochthonous tumors in animals, as well as in man (Table 6-1). Blocking factors in tumor-bearer serum (antigen–antibody complexes, antigen, and, perhaps, also free antibodies) can inhibit the cytotoxic lymphocyte effect. Certain immune sera, including some human convalescent sera, contain "unblocking" antibodies, i.e., antibodies that can abrogate the blocking effect of tumor-bearer sera. Other such sera are cytotoxic in the presence of complement and/or contain lymphocyte dependent antibodies "arming" non-T cells.

Since we have recently written an extensive review in this area (8), we do not feel that it is necessary too repeat here what has been already published. We have, instead, decided to discuss in this chapter some recent studies on the ability of lymphocytes from multiparous mice to kill cultivated syngeneic tumor cells. We believe that tumor antigens of an embryonic nature have acted as targets in the reactions we have studied, and we will refer to the antigens

Table 6-1 Some of the Factors Involved in the Immune Response to Tumor Antigens

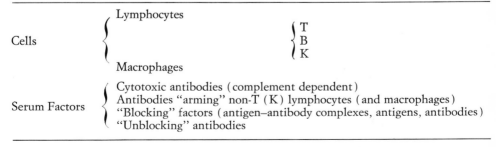

Fundamental Aspects of Neoplasia,
edited by A. Arthur Gottlieb, Otto J. Plescia, and David H. L. Bishop.
© 1975 by Springer-Verlag New York Inc.

as embryonic here, but there is no proof to date that they were really embryonic (e.g., the pregnant mice may have been sensitized to some viral antigens present in the tumors).

Our present approach was inspired by our conviction that work in animal model systems is needed to better define the role, *in vivo,* of those immune reactions that can be detected *in vitro* by the use of the microcytotoxicity test. It was also inspired by our feeling that immune reactions to embryonic tumor antigens must be much better understood, particularly with respect to the relevance, *in vivo,* of data obtained *in vitro.* Such understanding may have relevance for tumor prevention and therapy.

Correlation between *In Vivo* and *In Vitro* Findings

Previous studies have shown that there is, in many systems, a good correlation between the presence of specific, cell-mediated anti-tumor immunity together with the absence of serum blocking factors as detectable *in vitro* and the ability of animals to reject transplanted tumor cells *in vivo* (8). Similarly, detection of blocking serum factors has been found to correlate with a decreased resistance of animals to subcutaneously transplanted tumor cells. The blocking factors often appear in animals prior to their relapse after surgical removal of a growing neoplasm, and they are able to mediate enhancement of tumor growth *in vivo* (8,9).

There is also evidence, however, from studies on common embryonic tumor antigens, that some immune reactions detected against tumor antigens *in vitro* may be powerless to counteract tumor growth *in vivo* (1). This has been taken by some to imply that data from microcytotoxicity assays may not always reflect which immune responses are relevant for tumor rejection. One may speculate as to the reasons for the discrepancies between *in vivo* and *in vitro* findings (8). Embryonic tumor antigens may not be expressed *in vivo,* as a result, for example, of antigenic modulation, or they may be too loosely associated with (or too deeply buried within) the cell membrane for them to be useful targets in cytotoxic reactions, except when relatively very large numbers of immune lymphocytes are added, as in most *in vitro* studies. Alternatively, a blocking effect of embryonic tumor antigens, alone or complexed with antibodies, may be particularly efficient in preventing tumor cell destruction by immune lymphocytes. Since the tissue type-specific tumor antigens found among human neoplasms of the same histologic type might be similar to the embryonic antigens (1), there is a great need to investigate animal model systems involving this type of antigen.

Tissue Type-Specific and Common Embryonic Antigens

One animal system we have studied much in the past—and one we still continue to work with—involves mice and rats with chemically induced papillomas and carcinomas of the urinary bladder (10). Like human bladder tumors (8), such neoplasms have tissue type-specific antigens that are present in bladder papillomas and carcinomas but are absent from other tumors. Two years ago, we published work showing that immunization of rats with syngeneic bladder papilloma can delay the appearance of primary bladder papillomas (10), and this work has been recently repeated in our laboratory with similar results. We also have data, however, to indicate that mice immunized with bladder carcinoma cells develop transplantation resistance only against the particular tumor line used for immunization and not against other bladder carcinoma lines (11); this is the case in spite of the fact that these tumors have common antigens detectable by microcytotoxicity assay.

The recent interest in embryonic tumor antigens as possible targets for cytotoxic immune reactions was stimulated by the finding of Coggin et al. (6) that immunization of hamsters with embryonic cells can induce transplantation resistance to SV40 tumors. In 1970, Brawn (4) reported that lymph node cells from multiparous mice can be cytotoxic to cultivated syngeneic tumor cells but not to normal fibroblasts, and he postulated that this occurs because the lymphocytes are sensitized to some embryonic antigens present on the tumor cells (5). Extracts prepared from 10- to 13-day-old mouse embryos, but not extracts from normal mouse muscle, blocked the ability of the lymphocytes to kill; this is further evidence that an immune reaction to embryonic tumor antigens may have occurred (5).

Baldwin et al. (2), as well as Dierlam et al. (7), have confirmed the observation of a tumoricidal effect, *in vitro*, of lymphocytes from multiparous mice, and they have extended these findings by showing that the lymphocyte effect can be blocked by sera from multiparous mice and from mice bearing growing tumors of many kinds. There is not much new evidence, however, beyond Coggin's original work, that immunity to embryonic antigens can interfere with tumor growth *in vivo*, and there are several reports to the contrary (see, e.g., ref. 1). It has also been shown that lymphocytes adoptively transferred from multiparous mice do not protect recipients against the transplantation of small doses of syngeneic tumor cells (although they are sensitive to similar lymphocytes on exposure *in vitro*).

With this background, we will now present our own findings in this area.

Results and Discussion

Tumor Cells Can Be Killed by Lymphocytes from Multiparous Donors

Table 6-2 is a summary of experiments showing that lymph node cells from multiparous BALB/c mice can kill cultivated neoplastic cells derived from chemically induced sarcomas (#1315 and 1321), as well as neoplastic cells

Table 6-2   Cytotoxic Effect of 150,000 Lymph Node Cells/Well from
            Multiparous BALB/c Mice on BALB/c Target Cells, Plated in
            Microtest II (Falcon #3040) plates

Lymph Node Cells from Age-Matched Virgin BALB/c Females Were Used as Controls.

Target cells	Number of experiments performed	Lymphocyte-mediated cytotoxicity (%) (M±SE)
MCA sarcoma #1315	26	36.4±2.4
MCA sarcoma #1321	7	26.8±3.1
3T3 MSV transformed	12	49.6±3.5
3T3 spontaneously transformed	1	30.6
3T3 SV40 transformed	1	42.4
3T3 control	12	−8.2±4.1
Adult BALB/c fibroblast	5	−7.3±4.8

transformed *in vitro* from one clone of non-transformed 3T3 cells of BALB/c origin. The transformed lines studied were 3T3 cells transformed with Moloney sarcoma virus, 3T3 cells spontaneously transformed, and 3T3 cells transformed with SV40 virus. Normal BALB/c fibroblasts from newborn mice, and non-transformed (control) 3T3 cells were not killed by the same lymphocyte suspensions. Age-matched virgin BALB/c females were used as control lymphocyte donors.

Spleen cells from multiparous mice were no longer toxic following their treatment with mouse anti-θ serum and complement, but these cells were still toxic after passage through immunoglobulin-coated columns, which resulted in the removal of cells with surface immunoglobulins and cells forming plaques in the Jerne assay (Table 6-3). These findings argue against the cytotoxic effect seen against neoplastic (and *in vitro* transformed) cells being caused, for example, by activated macrophages present in lymphoid cell suspensions from multiparous mice, in greater numbers than in controls, which would exert a toxic effect on all kinds of target cells. They indicate, instead, that the reacting cells are T cells or that the killing is, at least, dependent on a T cell function (such as the production of a T dependent antibody, capable of arming lymphocytes or macrophages). The data do not exclude, however, the possibility that, under slightly different conditions, a non-T dependent killing of cells with embryonic tumor antigens may also occur.

We conclude from these data that the lymphocytes present in lymph nodes and spleens of multiparous mice exert a cytotoxic effect on cultivated neoplastic (or transformed) cell, as compared to non-neoplastic (or non-transformed) cells. Our findings indicate that this phenomenon is fairly general, a view that

Table 6-3   Cytotoxic Effect of 150,000 Purified Spleen Cells/Well from
Multiparous BALB/c Mice on BALB/c Target Cells

Similarily Purified Spleen Cells from Age-Matched Virgin BALB/c Females
Were Used as Controls

	Target Cells		
	---	---	---
Spleen cell suspension	#1315 (5 exps.)	3T3-MSV (3 exps.)	3T3 control
Untreated	27.1±5.5	59.8±3.0	−18.4
Column passed (−Ig control cells)	29.0±7.0	47.7±5.6	0
Complement treated	30.6±2.7	58.1±3.3	−11.9
Anti θ treated	49.1±8.4		
Anti θ +complement treated	14.0±4.6	5.4±15.9	−13.3

is supported by other published work (1,8). This must not be taken to mean, however, that embryonic tumor antigens are necessarily present on *all* mouse tumors; attempts to detect universal tumor antigens in the past have generally been futile.

Cytotoxic Effect of Lymphocytes from Multiparous Mice
Is Blocked by Serum from Multiparous and Tumor-Bearing Mice

Data from many experiments, two of which are summarized in Table 6-4, indicate that serum from multiparous mice (pregnant at the time of serum harvest) could block the cytotoxic effect of lymphocytes from multiparous mice. Sera from tumor-bearing mice had a similar effect. A blocking effect could often be seen even at high serum dilutions (1:320).

In order to test whether this blocking effect had any tumor specificity, or

Table 6-4   Blocking Activity of Serum Tested on MCA Sarcoma #1321
Cells (BALB/c) in Combination with Lymphocytes from
Multiparous BALB/c Mice (Giving Approximately 40 percent
Killing in the presence of Control Serum

Data Pooled from Two Experiments with Similar Results.

	Blocking activity (%) at serum dilution				
	---	---	---	---	---
Serum source	1:10	1:20	1:40	1:80	1:320
Multiparous BALB/c	194	129	134	167	−72
BALB/c with tumor #1315	24	203	94	244	
BALB/c with tumor #1321	63	120	62	130	124

K. E. Hellström and I. Hellström

whether it was due, for example, to the presence of some hormones or to any type of antigen–antibody complex present in serum from pregnant mice, experiments were performed to remove the blocking activity by specific absorption. Table 6-5 contains data from four such experiments, showing that removal of blocking activity by absorption with tumor (but not with control) cells could, indeed, be achieved.

Our data are compatible with the notion that the blocking factors detected in serum from multiparous and tumor-bearing mice have antibody specificity and that they are similar to blocking factors seen in other systems (8). It remains to be determined whether they are antigen–antibody complexes or just antibodies and to what extent circulating free antigens with blocking activity occur in this system.

Blocking factors to common embryonic antigens are detected at times when mice have an effective immunity to individually unique tumor antigens but are suspectible to challenge with other tumors sharing embryonic antigens with the immunizing tumor. Studies were performed with two methylcholanthrene-induced BALB/c sarcomas (#1315 and 1321), which demonstrate individually unique but no common antigens when assayed by regular transplantation tests (Table 6-6), and whose cells can be killed *in vitro* by exposure to lymphocytes from multiparous mice (Table 6-2). As shown in Table 6-7, mice in which transplantation immunity to sarcoma #1315 had been induced in

Table 6-5 Removal of the Blocking Effect of Serum from Multiparous Mice by Absorption with Tumor Cells (or Cells Transformed *In Vitro*), as Compared to Control Cells

Lymphocytes from Multiparous BALB/c Mice Giving Approximately 40 Percent Killing in the Presence of Control Serum Were Used as Effector Cells.

Target cells	Serum absorbed with:	Blocking activity (%)
MCA sarcoma #1315	MCA sarcoma #1315	−16.8
	MCA sarcoma #1321	33.1
	Adult BALB/c fibroblasts	92.1
MCA sarcoma #1321	MCA sarcoma #1315	40.3
	MCA sarcoma #1321	20.8
	Adult BALB/c fibroblasts	115.8
MCA sarcoma #1315	3T3 MSV transformed	14.7
	3T3 control	64.7
3T3 MSV transformed	3T3 MSV transformed	−1.0
	3T3 control	73.0

94

Table 6-6 Effective Sensitization of BALB/c Mice to Individually Distinct But Not to Common Antigens of Sarcomas #1315 and 1321 (by Tumor Transplantation, followed by Removal)

Immunization	Challenge[a]	Mice dead of tumor
1315	1315	7/16
1315	1321	18/19
1321	1315	20/20
1321	1321	7/20
—	1315	20/20
—	1321	20/20

[a] Mice were challenged with 10^4 or 5×10^4 sarcoma cells. The results reported include both.

Table 6-7 Detectable Blocking Factors to Common Embryonic Tumor Antigens at a Time When Mice Have Been Made Resistant to Tumors Carrying Unique Antigens But Accept Tumor Grafts Carrying Common Embryonic Antigens

Serum donor	Blocking activity (%) in combination with lymph node cells from:	
	Multiparous BALB/c	BALB/c immunized to #1315
BALB/c with growing #1315	53	106
Balb/c with #1315 tumor removed; 10 days later challenged with #1315; serum harvested 8 days after challenge; mice resistant to #1315	48	5
BALB/c with #1315 tumor removed; 10 days later challenged with #1321; serum was harvested 8 days after challenge; mice accepted grafted #1321 cells	37	NT

the classic way (tumor transplantation followed by removal), and which showed resistance to challenge with this tumor (but not to sarcoma #1321), had blocking factors canceling reactivity against the common embryonic antigens but not against the specific antigens of sarcoma #1315.

These findings suggest that the blocking mechanism may be very effective with respect to the common embryonic antigens, and they indicate that this mechanism may be more effective with respect to the common antigens than with respect to the individually unique ones. More work in this area is needed to clarify this issue.

Unblocking Sera Raised against Embryonic Antigens and Tested *In Vitro* as well as *In Vivo*

We are presently trying to raise unblocking sera by immunizing rabbits with embryonic cells and then absorbing the sera extensively, both *in vitro* and *in vivo*; the procedures developed to obtain unblocking antibodies to rat polyoma tumors (3) are being used. This way, we hope ultimately to be able to assess whether counteraction of the blocking serum effect will influence tumor growth *in vivo*.

The data shown in Table 6-8 suggest that unblocking sera to embryonic

Table 6-8 Unblocking Effect of Rabbit Antiserum to 12 to 15 Day BALB/c Mouse Embryos ("Immune rabbit"), *In Vitro* and *In Vivo* and Tested in the Presence of Serum from Multiparous or Control BALB/c Mice

Serum	Lymphocytotoxicity[a] (%)	Blocking (%)
Normal rabbit (1:10)+normal BALB/c (1:10)	50	Control 1
(1:50)	42	Control 2
(1:100)	40	Control 3
Normal rabbit (1:10)+multiparous BALB/c (1:10)	20	61
(1:50)	−6	111
(1:100)	3	93
Immune rabbit (1:10)+normal BALB/c (1:10)	54	−7
(1:50)	37	29
(1:100)	51	−28
Immune rabbit (1:10)+multiparous BALB/c (1:10)	61	−21
(1:50)	47	11
(1:100)	41	−3

a Lymph node cells from multiparous or control BALB/c mice were used, giving about 40 percent killing in the presence of control serum.

Table 6-9 Preliminary Data from an Experiment Performed by Inoculating Immunized Mice with Unblocking Serum (Table 9-8), 0.1 ml/mouse, Immediately before Tumor Challenge and 3 Days Later

Immunization[a]	Mice with tumor[b] (11 days after inoculation)	Mice with tumor (14 days after inoculation)[c]	Mice dead of tumor (30 days after inoculation)
#1315+control serum	4/10	5/10 (3.4)	7/10
+unblocking serum	0/9	6/9 (3.9)	4/9
Embryo+control serum	6/10	7/10 (4.6)	3/10
+unblocking serum	1/10	3/10 (2.2)	0/10
Adult kidney+control serum	6/10	6/10 (4.7)	4/10
+unblocking serum	2/10	7/10 (4.6)	2/9
Total control serum	16/30	18/30 (4.2)	14/30
Total unblocking serum	3/29	16/29 (3.6)	6/28

[a] Mice had been immunized with 10- to 15-day-old BALB/c embryos, with tumor #1315 or with adult kidney, as in experiment shown in Table 6-6.

[b] Mice were challenged with 10^4 sarcoma cells #1321, whose growth was measured.

antigens can, indeed, be raised. Table 6-9 presents the first (and only) *in vivo* experiment performed, which tested whether serum that is unblocking *in vitro* can affect the ability of transplanted cells from sarcoma #1321 to grow out *in vivo*. As shown in Table 6-9, there is some indication that it can. We are most anxious, however, to point out the preliminary nature of this finding, both with respect to its reproducibility (only one experiment was performed) and its implications. If the difference observed is accepted as real, one must know whether an unblocking effect was, indeed, involved, or whether the serum contained lymphocyte-dependent antibodies or antibodies that were tumoricidal in the presence of complement or whether it was just some other, non-immunologic, mechanism leading to a somewhat delayed tumor growth *in vivo*.

Summary

Animal experiments must be performed to better delineate the *in vivo* role of various immunologic parameters studied *in vitro*. Because of recent findings that immune reactions to common embryonic tumor antigens can be detected *in vitro*, whereas these antigens do not appear to act as transplantation antigens at all or only weakly, *in vivo*.

We have presented evidence that lymphocytes from multiparous mice are cytotoxic to syngeneic tumor cells, but not to the corresponding normal cells, and that this cytotoxic effect can be blocked by serum factors specific for antigens present on the tumor cells. We have shown that these blocking factors are present in immunized animals in which evidence of effective transplantation immunity against tumors having common embryonic antigens is not shown. Finally, we have presented data indicating that unblocking sera may be raised against embryonic antigens and have included data from our first *in vivo* experiment with such a serum. We suggest that tests of such unblocking sera for possible anti-tumor effects *in vivo* may be useful to determine whether the failure of embryonic antigens to act as transplantation antigens *in vivo* is indeed due to a particularly effective blocking mechanism operating for such antigens.

ACKNOWLEDGEMENTS

This work was supported by Grants CA-10188 and CA-10189 from the National Institues of Health, by Grant IM–43E from the American Cancer Society, and by Contract NIH NCI 71–2171 from the Virus Program, National Cancer Institute. The skillful technical assistance of Ms. Judi Bamer and Ms. Linda Katzenberger is gratefully acknowledged.

REFERENCES

1. Baldwin, R. W. and Embleton, M. J. Neoantigens on spontaneous and carcinogen-induced rat tumors defined by *in vitro* lymphocytotoxicity assays. Int. J. Cancer, 13:433, 1974.

2. Baldwin, R. W., Glaves, D., and Vose, B. M. Embryonic antigen expression in chemically induced rat hepatomas and sarcomas. Int. J. Cancer, 10:233, 1972.

3. Bansal, S. C. and Sjögren, H. O. Counteraction of the blocking of cell-mediated tumor immunity by inoculation of unblocking sera and splenectomy: Immunotherapeutic effects on primary polyoma tumors in rats. Int. J. Cancer, 9:940, 1972.

4. Brawn, R. J. Possible association of embryonal antigen(s) with several primary 3-methylcholantherene-induced murine sarcomas. Int. J. Cancer, 6:245, 1970.

5. Brawn, R. J. Evidence for association of embryonal antigen(s) with several 3-methyl-cholanthrene-induced murine sarcomas. *In* Anderson, N. G. and Coggin, J. H., Jr., eds., Proceedings of the First Conference and Workshop on Embryonic and Fetal Antigens in Cancer. Oak Ridge, Tenn., Oak Ridge National Laboratory, 1971, p. 143.

6. Coggin, J. H., Ambrose, K. E., Bellamy, B. B., and Anderson, N. G. Tumor immunity in hamsters immunized with fetal tissues. J. Immunol., 107:526, 1971.

7. Dierlam, P., Anderson, N. G., and Coggin, J. H., Jr. Immunization against tumors with fetal antigens: Detection of immunity by the colony inhibition test and by adoptive transfer. *In* Anderson, N. G. and Coggin, J. H., Jr., eds., Proceedings of the First Conference and Workshop on Embryonic and Fetal Antigens in Cancer. Oak Ridge, Tenn., Oak Ridge National Laboratory, 1971, p. 203.

8. Hellström, K. E. and Hellström, I. Lymphocyte-mediated cytotoxicity and blocking serum activity to tumor antigens. Adv. Immunol., 18:209, 1974.

9. Sjögren, H. O. and Bansal, S. C. Antigens in virally induced tumors. *In* Amos, B., ed. Progress in Immunology. 1971, p. 921.

10. Taranger, L., Chapman, W. H. Hellström, I., and Hellström, K. E. Immunological studies on urinary bladder tumors of rats and mice. Science, 176:1337, 1972.

11. Wahl, D. V., Chapman, W. H., Hellström, I., and Hellström, K. E. Transplantation immunity to individually unique antigens of chemically induced bladder tumors in mice. Int. J. Cancer, 14:114, 1974.

7

Escape from Immune Control by the Shedding of Membrane Antigens: Influence on Metastatic Behavior of Tumor Cells

P. Alexander

Introduction

Whether a tumor gives rise to distant metastases depends on many factors. That the immune response of the host to the tumor-specific, transplantation-type antigens (TSTA) present in the plasma membrane of tumor cells plays a part in determining the fate of malignant cells released into the circulation is suggested by the findings (5,6) that some experimentally induced animal tumors metastasize more readily when transplanted into an immunologically suppressed host (Fig. 7-1). The immunologic effector arm responsible for preventing bloodborne malignant cells from becoming established as lung metastases involve antibody. This became apparent from experiments (9) in which rats bearing sarcomas that did not cause spontaneous metastases were made to develop lung metastases following the prolonged draining of thoracic duct lymphocytes (see Table 7-1). This procedure drastically depletes the pool of circulating lymphocytes, and rats treated in this way are unable to mount primary immune responses (e.g., allografts are not rejected); yet immunologic memory was not impaired, and secondary immune responses were normal (8). During the course of thoracic-duct drainage, large amounts of lymph plasma are removed, this leads to the loss of circulating proteins, and the level of immunoglobulin in the blood is greatly reduced (13). The experiments illustrated in Table 7-1 show that the occurrence of metastasis following thoracic-duct drainage is due to the loss of a specific humoral factor and not to the removal of circulating lymphocytes. In the serum of rats with well-established sarcomas, antibody activity cannot be detected, and the antibody is bound to antigen in a complex (10,12). Such complexes can bind to monocytes and macrophages and thereby render them specifically cytotoxic to cells bearing on their surface the antigen present in the complex (7). These and other data led

Fundamental Aspects of Neoplasia,
edited by A. Arthur Gottlieb, Otto J. Plescia, and David H. L. Bishop.
© 1975 by Springer-Verlag New York Inc.

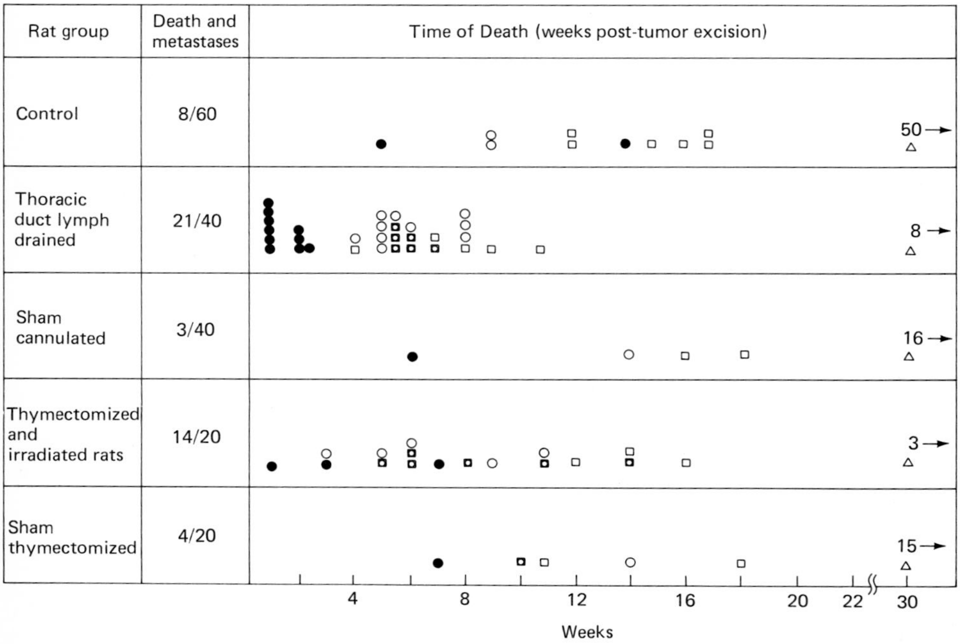

Rat group	Death and metastases	Time of Death (weeks post-tumor excision)
Control	8/60	
Thoracic duct lymph drained	21/40	
Sham cannulated	3/40	
Thymectomized and irradiated rats	14/20	
Sham thymectomized	4/20	

Figure 7-1. Effect of immune suppression on incidence of metastases after excision of chemically induced rat sarcoma (HSBPA). HSBPA tumors were grown intramuscularly in hind limbs of various groups of immuno-suppressed syngeneic rats and appropriate controls for 14 days. The tumor-bearing limbs were then amputated, and the animals kept for observation on the development of metastases for up to 30 weeks. Key: (●) deaths with no evidence of metastases, (○) deaths with lymph node metastases, (□) deaths with lung metastases, (■) deaths with lymph node and lung metastases, (△) survivors.

to the suggestion that the immune component responsible for eliminating bloodborne cancer cells is both antibody and antibody-antigen complex.

Escape and Immunogenicity

The point then arises as to why some tumors metastasize spontaneously, whereas others do not. An attractive hypothesis is that there are differences in the antigenicity of the tumors being compared; that is, that TSTA of metastasizing tumors is "weak" and does not invoke as strong a host reaction as does TSTA from non-metastasizing tumors. This concept appears to be supported by a number of investigations (e.g., ref. 5) in which it was found that

Table 7-1   Effect of Removing Thoracic Duct Lymph on Spontaneous
            Lung Metastases

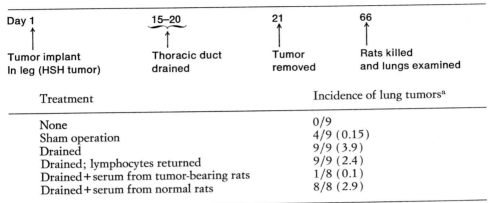

Treatment	Incidence of lung tumors[a]
None	0/9
Sham operation	4/9 (0.15)
Drained	9/9 (3.9)
Drained; lymphocytes returned	9/9 (2.4)
Drained + serum from tumor-bearing rats	1/8 (0.1)
Drained + serum from normal rats	8/8 (2.9)

[a] Numbers in parentheses are average weight (grams of lung tumors).

the number of tumor cells that can be rejected by suitably immunized animals
is greater for non-metastasizing than metastasizing tumors (Table 7-2).
But, this test measures an end effect—the rejection of tumor cells—determined both by the magnitude of the host reaction (i.e., the amount of antibody
and the number of cytotoxic cells produced by the host) as well as by the
facility with which injected tumor cells avoid destruction by the effector

Table 7-2   Relationship between Immunogenicity and Incidence
            of Metastases

Macrophage content, incidence of metastases, and immunogenicity of a variety of
chemically induced rat fibrosarcoma transplanted into syngeneic recipients. The incidence
of metastases was measured after excision of tumors, which had been growing
intramuscularly in hind limbs for 14 days.

Tumor	Macrophages (%) mean (and range)	Incidence of metastases (%)	"Immunogenicity"[a]
MC-3	8 (2–12)	100	$<10^3$
HSH	12 (10–15)	100	10^3–2×10^4
ASBPI	22 (18–26)	50–55–	10^5
MCI-M	38 (36–42)	20–30	10^6
HSN	40 (34–44)	30–35	5×10^6–10^7
HSBPA	54 (42–63)	10–12	10^7–5×10^7

[a] Assessed as number of cells required for tumor growth in rats immunized by excision of intra-
muscular tumors 14 days previously.

processes developed by the host. This last phenomenon is aptly described as "escape" and can occur in many different ways. We have found in the experimentally induced rat tumors that the inverse correlation between immunogenicity and capacity to metastasize is due to the fact that metastatic tumors escape more readily than do non-metastatic tumors. One of the most effective forms of escape is the release of TSTA in a soluble form into the environment of the tumor (3). Soluble TSTA combines with some of the effector arms of the immune response in a way that renders them incapable of subsequently attacking the tumor through interaction with the same antigen on the tumor cell surface.

Mechanisms of Antigen Release

There is convincing evidence of the presence, in the serum of patients with cancer and of rats with sarcomas, of a macromolecule that specifically inhibits mononuclear cells that are cytotoxic to tumor cells by *in vitro* tests. This substance has the expected properties of soluble TSTA, and material with the same properties can be isolated from the membranes of tumors (1,11,12). There are several ways (Table 7-3) in which TSTA is released from tumors and appears in the circulation of the tumor-bearing host in a soluble form capable of inhibiting the effector arms of the immune response.

For a chemically induced, transplantable rat sarcoma (MC-1), Thomson et al. (11) developed a radioimmunoassay for TSTA in serum. They demonstrated that when 10^6 tumor cells are inoculated into a normal rat, there is a rapid but transient appearance of TSTA in the serum. This occurs because the majority of the injected cells autolyze upon injection and then release TSTA. The surviving cells grow, and, 10 days after the inoculation, there is a palpable tumor, and the level of soluble TSTA in the serum rises progressively with tumor growth. When the tumor is surgically removed, TSTA in the serum disappears rapidly. For this tumor (i.e., the MC-1 sarcoma) the circulating TSTA released during tumor growth is not due to a spontaneous shedding of antigen but is a by-product of the immune reaction of the host to the tumor. In animals with immune systems suppressed by total body X-irradiation, no

Table 7-3   Mechanisms of Release in a Soluble Form
of Tumor-Specific Antigens (TSTA)
from Tumor Cells

1.	During tumor necrosis
2.	In consequence of immune reaction of host against the tumor
3.	Spontaneous release during normal growth

circulating TSTA of the MC-1 tumor can be detected after the intial burst, due to the autolysis of some of the inoculated cells. Yet the injected sarcoma cells do grow to cause a rapidly proliferating tumor in the X-irradiated host.

Spontaneous Shedding and Metastasis

This, however, is not a universal finding, and, with another chemically induced rat sarcoma (MC-3), circulating TSTA can be detected in the serum of both normal and immunosuppressed rats bearing growing tumors (2). In terms of the host reaction to the tumor, there is little difference between the MC-1 and the MC-3 sarcoma, and the cells in the node draining such growing tumors are approximately equally effective in killing specific target cells (i.e., MC-1 and MC-3 sarcoma cells, respectively) in culture (2,4). The key difference between the MC-3 and the MC-1 sarcomas is that the cells of the former shed TSTA spontaneously in tissue culture to a much greater extent than do the MC-1 sarcoma cells. This was shown by determining the level of TSTA in culture supernatants. The amount of specific soluble TSTA is much lower in the supernatants of cultures of MC-1 cells than of MC-3 cells. It is tempting to correlate the *in vivo* finding for shedding of antigen from the MC-3 tumor immunosuppressed animals and the *in vitro* finding of the greater shedding of TSTA from the MC-3 tumor in tissue culture with the difference in metastatic behavior of these two sarcomas. The biologic properties of the MC-1 and MC-3 sarcomas are contrasted in Table 7-4. Currie and I propose that the much greater tendency of the MC-3 sarcoma to metastasize is due to the release of soluble TSTA in amounts sufficient to protect micro foci at extracellular sites from destruction by the immune effector arms of the host (Table 7-5).

Similar correlations have been seen when a non-metastasizing tumor changes into a metastasizing one, following prolonged passage. In the examples we have studied, changes in the growth pattern of tumors following prolonged passage have not been accompanied by a loss of TSTA from the tumor cell membranes but by the greater facility with which TSTA is shed spontaneously.

The reasons why some tumors shed TSTA more readily than others are not known. It could be related to the plasticity (or rate of turnover) of the cell membrane or, more likely, to an overproduction of TSTA in the cell leading to its release from the cell membrane.

Conclusion

It must be emphasized that the efficiency of escape from the immune defences of the host can at best be only one of several factors that determine whether cells that are continually released from the primary tumor into the circulation

Table 7-4   Comparison of Two Chemically Induced Transplantable
              Rat Sarcomas

	MC-1 sarcoma	MC-3 sarcoma
Growth pattern *in vivo*	Local only; curable by surgery	Metastasizes to nodes and lung
Resistance to challenge following hyperimmunization with X-irradiated sarcoma cells	Powerful protection	No protection
Specific *in vitro* cytotoxicity of lymphoid cells from nodes draining the tumor	+ + +	+ + +
Soluble TSTA in serum of tumor bearers:		
normal	+ +	+ +
immunosuppressed	±[a]	+ +
Soluble TSTA detected in tissue culture supernatant	±[a]	+ +

[a] None or very little detected.

Table 7-5   Relationship of Metastasis to Shedding of TSTA

	Concentration of soluble antigen surrounding:	
Rate of spontaneous shedding of tumor antigens by tumor cells	Macroscopic primary tumor	Microfoci of metastized tumor
Low (nonmetastatic)	Sufficient to permit escape	Insufficient to avoid destruction by effector processes
High (metastatic)	Sufficient to permit escape	Sufficient to permit escape

give rise to metastases. We know that circulating tumor cells are also destroyed by nonimmune mechanisms and that they must have the proper armamentarium of enzymes necessary to extravasate and to implant if they are to give rise to metastases. Such factors may well be more important than immune parameters in determining metastatic behavior.

Summary

In the serum and urine of patients and rats with growing tumors, macromolecules with all the properties of tumor-specific membrane antigens in soluble form have been detected. These soluble antigens provide a powerful escape mechanism for antigenic tumors, since they are of very low immunogenicity and yet combine and inhibit the action of several of the effector arms of immunity. Depending on the extent of disease, these antigens may be present, in part, as antigen/antibody complexes. It is, however, quite clear that the prime mover in the interference with the effector aims of the immune response is the antigen moiety and not the antibody moiety of such a complex. Three mechanisms have been elucidated by which such antigens appear in soluble form in the circulation: (a) As a result of tumor necrosis, (b) as a by-product of an immune reaction directed against the tumor, and (c) by spontaneous shedding from viable tumor cells (this does not require antibody). Recent experiments have shown that tumors vary widely in their capacity to shed tumor-specific antigens spontaneously, and the metastatic behavior of tumors can be correlated with the readiness with which they release antigens into the culture supernatant. The available evidence suggests that a factor in determining whether tumors metastasize or not is the extent to which they release tumor-specific antigens in a soluble form in their environment. If the rate of release is high, then even micro foci of tumors are protected against many forms of the host's immune defences because the "smoke screen" of soluble antigens is sufficient to guard such micro foci. If, however, the rate of spontaneous release is low, then only around large tumors is there a sufficient concentration of antigen to guard them against attack, whereas micro foci arising from bloodborne dissemination are vulnerable to destruction by the host's immune defenses.

REFERENCES

1. Currie, G. A. The role of circulating antigen as an inhibitor of tumour immunity in man. Br. J. Cancer, 28 (Suppl. I):153, 1973.

2. Currie, G. A. and Alexander, P. Spontaneous shedding of tumour-specific antigens by viable sarcoma cells: Its possible role in facilitating metastatic spread. Br. J. Cancer, 29:72, 1974.

3. Currie, G. A. and Basham, C. Serum-mediated inhibition of the immunological reactions of the patient to his own tumour: A possible role for circulating antigen. Br. J. Cancer, 26:427, 1972.

4. Currie, G. A. and Gage, J. O. Influence of tumour growth in the evolution of cytotoxic lymphoid cells in rats bearing a spontaneously metastasizing syngeneic fibrosarcoma. Br. J. Cancer, 28:136, 1973.

5. Eccles, S. A. and Alexander, P. The macrophage content of tumours in relation to the immune reaction of the host and metastatic spread. Nature, 250:667, 1974.

6. Fisher, B., Soliman, A., and Fisher, E. R. Effect of anti-lymphocyte serum on parameters of tumor growth in a syngeneic tumor host system. Proc. Soc. Exp. Biol. Med., 131:16, 1969.

7. Greenberg, A. H., Shen, L., and Roit, I. M. Characterization of the antibody dependent cytotoxic cell. Clin. Exp. Immunol., 15:251, 1973.

8. McGregor, D. D. and Gowans, J. L. The antibody response of rats depleted of lymphocytes by chronic drainage from the thoracic duct. J. Exp. Med., 117:303, 1963.

9. Proctor, J. W., Rudenstam, C. M., and Alexander, P. A factor preventing the development of lung metastases in rats with sarcomas. Nature, 242:29, 1973.

10. Thomson, D. M. P. and Alexander, P. A cross-reacting embryonic antigen in the membrane of rat sarcoma cells which is immunogenic in the syngeneic host. Br. J. Cancer, 27:35, 1973.

11. Thomson, D. M. P., Sellens, V., Eccles, S., and Alexander, P. Radioimmunoassay of tumour-specific transplantation antigen of a chemically-induced rat sarcoma: Circulating soluble tumour antigen in tumour bearers. Br. J. Cancer, 28:377, 1973.

12. Thomson, D. M. P., Steele, K., and Alexander, P. The presence of tumour-specific membrane antigen in the serum of rats with chemically-induced sarcomata. Br. J. Cancer, 27:27, 1973.

13. Wistar, R. and Shellam, G. R. Immunoglobulin levels during thoracic duct drainage in the rat. Int. Arch. Allergy, 36:323, 1969.

8

Expression of HL-A Antigens on Lymphoblastoid Cells

R. A. Reisfeld, M. A. Pellegrino,
S. Ferrone, and S. Oh

Introduction

In recent years it has become increasingly evident that the cell surface membrane plays a crucial role in almost all cellular activities and is, thus, of great importance in defense against neoplastic disease. Changes in the structure of the cell membrane are of particular interest because alterations in the properties of the cell surface are believed to contribute to the disordered proliferations that characterize malignant cells. Human histocompatibility (HL-A) antigens have proved to be a particularly useful tool in studying these changes on the cell membrane, since these genetically segregating antigenic components are present on the surface of all nucleated cells. These individuality markers can readily be defined since grafts exchanged between individuals who differ with respect to these antigens are promptly rejected by the immune system of the recipient. Furthermore, the association of some HL-A antigens with susceptibility to neoplastic disease has given an additional impetus to the characterization of these cell surface markers at the cellular and molecular levels in order to acquire a better understanding of the allograft rejection phenomenon and to gain further insight into the pathogenesis of the neoplastic process. In an effort to gain some further insight into these phenomena, we have attempted to evaluate cultured human lymphoid cells, derived from donors with and without lymphoid malignancies during different phases of their growth cycle, with regard to (a) cell surface expression of HL-A antigens and (b) susceptibility to lysis mediated by HL-A alloantisera and complement. In addition, we have tried to determine some of the chemical properties and molecular characteristics of these antigenic cell surface markers.

Expression of HL-A Antigens during the Cell Growth Cycle

A quantitative microabsorption technique was utilized to determine whether there was any fluctuation in cell surface expression of HL-A antigens during the growth cycle of human lymphoid cell lines derived from a donor with a

Fundamental Aspects of Neoplasia,
edited by A. Arthur Gottlieb, Otto J. Plescia, and David H. L. Bishop.
© 1975 by Springer-Verlag New York Inc.

lymphoid malignancy (RPMI 8866; HL-A2,3,7,12) and a normal individual (WI-L2; HL-A1,2,5,17). The life cycles of these cells, maintained in continuous culture, were synchronized by measuring the extent of DNA synthesis and cell viability. When the rate of DNA synthesis, ascertained by incorporation of [^{3}H]thymidine, reached 2 percent of maximum (G_0 phase), the resting cells were harvested and resuspended in fresh medium. The course of DNA synthesis was then ascertained to determine G_1 and S phases, respectively (13). The quantitative microabsorption technique utilized to assess the relative amount of HL-A surface antigen consists of the absorption of an appropriate HL-A alloantiserum at a given concentration, with progressive numbers of cells followed by a measurement of its residual cytotoxicity against selected target cells. To quantitate the expression of cell surface antigens, the absorption dosage (AD_{50}) is utilized; this parameter represents the number of cells required for 50 percent absorption of an antiserum's cytotoxic activity (14).

Cultured human lymphoid cells WI-L2 and RPMI 8866 display less than half the absorbing capacity in G_1 than in S phase (Fig. 8-1) (13,16). Cells in G_1 have a slightly higher absorbing capacity than cells in resting phase, whereas cells in log phase show a lower absorbing capacity than those in S phase. The volume of WI-L2 cells, however, changes approximately 1.4 fold between the G_1 and S phases. If one takes these findings into consideration and corrects the AD_{50} values appropriately, then it must be concluded that there are essentially equal numbers of HL-A determinants per cell volume in G_1 and S phases, especially if one considers that cells in S phase have considerably more microvilli and thus, possess a more irregular and larger surface area than cells in resting phase. Consequently, it appears that the actual difference in cell surface area is greater than that indicated by cell volume measurements. In cultures kept for 2 days after the cells had reached stationary phase, which consequently contained a large number of dead cells, a decrease in absorbing capacity was detected that may have been caused by the progressive disintegration of cells (14).

It is of some interest that both cell lines, i.e., WI-L2 derived from a donor free of malignancy and RPMI 8866 derived from a patient with myelogenous leukemia, displayed essentially a constant expression of HL-A antigens throughout the cell cycle. These findings were in contrast to those in our own laboratory with a murine leukemia (L1210) cell line. Thus, when the same quantitative microabsorption technique is utilized, the expression of H-2 antigens was found to vary during the cell cycle, being maximal in G_1 and decreasing during the G_1–S period (9). In addition, work by others also indicated that the H-2 expression of murine tumor cell lines YCAB and L1210 fluctuates during the cell cycle and appears to be maximal in G_1 (for review, see ref. 8). Similar results have also been obtained with the human lymphoblastoid lines Daudi

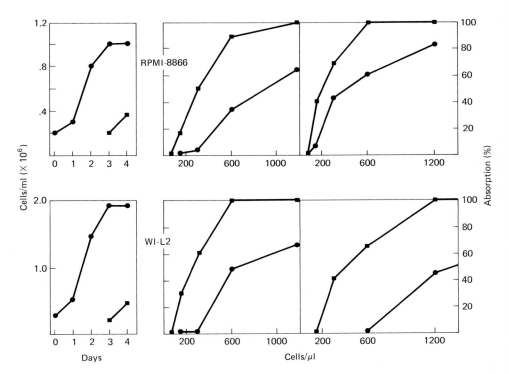

Figure 8-1. Relationship between the growth curve of cultured human lymphoid cells RPMI 8866 and WI-L2 and their absorbing capacity for HL-A alloantisera: (■) 1-day-old cells RPMI 8866 in logarithmic phase, and (●) 4-day-old cells in resting phase, were utilized to absorb anti-HI-A2 (middle graph) and anti-HL-A7 alloantisera (right graph); WI-L2 cells in the same stages of their growth cycle were utilized to absorb anti-HL-A2 (middle graph) and anti-HL-A5 alloantisera (right graph).

and P3J derived from the Burkitt tumor of African patients (5,10), where in each case, HL-A antigens were reported to be maximally expressed in G_1 phase.

Growth Cycle and Susceptibility to Lysis Mediated by Antisera to Histocompatibility Antigens

Several investigators showed that both non-synchronized and synchronized cultures of cultured murine tumor cells had a cyclic variation in their sensitivity to the cytolytic activity of complement and H-2 alloantisera. Susceptibility to lysis was found to be maximal during the G_1 phase of the cell cycle, it decreased during the S and G_2 phases, and it increased again when the majority of cells divided and entered the G_1 period of the next cycle (for review, see ref. 9).

In contradistinction, investigations with cultured human lymphoid cells showed that WI-L2 (8) and also RPMI 1788 and RPMI 4098 cells (our unpublished results) did not vary in their susceptibility to lysis throughout the cell cycle, as shown by the fact that they elicited similar titers of HL-A alloantisera directed against antigenic determinants of the first and second segregant series when cells in either G_1 or S phase were the targets. These data are in agreement with those from WI-L2 cells (see above), in which the surface expression of HL-A was constant throughout the growth cycle. Since RPMI 8866 cells derived from a donor with myelogenous leukemia also showed no fluctuation in HL-A expression throughout the cell cycle, we assumed that a priori, these cells would not vary in their susceptibility toward HL-A antibody- and complement-mediated lysis during different phases of the cell growth cycle. Much to our surprise, however, we found that RPMI 8866 (HL-A 2,3,7,12) cells indeed vary in their sensitivity to lysis. Thus, cells in the G_1 phase were approximately twofold less sensitive than those in G_0 or S to the cytolytic potential of alloantisera directed against HL-A2 (16). Similar results were obtained with alloantisera directed against HL-A7, a specificity of the second segregant series (Fig. 8-2). Rabbit serum is known to contain natural antibodies directed against a polymorphic system of antigens present on human lymphoid cells (7). To eliminate the possibility that the variation in the lysis obtained with HL-A alloantisera and rabbit complement was due only to changes in the expression of the antigenic determinants toward which these natural rabbit antibodies are directed, we repeated the cytotoxic test with human and guinea pig sera, which do not contain antibodies directed against cultured human lymphoid cells, as the sources of complement. Although both of these complement sources were cytolytically less efficient than rabbit complement, the lytic pattern observed was identical to that found with rabbit complement and HL-A alloantisera. To determine whether variable susceptibility to lysis applied also to other antigen systems, RPMI 8866 cells at various phases of the growth cycle were reacted with rabbit IgM, which contains the natural antibodies directed against human lymphocytes and human complement. Cells in the G_1 phase were again found to be least sensitive to cytotoxicity. These results indicate that RPMI 8866 cells change in susceptibility to immune lysis throughout their growth cycle, with cells in the G_1 phase being about twofold more resistant than cells in other portions of the cell cycle to the lytic activity of HL-A alloantisera and/or rabbit natural antibodies in conjunction with complement supplied in rabbit, human, or guinea pig serum.

In an attempt to explain this variability in lytic susceptibility, we performed, in addition to the quantitative microabsorption mentioned above, two independent tests to assess the density of HL-A antigens on the surface of RPMI

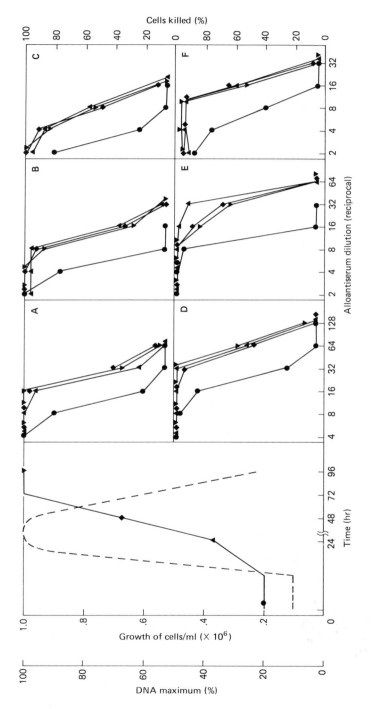

Figure 8-2. Relationship between the growth cycle and susceptibility to lysis of lymphoid cells RPMI 8866 by HL-A alloantisera and complement. On the left, (——) the growth curve and (-----) DNA synthesis of the cells is depicted. The small graphs plot the susceptibility of RPMI 8866 cells against the lytic activity of anti-HL-A2 (upper) and anti-HL-A7 (lower) in conjunction with rabbit (A), (D), human (B), (E), and guinea pig (C), (F) complement. The growth phase of the target cells is indicated by the corresponding symbol in the growth curve.

113

8866 cells in synchronous growth. First, cells were reacted with HL-A allo-antisera followed by incubation with radiolabeled antihuman IgG in an isotopic antiglobulin test. Specific binding of the second radiolabeled antibody is a function of the number of bound HL-A antibodies and thus, indirectly of the number of accessible antigenic sites. This test failed to reveal any significant difference in antigenic density between G_0, G_1, or S phases of the cycle when the (1.5 to 2 times) greater volume of S cells was taken into account. Second, soluble HL-A anitgens were extracted from RPMI 8866 cells with 3 M KCl during different stages of cell growth. No difference was detected in the total amount of HL-A antigenic activity solubilized throughout the cell cycle (16). As shown in Table 8-1, however, twice as much protein was solubilized from cells in G_0 phase than from those in G_1 or S phase, which simply suggests greater solubilization of contaminating proteins in G_0 phase. Finally, to rule out the possibility that the fluctuation in susceptibility to lysis during the growth cycle of RPMI 8866 cells was not due to differences in interaction with the complement system, we assessed the binding of radiolabeled complement components by sensitized lymphoid cells. Cells sampled in G_0, G_1, and S phase were equivalent in their ability after sensitization with various HL-A alloantisera to activate the complement system and to bind radiolabeled C3, C4, and C8 incorporated in the complement source (16). Furthermore, additional studies revealed that the pathway of complement activation, whether alternate or classic, depending on the source of complement employed, did not change during the cell cycle (16).

Much like RPMI 8866 cells, murine tumor cells YCAB (4,12) and L1210 (10) vary in suceptibility to complement-mediated lysis during the cell cycle, but these human cells differ from the murine cells both in the phase of the growth cycle during which they are least susceptible to lysis and in the unchanged antigen density during the growth cycle. Thus, YCAB and L1210 cells were found to be most sensitive to complement-mediated cytolytic damage initiated by H-2 antibodies in the G_1 phase of the cell cycle, when the quantitative expression of antigen as determined by absorption tests and extractibility was most pronounced. Along with the results from other investigators, these studies suggest that there is no direct correlation between susceptibility to lysis and the expression of membrane-associated antigens. The evidence thus far accumulated also suggests that variability in lytic susceptibility is not directly related to the ability of target cells to activate complement, to bind activated complement components, or to sustain complement-dependent ultrastructural lesions (6,11,12). In all probability, therefore, the differential susceptibility to lysis is due to changes in the properties of the cell membrane during the cell cycle. This is not unlikely in that many parameters of membrane function and structure are known to vary during cell growth, including turnover of mem-

114

Table 8-1 Solubilization of HL-A Antigens from Cultured Lymphoid Cells (WI-L2) in Different Stages of Cell Growth

Cells/ml ($\times 10^6$)	Cell growth stage	AD_{50} units[a]		Protein (mg/10^9 cells)	ID_{50} units[b]		HL-A2[c] specificity ratio	Recovery (%)[d]	
		HL-A2	HL-A5		HL-A2	HL-A5		HL-A2	HL-A5
0.80	Early log	2.0×10^6	1.1×10^6	50	2.5×10^5	1.0×10^5	100	12.5	9
1.90	Late log	1.0×10^6	0.6×10^6	20	1.0×10^6	0.5×10^6	190	100	83
2.46	Resting	1.0×10^6	0.6×10^6	20	1.0×10^6	0.5×10^6	200	100	83
1.8[e]	Late resting	6.2×10^5	3.7×10^5	19	3.1×10^4	4.0×10^3	50	5	1

a $AD_{50}/10^9$ cells.

b Number of ID_{50}/mg protein obtained from 10^9 viable cells.

c Ratio between the reciprocal of amount of the soluble antigen inhibiting the indifferent antiserum Cutten (anti-HL-A7) and that required for the inhibition of the homologous antiserum Eriksson (anti-HL-A2).

d Recovery equal to (ID_{50}/AD_{50}) $\times 100$ represents the percent absorbing capacity of cells recovered as soluble antigen.

e In the late resting phase there were 50 percent dead cells, whereas, in all other stages, there was full cell viability.

brane components (20), synthesis of immunoglobulins (3,19), and susceptibility to infection by virus (1) and to oncogenic transformation by chemicals
(2). Alternatively, it may be that the cell membrane possesses the capacity to
repair complement-induced damage at certain intervals during the cell cycle.

The clinical relevance of these *in vitro* findings becomes apparent when we
wish to plan an immunotherapy regimen to combat neoplastic disease, e.g.,
when there is tumor cell growth while circulating antibodies are detected in
a patient's serum. The length of the G_1 phase of the cell cycle varies with the
cell line; such tumor cells as RPMI 8866, with a long G_1 phase, which are thus
less susceptible to lysis, have an increased chance of escaping destructive
activity by antibody and complement. If this is indeed the case *in vivo*, the
efficacy of immunotherapy regimens could be greatly increased by planning that
takes this into account.

Isolation and Characterization of HL-A Antigens

The elucidation of the chemical properties and molecular characteristics of
HL-A antigens solubilized from the surface of lymphoid cells has proved to be
a considerable challenge. Although an array of extraction procedures was developed during the last decade, it is now fairly evident that none of these methods
utilizing detergents, proteases, low-frequency sound or simple salts has been
optimally effective, because they are all quite non-selective, i.e., they solubilize
relatively small amounts of antigen together with vast quantities of contaminants.

Most of the effective methods used to isolate naturally soluble serum proteins
or enzymes proved to be inadequate for solubilizing histocompatibility (H)
antigens, which most likely are embedded in a sea of hydrophobic materials
on the cell membrane, e.g., lipids and complex glycolipids. The above mentioned
procedures have, however, all yielded H-antigenic substances, which, although
varying somewhat in molecular size and charge, were capable of evoking
humoral and/or cellular immune responses characteristic of H or transplantation antigens (for review, see ref. 18).

Finding a source from which to extract soluble HL-A antigens presented a
particular problem, since only small quantities of antigens could be solubilized from spleen cells, peripheral lymphocytes, and platelets. Although
cultured human lymphoid cells yield relatively larger amounts of soluble HL-A
antigens, the amount of cells required ($>10^{10}$ cells) involves a considerable
expense. In addition, only a limited number of HL-A phenotypes are available
from these cultured cell lines. Regardless of these strictures, HL-A antigens
have been isolated from this source, and very small amounts of highly purified
antigens have been partially characterized by biologic and chemical means. Data

116

reported from different laboratories are at variance regarding the molecular size, amino acid and carbohydrate composition, and electrophoretic mobility of these antigens. These differences are most likely due to the vastly different extraction methods employed (for review, see ref. 17). Initially using low-frequency sound and, later, hypertonic salt extraction (3 M KCl) of cultured human lymphoid cells, we were able to isolate highly purified HL-A antigens with a molecular size of ~33,000 lacking neutral carbohydrates detectable at levels greater than 1 percent (17).

Nature has overcome these problems by providing soluble HL-A antigens in serum and in due time, several investigators, including ourselves, discovered this fact (for review, see ref. 9). Consequently, human serum is now being used as an inexpensive, readily available source of H-antigens, extractable without tedious and nonselective procedures.

While screening sera from individuals with known HL-A phenotypes by determining their capacity to inhibit the cytotoxic activity of HL-A alloantisera against selected target cells, it became evident that, in contrast to all other major HL-A specificities, HL-A9 could always be detected, since it seems to be present in substantially larger amounts in serum. However, all major HL-A specificities could be detected in sera following their concentration by salt fractionation with ammonium sulfate at 0.5 and 0.8 saturation. Interestingly enough, all but HL-A9 and 5 specificities precipitated at 0.5 saturation, whereas these two specificities precipitated at 0.8 saturation. While isolating HL-A antigens from the serum of donor C.H. (HL-A3,5,7,9), we achieved additional purification of these salted-out fractions by gel exclusion chromatography on Sephadex G-100, resulting in a 10- to 20-fold increase in specific blocking activity (Table 8-2). Futher purification was achieved by ion exchange chromatography on cellulose phosphate, employing a straight line gradient (0.01 to 0.2 M phosphate buffer, pH 6.0). When fractions enriched in HL-A9 and 5 were used, it was found that they readily eluted at 0.01 M phosphate concen-

Table 8-2   Purification Scheme of HL-A9 Antigen Isolated from Serum

	ID_{50} units/mg[a]	Recovery (%)	Times purification
Whole serum	660	100	
50 to 80 percent ammonium sulfate	1,100	88	2
Sephadex G-100	4,200	78	6
Cellulose phosphate	10,000	60	15
PAGE	50,000	36	75

[a] The reciprocal of the soluble antigen dose that blocks 50 percent of the cytotoxic activity of a specific HL-A alloantiserum.

tration, whereas fractions enriched in HL-A7 eluted at 0.1 M phosphate concentration, which suggested that these molecules have considerable charge differences. Indeed, upon isoelectric focusing, it was apparent that HL-A9 and HL-A7 have different isoelectric points, i.e., pH 5.0 and 5.8, respectively. Finally, after cellulose phosphate chromatography, HL-A9 antigen was purified by semipreparative acrylamide gel electrophoresis at pH 9.6. A single electrophoretic component was resolved under these conditions with a relative electrophoretic mobility of 0.22. When eluted from the gel, this material had excellent antigenic activity, as evaluated in the blocking assay. On the average, overall purification of antigenic activity was about 75-fold, with 36 percent recovery (Table 8-2). In the best case, purification was about 150-fold, with an overall 60 percent recovery of HL-A9 antigenic activity.

From gel exclusion chromatography on Sephadex G-100, the HL-A9 antigen appeared to have a molecular weight over 100,000. Since it was suspected that the hydrophobic antigen was in an aggregated form in the aqueous buffer system, the molecular weight was determined by SDS polyacrylamide gel electrophoresis. The antigen, which appeared as a single component (R_m 0.22) upon analytic polyacrylamide gel electrophoresis at pH 9.6, now completely resolved into a single moiety with a molecular weight of 33,000, without any previous reduction (Fig. 8-3). The same pattern was obtained following prior reduction and carboxamidomethylation in 5 M urea. Like HL-A antigen isolated by 3 M KCl extraction from lymphoid cells, HL-A antigen isolated from serum also has a molecular weight of about 33,000. Similarly, gas chromatographic analyses of the HL-A9 antigen isolated from serum did not reveal any detectable neutral carbohydrates or hexosamines. Thus, it appears that HL-A antigens in serum are quite similar in their physicochemical characteristics to HL-A antigens solubilized from cells by 3 M KCl extraction and subsequently purified by preparative polyacrylamide gel electrophoresis. The HL-A antigens isolated from both sources were shown to be immunologically potent, since they specifically inhibited the cytotoxic activity of HL-A alloantisera. Also, HL-A9 antigen isolated from serum elicited the production of a monospecific, high titer (1:128) HL-A xenoantibody in rabbits, which means that it is indeed immunogenic.

As far as the molecular nature of HL-A antigens is concerned, it appears from our data that each antigenic determinant within a given phenotype of an individual is located on a single polypeptide chain and that these chains are not covalently linked. Furthermore, it seems that these polypeptides have a molecular weight of 33,000, lack carbohydrate, and can be distinguished by charge differences. Polypeptide chains bearing different HL-A determinants most likely will vary in amino acid sequences. On cell surfaces these individual polypeptides, each bearing a single HL-A determinant, are probably linked by hydrophobic bonds, since they are likely to be, at least in part, buried within complex

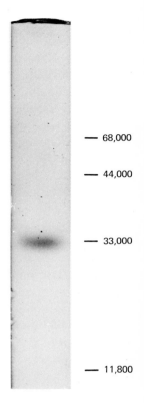

— 68,000

— 44,000

— 33,000

— 11,800

Figure 8-3. SDS-polyacrylamide gel electrophoresis profile of highly purified HL-A9 antigen isolated from serum. Positions of molecular weight markers are indicated on this gel. Protein molecular weight standards used were human serum albumin (68,000), ovalbumin (44,000), bovine carboxypeptidase A (33,000) and cytochrome c (11,800).

hydrophobic lipoprotein lattices. Indeed, if the HL-A genetic model of a set of factors expressed within mutually exclusive segregant series is correct, one might expect the histocompatibility genes to translate their messages in the synthesis of individual polypeptide chains, one each for the segregant series factors of a heterozygous individual.

Only sequence analyses will reveal whether, like immunoglobulin molecules, HL-A antigens contain extensive and sharply divided regions of variability and constancy, with the latter containing amino acid sequence differences attributed to HL-A allotypes. In this case, functional specialization of the molecule independent of the histocompatibility system would be represented in the variable region, where the antibody-combining sites of immunoglobulins are reported to be. On the other hand, single regions of constant amino acid sequence might have only small differences, i.e., point mutations, attributable to HL-A specificity. In this case, there would be no extended variable region on the HL-A molecule. This latter model seems most consistent with present data, since isolated, purified HL-A antigens appear to have minimal heterogeneity as shown by electrophoretic and peptide mapping techniques (17).

R. A. Reisfeld, M. A. Pellegrino, S. Ferrone, and S. Oh

The fact that simple ammonium sulfate fractionation concentrates all major HL-A specificities in serum, to an extent where they can be readily identified by blocking assays, suggests that it may be feasible to utilize human serum for direct HL-A typing. This approach would eliminate the variability constituted by peripheral lymphocyte target cells in the direct microcytotoxic test used for routine HL-A typing. Correlations between HL-A antigens and susceptibility to disease will be simplified, particularly when the disease in question produces structural alterations within the cell membrane and, thus, an abnormal reactivity of the lymphocytes in the cytotoxic test. The availability of soluble, purified HL-A antigens from serum will also make it feasible to develop meaningful radioimmunoassays for their detection in serum. Most important, the availability of purified HL-A antigens isolated from serum will make it possible to (a) follow their quantitative and qualitative changes during the course of neoplastic disease, (b) determine the effect of therapy on the expression of these cell surface markers, and (c) assess whether neoplasia induces any changes in their immunogenicity and molecular structure.

Evaluation of the cell surface expression of HL-A antigens during the cell growth cycle yields information concerning the antigenic constitution of the host which plays a key role in the defense against neoplasia. Since some HL-A antigens have been associated with susceptibility to neoplastic disease, the characterization of these genetically segregating cell surface markers at the cellular and molecular level may provide further insight into the pathogenesis of the neoplastic process.

ACKNOWLEDGMENTS

This is publication number 841. This work was supported by USPHS Grants AI-10180, AI-07007, and CA-16071 from the National Institutes of Health, California Division of the American Cancer Society Senior Fellowship #D221, and Grant 70-615 from the American Heart Association, Inc.

REFERENCES

1. Basilico, C. and Marin, G. Susceptibility of cells in different stages of the mitotic cycle to transformation by polyoma virus. Virology, 28:429, 1966.
2. Bertram, J. S. and Heidelberger, C. Cell cycle dependency of oncogenic transformation induced by N-methyl-N'-nitronitrosoguanidine in culture. Cancer Res., 34:526, 1974.
3. Buell, D. M. and Fahey, J. L. Limited periods of gene expression in immunoglobulin synthesizing cells. Science, 164:1524, 1969.
4. Cikes, M. Relationship between growth rate, cell volume, cell cycle kinetic and antigenic properties of cultured murine lymphoma cells. J. Nat. Cancer Inst., 45:979, 1970.

5. Cikes, M. Expression of surface antigens on cultured tumor cells in relation to cell cycle. Transplant. Proc., 3:1161, 1971.

6. Cooper, N. R., Polley, M. J., and Oldstone, M. B. A. Failure of terminal complement components to induce lysis of Moloney virus transformed lymphocytes. J. Immunol., 112:866, 1974.

7. Ferrone, S., Cooper, N. R., Pellegrino, M. A., and Reisfeld, R. A. The lymphocytotoxic reation: The mechanism of rabbit complement action. J. Immunol., 107:939, 1971.

8. Ferrone, S., Cooper, N. R., Pellegrino, M. A., and Reisfeld, R. A. Interaction of histocompatibility (HL-A) antibodies and complement with synchronized human lymphoid cells in continuous culture. J. Exp. Med., 137:55, 1973.

9. Ferrone, S., Pellegrino, M. A., Dierich, M. P., and Reisfeld, R. A. Expression of histocompatibility antigens during the growth cycle of cultured lymphoid cells. *In* Koprowski, H., ed., Current Topics in Microbiology and Immunology. New York, Springer-Verlag, 1974, Vol. 66, p. 1.

10. Götze, D., Pellegrino, M. A., Ferrone, S., and Reisfeld, R. A. Expression of H-2 antigen, during growth of cultured tumor cells. Immunol. Comm., 1:533, 1972.

11. Karb, K. and Goldstein, G. Combination autoradiography and membrane fluorescence in studying cell cycle transplantation antigen relationship. Transplantation 11:569, 1971.

12. Lerner, R. A., Oldstone, M. B. A., and Cooper, N. R. Cell cycle-dependent immune lysis of Moloney virus-transformed lymphocytes: Presence of viral antigen, accessibility to antibody and complement activation. Proc. Natl. Acad. Sci. USA, 68:2584, 1971.

13. Pellegrino, M. A., Ferrone, S., Natali, P., Pellegrino, A., and Reisfeld, R. A. Expression of HL-A antigens in synchronized cultures of human lymphocytes. J. Immunol., 108:573, 1972.

14. Pellegrino, M. A., Ferrone, S., and Pellegrino, A. A simple microabsorption technique for HL-A typing. Proc. Soc. Exp. Biol. Med., 139:484, 1972.

15. Pellegrino, M. A., Ferrone, S., Pellegrino, A., and Reisfeld, R. A. The expression of HL-A antigens during the growth cycle of cultured human lymphoid cells. Clin. Immunol. Immunopathol., 1:182, 1973.

16. Pellegrino, M. A., Ferrone, S., Cooper, N. R., Dierich, M. P., and Reisfeld, R. A. Variation in susceptibility of a human lymphoid cell line to immune lysis during the cell cycle: Lack of correlation with antigen density and complement binding. J. Exp. Med., 140:578, 1974.

17. Reisfeld, R. A. and Kahan, B. D. The molecular nature of HL-A antigens. *In* Kahan, B. D. and Reisfeld, R. A., eds. Chemical Markers of Biological Individuality: The Transplantation Antigens. New York, Academic Press, 1972, pp. 489–501.

18. Reisfeld, R. A., Ferrone, S., and Pellegrino, M. A. Isolation and serological evaluation of HL-A antigens solubilized from cultured human lymphoid cells. *In* Korn, E. D., ed. Methods in Membrane Biology. New York, Plenum Press, 1974, Vol. 1, pp. 143–92.

19. Takahashi, M., Yagi, Y., Morre, G. E., and Pressman, D. Immunoglobulin production in synchronized cultures of human hematopoietic cell lines. J. Immunol., 103:834, 1969.

20. Warren, L. and Glick, M. D. Membranes of animal cells. II. The metabolism and turnover of the surface membrane. J. Cell. Biol., 37:729, 1968.

9

Inhibitory Action of Poly A:Poly U on Tumor Growth: Enhancement of Host Immune Response?

F. Lacour, G. Delage, E. Fenster, and J. Harel

Introduction

The relationship between immunity and malignancy is well documented in studies on experimental animals. The study of this relationship in humans is now an area of rapid development. It is known that serious congenital deficiencies of the immune system are usually associated with an abnormally high incidence of neoplastic disease, particularly of the lymphoid system. In addition, there has been much concern recently regarding the undue incidence of such conditions in recipients of transplanted organs who are subjected to prolonged immunosuppressive therapy. Another interesting relationship between immunity and malignancy is revealed in studies of aging. With aging, in animals and in man, there is a decline in cellular immunity. More studies to extend and evaluate these quantitative relationships seem warranted in light of the frequent occurrence of certain forms of malignancy with age (8). Also it is already known that cancer patients show a sharply diminished capacity to reject grafts of human skin or other human cultured cells (18). It is not clear whether this low reactivity in part precedes the appearance of cancer or is wholly a manifestation of processes related to the malignancy.

A working hypothesis which, in principle, is susceptible to experimental verification, is that appropriate immunologic stimulation would improve the success of the conventional treatment of operable cancers. Positive experimental results would provide a basis for their application at the clinical level. Also, immunologic stimulation prior to the appearance of a tumor could lead to partial prophylaxis against neoplasia.

Unless unexpected new developments arise, we cannot currently foresee, with any degree of assurance, that specific immune stimulation with tumor antigens will correct the immunodeficiencies of the cancer patient. We have focused our attention, therefore, on procedures that might modify host responsiveness by nonspecific stimulation of antigenic responses in general. Such an approach is no longer unique, and there is a large body of data in the literature

Fundamental Aspects of Neoplasia,
edited by A. Arthur Gottlieb, Otto J. Plescia, and David H. L. Bishop.
© 1975 by Springer-Verlag New York Inc.

that nonspecific stimulators of the immune response (generally bacterial products) increase host resistance to transplantable or autochtonous tumors. In occasional experiments, these substances caused increased tumor growth rather than increased host resistance. When it was discovered that double-stranded polynucleotides could stimulate immunologic responses (1), studies were initiated both to define the various parameters of the immune response system and to determine the capacity of the host to develop increased resistance to tumors.

It was shown that antibody formation and cellular immunity can be stimulated by poly A:poly U. Red blood cells, bovine gamma globulin (BGG), synthetic polypeptides, keyhole limpet hemocyanin, ferritin, and viruses have been successfully employed in tests of the stimulatory effect of synthetic polynucleotide complexes on antibody formation.

Shortening of the induction period of antibody formation by the injection of poly A:poly U, together with a single injection of the immunogen BGG, has also been shown and both 19 S and 7 S antibody levels were found to increase. A dramatic effect of poly A:poly U in rendering minute amounts of BGG immunogenic has been described (10). These findings suggest the potential practical value of utilizing polynucleotides as adjuvants when employing immunogens that are weakly antigenic, such as autochtonous tumors or auto-antigens.

The polynucleotide duplex also acts on newborn mice to provoke high levels of antibody production. Poly A:poly U not only enhances antibody formation in normally responding animals, but it can act in genetically low responding strains to restore normal levels of antibody production. In addition, poly A:poly U has been shown to restore responsiveness in aging C57 mice which normally display impaired antibody responses (2).

The stimulatory effect of poly A:poly U on the cell-mediated immune response is evident in the shortening of the induction period of delayed hypersensitivity to tuberculin in guinea pigs (2), in the hastening of the immune process involved in graft rejection in mice and in the adjuvant effect on mixed leukocyte interactions. Finally, the complex has been used to improve markedly the capacity of neonatally thymectomized mice to respond to skin homografts (10).

The basic mechanism of the effect of double-stranded polynucleotides on the immune response is still not understood. It has been suggested, however, that polynucleotides act on systems that utilize cAMP as an intermediary, either by magnifying membrane signals or, possibly, by furnishing, through their derivatives, appropriate precursors for cyclic nucleoside monophosphates (2).

The capability of poly A:poly U to affect the growth of animal tumors and to prevent the occurrence of spontaneous tumors was therefore investigated by us. Poly A:poly U is a well-defined substance that offers the possibility of a molecular and pharmacologic approach. In these studies we were able to demonstrate cell penetration and localization of poly A:poly U and the effects of this compound on nucleic acid biosynthesis in human lymphocytes.

Effect of Poly A:Poly U on Tumor Growth in Normal Animals and in Animals Following Tumor Excision

The lack of toxicity of poly A:poly U was the reason for using it in our studies. Stimulation of immunologic responses can be induced by two different synthetic polynucleotide duplexes, namely, poly I:poly C and poly A:poly U, but the former was reported to be toxic by several authors. Pharmacologic studies of poly A:poly U in our laboratory showed that 250 mg/kg injected intraperitoneally into mice in a single dose, or in five successive daily doses of 50 mg/kg/day is not toxic and no fatalities occurred. In the study by Philips et al. (14), a single injection of 100 mg/kg of poly I:poly C was lethal for mice and fatalities were observed between 9 and 20 hr following injection. Moreover, in the latter study, rabbits proved to be the most susceptible to the lethal action of poly I:poly C and the median lethal intravenous dose was 0.1 to 0.3 mg/kg/day. In contrast, neither fatalities nor pyrogenicity was found in our experiments upon injecting 2 mg/kg intravenously into six rabbits, each of which was observed for a period of 2 months. The difference in the configurations of the two double-stranded complexes may explain the difference in their toxicities.

We chose spontaneous mammary carcinoma in C3H/He mice for a study of the effect of poly A:poly U on tumor growth since it can be correlated with a human cancer. A transplantable melanoma of the hamster, which metastasizes to the lymph nodes in 96 percent of the tumor-bearing animals, was used to study the action of poly A:poly U on metastases. A murine leukemia, in ascitic form, was also used in our experiments.

The effects of poly A:poly U on spontaneous mammary carcinoma of mice are shown in Table 9-1. The mean survival time of animals treated with poly A:poly U alone was not appreciably different from that of the controls, but it was significantly increased (31 percent) by surgery alone. But the best results were obtained by combining surgery with poly A:poly U treatment. The mean survival time in this combined group was strikingly increased (69 percent) as compared with the controls, and it was 29 percent greater than the surgery group. Also, the incidence of detectable metastases was lower in mice treated by surgery + poly A:poly U than in the other groups, but the number of cases involved was too small to make this difference significant.

In hamsters bearing a transplantable melanoma, local cures were obtained

Table 9-1   Effect of Poly A:Poly U on the Survival of Mice Bearing Spontaneous Mammary Carcinoma or Mice from Which the Tumor Was Surgically Removed[a]

Groups	Number of mice	Metastases		Mean survival time after onset of tumor (days)
		Number	Percent	
1. Controls	41	13	32	78
2. Poly A:U[b]	33	14	42	83
3. Surgery[c]	25	8	32	102[d]
4. Surgery + Poly A:U[b]	23	5	22	132[e]

[a] Lacour et al., ref. 11.
[b] Poly A:poly U (250 μg) was given intravenously once a week for 6 weeks.
[c] A simple mastectomy was performed under aseptic conditions.
[d] Surgery vs. controls, $p < 0.02$, calculated by Student's t test.
[e] Surgery + poly A:poly U vs. surgery alone, $p < 0.02$.

by surgery. The survival time increased when poly A:poly U was used with surgery (Table 9-2), but metastases were observed in all three groups. But, in clinical observations we noticed that metastases occurred later in group 3 than in the other two groups. This observation was confirmed in another experiment. In this experiment, 72 hamsters were inoculated intradermally with 10^5 viable tumor cells. When palpable tumors, 4 to 6 mm in diameter, appeared, the hamsters were randomized into three groups: group 1, control; group 2, surgery; group 3, surgery and poly A:poly U. Starting on day 9 after surgery, and every other day until day 19, four hamsters from each group were sacrificed, and histologic examinations of the axillary and inguinal lymph nodes were systematically performed. One-half as many metastases were found in hamsters

Table 9-2   Effect of Poly A:Poly U Treatment on the Survival of Surgically Treated Hamsters Bearing T 1196 Transpantable Melanomas[a]

Groups	Number of hamsters	Mean survival time (days)
I Control[b]	10	51.6
II Surgery[c]	10	70.9
III Surgery + poly A:poly U[d]	10	79.9

[a] From Lacour et al., ref. 11.
[b] Randomized golden Syrian hamsters were inoculated intradermally with 10^5 viable tumor cells.
[c] The animals were anesthetized, and all grossly detectable tumor and surrounding tissue was excised.
[d] Following surgery, 200 μg poly A:poly U was given intraperitoneally on alternate days for 2 weeks.

treated by surgery + poly A:poly U, compared with the other groups, the difference being highly significant ($p < 0.01$) and, in addition, the appearance of metastases was delayed (Table 9-3) (10).

No inhibitory effect of poly A:poly U was observed on the growth of leukemia ascites cells L 4946. Twenty Swiss mice inoculated intraperitoneally with 4×10^5 cells, were separated at random into two groups. Intravenous poly A:poly U was administered, 250 μg every 3 days, to 10 mice. The second group served as a control. The mean survival time was 22 days in the control group, and 2 days longer in the experimental group. This difference is not statistically significant.

It is important that there was no evidence of hematologic or systemic toxicity either in the mice or in the hamsters treated with poly A:poly U. In addition, no early deaths were observed in the animals treated by surgery and poly A:poly U.

Thus, in mice bearing spontaneous mammary adenocarcinoma, treatment with the double-stranded polynucleotide complex poly A:poly U was a potent adjunct to surgery in that it reduced the rate of tumor growth and increased the mean survival time significantly. In hamsters bearing a highly metastatic transplantable melanoma, poly A:poly U reduced the appearance of early metastases by 50 percent, as compared with untreated animals or animals treated by surgery alone.

Table 9-3   Effect of Poly A:Poly U Treatment, as a Supplement to Surgery, on Appearance and Incidence of Metastases in Hamsters Inoculated with T 1196 Transplantable Melanoma[a]

	Number of animals with metastases		Number of animals sacrificed
Days following treatment	Controls	Surgery	Surgery + poly A:poly U[b]
9	2/4	4/4	1/4
11	2/4	3/4	1/4
13	3/4	2/4	2/4
15	4/4	4/4	2/4
17	4/4	3/4	3/4
19	4/4	4/4	1/4
Totals	19/24	20/24	10/24[c]

[a] From Lacour et al., ref. 11.

[b] 200 μg poly A:poly U was given intraperitoneally on alternate days until the hamsters were sacrificed.

[c] $p < 0.01$.

F. Lacour, G. Delage, E. Fenster, and J. Harel

Reduced Incidence of Spontaneous Mammary Tumors in C3H/He Mice Following Prophylactic Treatment with Poly A:Poly U

Mammary tumors that appear in mature C3H/He female mice represent a viral (MTV) infection occurring at birth. The RNA MTV virus is transmitted by the mother through the milk, and this infection leads to high tumor incidence in mature female. It is now known that, despite this neonatal infection, the C3H mouse can respond immunologically to MTV. Also, the inoculation of MTV, together with complete Freund's adjuvant, into neonatally infected mice enhances mammary tumor development (9). This suggests the existence of some "underground" immunity to MTV, both at the cellular and the humoral level, in these mice. Mammary carcinoma in mice today appears as a system that can serve as a tool for many investigators, despite, or perhaps because of, the very great complexity of interacting host and tumor factors.

Since the double-stranded synthetic polyribonucleotide complex poly A:poly U acts on newborn mice to produce high levels of antibody at a time when such a response is normally very weak, we administered this complex in the neonatal period to see if we could reduce tumor incidence later in life. Newborn C3H/He females received three intraperitoneal injections of 15 μg of poly A:poly U on days 1, 3, and 5 after birth. The mice were weaned 3 weeks later. To avoid any possible change in the hormonal milieu necessary for development, the females were caged with males. They were maintained on a diet of pellets and tap water, and, once a week, they received carrots and lettuce. A control group of untreated mice was kept under the same conditions.

The animals in both groups were observed for 380 days, and autopsies were performed on all the mice that died. The nature of the tumors found were confirmed by histologic examination. During this 380-day experimental period, 80 of the 127 control mice, or 63 percent, developed mammary tumors. Among the animals in the group that had received neonatal injections of poly A:poly U, 35 of the 83 treated mice, or 42 percent, developed tumors in that same time period. The difference of 21 percent in tumor incidence between the experimental and control groups is statistically very significant, with a chi square between 0.01 and 0.001 (Table 9-4).

Not all the animals survived the full experimental period; but all tumors were recorded and have been included in the calculations. In the treated group, there were 61 death before the end of the experiment. Of these animals, 30 had mammary tumors, and 31 were free of tumors. Some of the latter had died from obvious extraneous infections. The 22 surviving mice at day 380 were sacrificed, and, upon autopsy, five were found to bear tumors. The remaining 17 were tumor free.

128

Table 9-4   Analysis of Autopsy Observations of C3H/He Mice During a
380-Day Experimental Period

Observations	Number of mice	Tumor bearing mice	Non tumor–bearing mice
Controls			
Deaths	84	55	29
Survivors	43	25	18
Total	127	80	47
Poly A:Poly U-treated			
Deaths	61	30	31
Survivors	22	5	17
Total	83	35	48

In the control group, 84 of the mice died before the 380th day; of these, 55 had mammary tumors and the remaining 29 died from unrelated causes. Among the surviving 43 mice, 25 were found to bear tumors at autopsy, and 18 were tumor free. The tumor-free mortality rates in the two groups, treated and control, were not significantly different.

The tumor incidence among the animals surviving 380 days is seen to be 58 percent in the control group and 23 percent in the treated group, a significant difference with a chi square of less than 0.01. From these experiments, then, it can be concluded that a significant reduction in the occurrence of mammary tumors was obtained when poly A:poly U was given newborn C3H/He female mice.

Nuclear Penetration and Stimulation of Nucleic Acid Synthesis in Mammalian Cells by Poly A:Poly U

Nonspecific stimulation, by double-stranded synthetic polyribonucleotides, of resistance to autochtonous or transplantable tumors can most profitably be discussed and explored within the framework of the immunologic response. There are, however, other factors that may be partly or perhaps completely responsible for the anti-tumor effects of such complexes. Moreover, the mechanism of the stimulatory effect of poly A:poly U on humoral antibody formation and on cell-mediated immune response is not well understood. It was, therefore, of interest to study the early cellular events following treatment with poly A:poly U.

We can show the uptake of poly A:poly U by mouse ascites tumor cells and human lymphocytes in culture. We can also show that a large proportion of the incorporated double-stranded complex rapidly migrates into the cell nucleus, and it remains essentially intact for at least 2 hr. In addition, an early stimulation of both DNA and RNA synthesis is observed in human lymphocytes.

Experiments were performed with normal human lymphocytes, LHN 13, obtained from C. Rosenfeld (15) and maintained in suspension cultures in RPMI 1640 medium, or with FLS cells, an ascitic tumor removed 6 to 8 days after passage in Swiss mice. Poly A and poly U were synthesized with polynucleotide phosphorylase from the nucleoside diphosphates [³H]UDP, [¹⁴C]UDP, or [¹⁴C]ADP (The Radiochemical Center, Amersham) by A. M. Michelson, and each was mixed in an equimolar ratio with the non-radioactive complementary polymer. The activity of poly-[¹⁴C]A:poly U was 97,000 cpm/μg; of poly A:poly-[¹⁴C]U, 399,000 cpm/μg, and of poly A:[³H]poly U, 60,000 cpm/μg.

Figure 9-1 shows a typical radioautograph of an FLS cell exposed to poly A:poly-[³H]U for 30 min. Most of the grains appear in the nucleus. From Table 9-5, it can be seen that a small amount of polymer is taken up by both FLS and LHN 13 cells; the distribution in the cytoplasm and nuclei of acid-soluble and acid-precipitable materials is shown. We tested DEAE dextran for its ability to facilitate cell penetration of poly A:poly U, and, indeed, a very large apparent increase was found (Table 9-6). But the greater part of this facilitation represented adsorbed polymer, which could be removed by brief incubation of the cells in 100 to 200 μg dextran sulfate, but the other portion remained with the nuclear fraction after cell washing and removal of the cytoplasm. FLS cells, exposed to DEAE dextran, and washed and incubated for 2 min at room temperature with poly-[¹⁴C]A:poly U, retained 7,660 cpm after two TBS washes. Treatment with dextran sulfate removed all but 109 cpm. Finally, the effect of DEAE dextran, including subsequent dextran sulfate

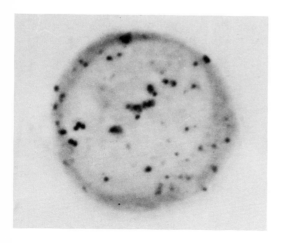

Figure 9-1. Radioautography of incorporated poly A:poly-[³H]U. Cells were exposed to poly A:poly-[³H]U in Eagle's medium for 30 min, washed, and resuspended in a drop of calf's serum; they were then spread on slides, fixed for 5 min with methanol, and coated with Ilford K2 emulsion. After a 15-day exposure, radioautographs were developed and stained with Giemsa.

Table 9-5   Penetration of Poly A:Poly U into Cells

Cells were washed with Eagle's medium, and resuspended in Eagle, incubated for 30 min with labeled poly A:poly U.FLS cells: 2 μg/ml, 2×10^5 cpm of poly-[^{14}]A:poly U, 5×10^6 cells/ml, 6 ml; LHN 13 cells: 0.46 μg/ml, 1.67×10^5 cpm of poly A:poly-[^{14}C]U, 8×10^6 cells/ml, 5 ml. The cells were then washed twice with TBS buffer, resuspended in cold TBS sucrose (0.2 M) containing 0.2 percent Nonidet p40, allowed to stand for 5 min in an ice bath; nuclei were then pelleted by low speed centrifugation. The nuclei were washed with TBS sucrose and resuspended at room temperature in 0.7 ml TBS sucrose, 0.2 ml (200 μg) DNase and 0.1 ml of 1 percent SDS. Lysis was rapid, and the preparation was incubated for 10 min at 37°C. An additional 0.2 ml of SDS was then usually added to assure complete lysis. (AS) acid-soluble; (AP) acid-precipitable.

	Cytoplasm		Nuclei	
Cell type	AS (cpm)	AP (cpm)[a]	AS (cpm)	AP (cpm)[a]
FLS	2,906	1,015 (0.0040)	224	878 (0.0035)
LHN 13	12,032	8,168 (0.0049)	16,079	18,563 (0.0097)

[a] The number in parentheses indicate the quantity of AP poly A:poly U incorporated in 10^7 cells (μg).

incubation, was to increase poly A:poly U penetration into nuclei about 20-fold (Table 9-6, II), after 30-min incubation.

The state of poly A:poly U in LHN 13 cells was determined by centrifugation of the nuclear lysate on a sucrose gradient. The cells were preincubated in DEAE dextran, and, after penetration of poly A:poly U, treated with dextran sulfate. Figure 9-2 shows that two controls, poly A:poly U alone (2a) and poly A:poly U added to a nuclear lysate (2b), and the poly A:poly U that had

Table 9-6   Effect of DEAE Dextran on Poly A:Poly U Penetration of FLS Cells

Cells were exposed to 50 μg/ml of DEAE dextran for 10 min. at room temperature and then washed. After poly A:poly U penetration, the cells were incubated for 5 min in 200 μg/ml dextran sulfate and then treated as indicated in the legend of Table 9-1.

Experiment[a]	DEAE dextran	Dextran sulfate	Nuclear AP material (μg/10^7 cells)
I	−	−	0.015
	+	−	5.23
II	+	+	0.34

[a] I: 22 μg/ml of poly-[^{14}C]A:poly U; II: 10 μg/ml of poly-[^{14}C]A:poly U. Nonradioactive polymer was added to achieve these concentrations. Cell concentrations was 10^7/ml.

penetrated into the nuclei (2c), all appear in the same position in the gradient. A gradient of a lysate prepared from cells exposed to poly A:poly U, treated with dextran sulfate after removal of the polymer and incubated an additional 2 hr shows that the peak is stable, although there is some increase in amount of lower molecular weight material (2d). Poly U is lighter than poly A:poly U (2e), and it is degraded in the presence of a nuclear lysate (2f). We conclude from these data that the material recovered from nuclei is double stranded. In LHN 13 cells pretreated with DEAE dextran, DNA and RNA synthesis increased shortly after poly A:poly U was added (Fig. 9-3). Similar results were obtained in three separate experiments.

In conclusion, our results show the rapid penetration of poly A:poly U into cell nuclei. Most of the poly A:poly U remains intact in the nuclei, for at least 2½ hr from the time the polymer complexes were added.

Discussion

Certain complexes of multi-stranded synthetic polynucleotides possess two different activities: induction of interferon (7) and stimulation of immunologic reactions. Consequently, there have been numerous attempts to determine whether such polynucleotides had any effect on neoplasia. Two double-stranded complexes of synthetic polynucleotides have been used: poly I:poly C and poly A:poly U. Poly I:poly C was initially employed because of its effectiveness in inducing interferon. Repeated injections of poly I:poly C have protected animals from virus- and chemically induced, transplantable syngeneic tumors and have prevented induction of leukemia or tumors by viruses (13,16). It has been clearly established, however, that the anti-tumor effect is not correlated

Figure 9-2. Density gradient centrifugation of poly A:poly U. The nuclear lysate was diluted with an equal volume of TBS layered on a 5 to 20 percent sucrose gradient (in TBS) and centrifuged for 18 hr at 23,000 rpm in an SW 25.1 rotor at 15°. One-milliliter fractions were counted in Aquasol (New England Nuclear). (A) Poly A:poly-[^{14}C]U alone; (B) poly A:poly-[^{14}C]U added to the nuclear lysate prepared from 10^7 LHN 13 cells; (C) poly A:poly-[^{14}C]U in the nuclear lysate obtained from 2×10^7 LHN 13 cells after 30-min penetration. The polymer concentration was 4.3 μg/ml. (D) LHN 13 cells (5×10^6/ml) were incubated for 40 min in 2.14 μg/ml poly A:poly-[^{14}C]U, washed, treated with dextran sulfate, rewashed, and resuspended in Eagle's medium for an additional 2 hr. Thirty minutes were consumed by the several centrifugations, giving a total time of 2½ hrs. (E) poly-[^{14}C]U; (F) poly-[^{14}C]U after a 10-min incubation at 37° with a nuclear lysate.

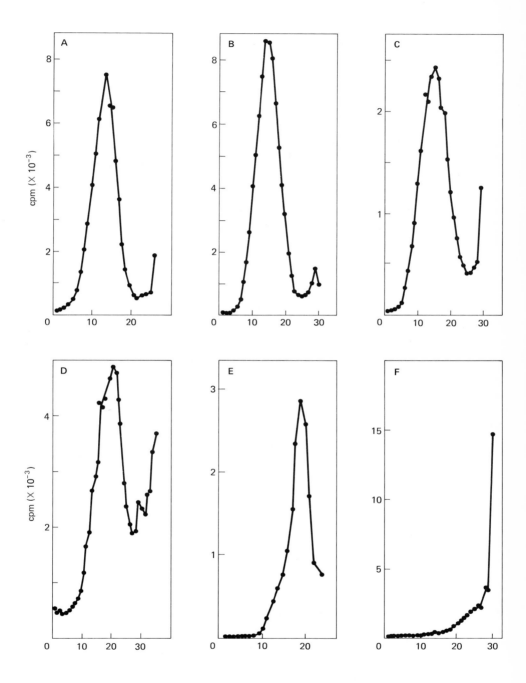

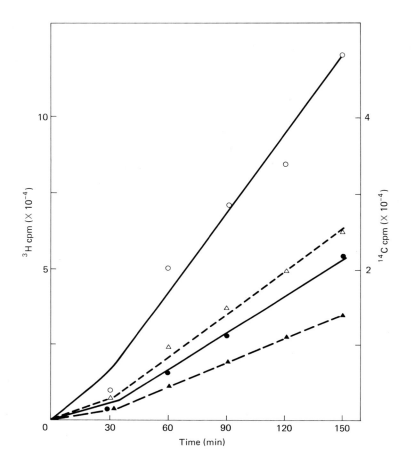

Figure 9-3. Nucleic acids synthesis. LNH 13 cells were washed with Eagle's medium, treated for 10 min with DEAE dextran, and resuspended at 1.2×10⁶ cells/ml with or without 100 μg/ml poly A:poly U, [³H] hymidine (3.5 μCl/ml) and [¹⁴C]Uridine (0.44 μCi/ml) were added to each sample. Cells were incubated at 37°C, and incorporation into acid-preciptable material was followed: (———) thymidine incorporation, (----) uridine incorporation (●,▲) no poly A:poly U, (○, △) with poly A:poly U.

with poly I:poly C-induced circulating interferon (21). In addition to its protective effects, poly I:poly C has shown such deleterious characteristics as toxicity, especially in rabbits and mice, and pyrogenicity, in rabbits. The non-toxic poly A:poly U is a poor inducer of interferon, but it has been utilized as a nonspecific stimulator of the immune system.

An important feature of the tumor rejection system is its inability to deal with more than a relatively small number of tumor cells. Although the described experimental results indicate that the polyribonucleotide duplex poly A:poly U has a definite inhibitory effect on tumor progression, this effect was observed only after surgical removal of the tumor. No effect was noted in the absence of surgical treatment, probably because of the presence of large numbers of tumor cells. The inhibitory effect was observed on a spontaneous mammary carcinoma of mice, as well as on a transplantable hamster melanoma after tumor removal. The conspicuous delay in the recurrence of virus-induced mammary tumors in mice is probably not due to some virus-mediated mechanism, triggered by poly A:poly U, since a similar effect was obtained with the hamster melanoma, which thus far is not known to contain any infectious oncogenic virus. From experiments with this latter tumor, the effect of poly A:poly U on metastases was clearly shown.

The benefit from surgery complemented by poly A:poly U administration may be due to a decrease in tumor cells, i.e., a decrease of the remaining tumor antigen and/or augmentation of the activity of antigen-reactive cells.

The benefit could also be due to a shortening of the immunologic eclipse period (12) and a stimulation of the immunologic reactivity of the host following the surgical removal of the tumor, but, a direct action of this complex on the tumor cells cannot be excluded.

With the same complex, Braun et al. reported a decrease in the recurrence of transplantable syngeneic tumors in mice in which the primary tumor had first been removed by surgery (3). This complex, injected with theophylline into BALB/C mice, also retards the rate of intradermal growth of ascites tumor cells induced by Rausher leukemia virus. Retardation of tumor development occurred particularly during the early period of tumor growth. Since the anti-tumor effect was also observed in irradiated mice, the hypothesis that a substantial part of the antitumor activity of these agents could be due to direct effects on the tumor cells was advanced (20).

A significant diminution of the incidence of spontaneous mammary tumors was observed when poly A:poly U was injected in C3H/He newborn female mice. The mechanism of this prophylactic effect has not yet been elucidated. It was shown that exogenous interferon given early in life can delay mammary tumor development. It should be noted, however, that in experiments utilizing large doses of exogenous interferon, the results indicated only a delay in the onset of the tumors rather than a reduction in tumor frequency (4). Even though poly A:poly U is known to be a poor inducer of interferon, we cannot exclude the possibility that a low dose of interferon was responsible for the observed reduction in mammary tumor incidence. On the other hand, evidence is now available that C3H can respond immunologically to MTV. It is tempting to speculate that poly A:poly U induced a nonspecific stimulation of the anti-

MTV immune response of the host. (Recently, Drake *et al.* (56) reported that poly A:poly U strikingly prolonged long-term survival in AKR mice.)

Since poly A:poly U is thought to stimulate immune response, and since we have demonstrated its inhibitory action on tumor growth, it was recognized that a study of the early cellular events following its uptake might cast some light on the biologic mechanisms involved. Thus far, there have been no extensive studies in this area.

The uptake of poly A:poly U has been demonstrated by Shell (17) in Ehrlich ascites tumor cells. We confirmed the entry of poly A:poly U into the cell by radioautography and showed that acid-precipitable material is found in both the cytoplasm and the nucleus.

In these experiments, we took advantage of the DEAE dextran facilitation of poly A:poly U uptake and re-isolated the polymer from nuclei, to show that it occurs as a symmetric peak at the same position as control poly A:poly U in sucrose gradients. Poly U is significantly lighter than poly A:poly U and is degraded by a nuclear lysate. This argues against both strand separation of penetrated poly A:poly U as well as its degradation and reincorporation into cellular RNA. Furthermore, the greater part of poly A:poly U incorporated into nuclei is not destroyed for at least 2½ hr.

Chess *et al.* (5) measured the ability of poly A:poly U to stimulate DNA synthesis in leukocytes and found that poly A:poly U alone gave variable results, but that, in combination with an antigenic stimulant, it uniformly increased thymidine incorporation. In no case, however, did they report any effect before the 4th day of incubation of the cells with poly A:poly U.

Teng *et al.* (19), on the other hand, found that poly A:poly U depressed DNA synthesis in HeLa cells to 60 percent of normal after just 4 hr of contact, but only when these cells were in late G_1 or S phase. We report here that lymphocytes, treated with DEAE dextran, show increased DNA and RNA synthesis shortly after the addition of poly A:poly U.

We cannot say whether this represents an effect on the synthetic process or whether it results from the increased permeability of nucleosides in the presence of poly A:poly U. Although we have no direct evidence, it is still possible that this early increase in nucleic acid synthesis is related to immune stimulation by poly A:poly U. This possibility is not unlikely, since antigenic stimulation of immunocompetent cells has a similar effect on the biosynthesis of nucleic acids. The inhibitory action on tumor growth could be related to polyA:poly U-induced stimulation of the immune response in treated animals. It is not excluded, however, that the elicited cellular reactions are nonspecific, and there may be a variety of cellular functions triggered, which subsequently affect tumor growth.

Further work is needed to decide whether the poly A:poly U possesses antitumor activity because it is a mediator of the immune response, or whether more direct effects, either on the malignant cells or on such causative agents as the oncogenic viruses, account for this activity.

REFERENCES

1. Braun, W. and Nakano, M. Stimulation of polyadenylic and polycytidylic acids. Science, 157:819, 1967.

2. Braun, W., Ishizuka, M., Yajima, Y., Webb, D., and Winchurch, R. Spectrum and mode of action of poly A:U in the stimulation of immune responses. *In* Beer, R. F., and Braun, W., Ed. Biological Effect of Polynucleotides. New York, Springer-Verlag, 1971, pp. 138–56.

3. Braun, W., Plescia, O. J., Rascova, J., and Webb, D. Basic proteins and synthetic polynucleotides as modifiers of immunogenicity of syngeneic tumor cells. Israel J. Med. Sci., 7:72, 1971.

4. Came, E. and Moore, D. H. Effect of exogenous interferon treatment on mouse mammary tumors. J. Natl. Cancer Inst., 48:1151, 1972.

5. Chess, L., Levy, C., Schmukler, M., Schmidt, K., and Mardiney, Jr., M. R. The effect of synthetic polynucleotides in immunologically induced tritiated thymidine incorporation. Transplantation, 14:748, 1972.

6. Drake, W. P., Cimino, E. F., Mardiney, M. R., and Sutherland, J. C., Prophylactic therapy of spontaneous leukemia in AKR mice by polyadenylic-polyuridylic acid. J. Natl. Cancer Inst., 52:941, 1974.

7. Field, A. K., Tytell, A. A., Lampson, G. P., and Hilleman, M. R. Inducers of interferon and host resistance II. Multistranded synthetic polynucleotides complexes. Proc. Natl. Acad. Sci. USA, 58:1004, 1967.

8. Good, R. A. Relations between immunity and malignancy. Proc. Natl. Acad. Sci. USA, 69: 1026, 1972.

9. Hilgers, J. O., Daams, J. H., and Bentvelzen, P. The induction of precipitating antibodies to the mammary tumor virus in several inbred mouse strains. Israel J. Med. Sci., 7:154, 1971.

10. Johnson, A. G., Cone, R. E., Friedman, H. M., Han, J. H., Johnson, R. J., and Stout, R. D. Stimulation of the immune system by homopolyribonucleotides. *In* Beer, R. F. and Braun, W., eds. Biological Effect of Polynucleotides. New York, Springer-Verlag, 1971, pp. 157–177.

11. Lacour, F., Spira, A., Lacour, J., and Prade, M. Polyadenylic-polyuridylic acid, an adjunct to surgery in the treatment of spontaneous mammary tumors in C3H/He mice and transplantable melanoma in the hamster. Cancer Res., 32:648, 1972.

12. Le Francois, D., Youn, K. J., Belehradek, J., and Barski, G. Evolution of cell mediated immunity in mice produced by a mammary carcinoma line. Influence of tumor growth, surgical removal and treatment with irradiated tumor cells. J. Natl. Cancer Inst., 46:981, 1971.

13. Levy, H. B., Adamson, R., Carbone, P., Devila, V., Gazdar, A., Rhim, J., Weinstein, A., and Riley, F. Studies on the antitumor action of poly I:poly C. *In* Beer, R. F. and

Braun, W., Eds. Biological Effect of Polynucleotides. New York, Springer-Verlag, 1971, pp. 55–65.

14. Philips, F. S., Fleisher, M., Hamilton, L. D., Schwartz, M. C., and Stenberg, S. S. Polyinosinic.polycytidylic acid toxicity. *In* Beer, R. F. and Braun, W., eds. Biological Effect of Polynucleotides, New York, Springer-Verlag, 1971, pp. 259–273.

15. Rosenfeld, C., Macieira-Coelho, A., Vemuat, A. M., Jasmin, C., and Trian, T. Q. Kinetics of the establishment of human peripheral blood cultures. J. Natl. Inst., 43:58, 1969.

16. Sarma, P. S., Shiu, G., Neubauer, R. H., Baron, S., and Huebner, R. J. Virus induced sarcoma of mice. Inhibition by a synthetic polyribonuclectide complex. Proc. Natl. Acad. Sci. USA, 62:1046, 1969.

17. Schell, P. L. Uptake of polynucleotides by intact mammalian cells. VIII. Synthetic homoribopolynucleotides. Biochem. Biophys. Acta, 240:472, 1971.

18. Southam, C. M., Moore, A. E., and Rhoads, C. P. Homotransplantation of human cell lines. Science, 125:158, 1957.

19. Teng, C., Chen, M. C., and Hamilton, L. D. Poly (inosinic acid) poly (cytidylic acid) inhibition of DNA synthesis in synchronized HeLa cells. Proc. Natl. Acad. Sci. USA, 70:3904, 1973.

20. Webb, D., Braun, W., and Plescia, O. J. Antitumor effects of polynucleotides and theophylline. Cancer Res., 32:1814, 1972.

21. Weinstein, A. J., Gazdar, A. F., Sims, H. L., and Levy, H. B. Lack of correlation between interferon induction and antitumor effect of poly I:poly C. Nature [New Biol.], 231:53, 1971.

10

The Problem of Cancer Immunotherapy in Perspective

O. J. Plescia, A. Smith, K. Grinwich, and C. Feit

Introduction

The basic premises underlying cancer immunotherapy are (a) that cancer cells possess cancer-specific transplantation-like antigens, and (b) that their host is capable of mounting an immune response to these antigens that results in the rejection of the cancer cells as a homograft.

Heretofore, emphasis has been on the cancer-specific antigens, the objectives being first to establish their existence and second to use them effectively as immunogens in inducing cancer immunity. The first objective has been reasonably achieved, but effective cancer vaccines have proved elusive (4). The problems seem to be (a) how to isolate and purify cancer-specific antigens, (b) how best to modify them to increase their immunogenicity, and (c) how best to administer them to induce a state of immunity rather than enhancement of tumor growth. Our approach to circumventing these problems has been to avoid the isolation step and, rather, to attenuate and modify tumor cells by biochemical means, using such altered cells directly as sources of functional specific antigens (6).

Preparing cancer-specific antigens is only the first step in cancer immunotherapy. Other obstacles must be overcome, inasmuch as cancer vaccines to date have not proved effective. Possible reasons for the apparent failure of cancer vaccines are listed in Table 10-1. In general, failure might be due to deficiencies in or peculiarities of the antigens, on the one hand, and to inadequacy of the host, on the other hand.

Recently the question of immunologic competence of the host has become paramount because of the consensus that immune surveillance is a major deterrent in cancer development. There are two possibilities that could account for the apparent inadequacy of the immune system of a cancer-bearing host. The host might be immunodeficient, as a result of genetic or environmental factors, prior to development of the cancer, or the cancer cells might themselves be immunosuppressive and, thus, subvert the immune system. In either case, the net result would be immunodeficiency on the part of the host, resulting

Fundamental Aspects of Neoplasia,
edited by A. Arthur Gottlieb, Otto J. Plescia, and David H. L. Bishop.
© 1975 by Springer-Verlag New York Inc.

Table 10-1   Possible Reasons for Failure of Immune Surveillance System against Cancer

I. Properties of Tumor Antigens
    A.   Antigens are weak and poorly immunogenic
    B.   Antigens are sheltered from immunocompetent cells of the host because of the location of the tumor
    C.   Antigens induce specific unresponsiveness depending on the concentration and distribution of the antigens
    D.   Antigens induce specific blocking factors that interfere with tumor immunity

II. Host Competence
    A.   Immunodeficiency prior to tumor formation
        1.   Genetic
        2.   Environmental
    B.   Immunodeficiency associated with tumorigenesis, i.e., tumor cells are generally immunosuppressive

in the host's failure to respond to cancer, especially a weakly immunogenic one, and thus facilitating the development of cancer.

Results reported herein will show that syngeneic mouse tumor cells, of both chemical and viral etiology, are indeed immunosuppressive *in vivo* and *in vitro*. This evidence, thus, brings to the fore the question of tumor immunosuppression as a critical and possibly decisive factor in cancer immunotherapy.

Results

Immunosuppression by Tumor Cells *In Vivo*

Groups of Balb/C mice were inoculated intraperitoneally with syngeneic Rauscher leukemia virus-induced ascites tumor cells (MCDV-12), and, at 2-day intervals thereafter, groups of mice were tested for immunologic responsiveness to sheep red blood cells (sRBC). The sRBC were administered intravenously. Untreated Balb/C mice served as controls for tumor-bearing mice. Four days following the administration of sRBC, the mice were bled to obtain serum and then sacrificed to obtain their spleens. Sera were assayed individually for hemagglutinating antibody, and the spleens were pooled and assayed for 19 S antibody-forming cells, using the Jerne plaque-forming assay (3). The results in Table 10-2 show that, by day 4, the tumor-bearing mice are becoming immunodeficient and, by day 6, they are essentially unresponsive to sRBC.

A similar experiment was carried out using a syngeneic tumor of chemical etiology. Mice of the C57Bl/6J strain were inoculated subcutaneously with a suspension of methylcholanthrene-induced fibrosarcoma cells (MC16), and, at 5-day intervals thereafter, groups of these mice were sacrificed, and their

Table 10-2   Immunosuppression Associated with Tumorigenesis in Balb/C Mice

Group	Syngeneic virus-induced tumor implanted on day 0	sRBC injected on day	Antibody response[a] (day 4 after sRBC) PFC/10^6 spleen cells	Hemagglutinin titer
1A	−	0	2,580	7.0
1B	+	0	1,960	7.5
2A	−	2	3,040	7.0
2B	+	2	3,240	7.0
3A	−	4	1,960	7.0
3B	+	4	348	5.5
4A	−	6	1,120	7.0
4B	+	6	450	1.0

[a] Four days after administration of sRBC, mice were bled to obtain serum and then sacrificed to obtain the spleen. Sera were assayed for hemagglutinating antibody, the titer expressed as $\log_2$ of dilution end-point. Spleens were assayed for antibody-forming cells, measured as plaque-forming cells.

spleens were assayed for immunologic responsiveness to sRBC in *in vitro* cultures. In each instance, spleens of untreated C57Bl/6J mice served as controls. From the results in Table 10-3, the tumor-bearing mice show evidence of immunodeficiency by day 5, and they are almost completely immunosuppressed by day 10.

Immunosuppression by Tumor Cells *In Vitro*

Tumor cells of the MC16 line were added to *in vitro* cultures of syngeneic mouse spleen cells and sRBC to assess the immunosuppressive property of the tumor cells. The tumor cells were kept in the culture throughout a period of 4 days, after which the cultures were examined for 19 S antibody-forming cells and for viable nucleated spleen cells. The results are shown in Figure 10-1. Clearly, direct interaction of tumor cells and spleen cells led to suppression of antibody response to sRBC by the spleen cells. There was complete suppression by 2×10^5 tumor cells, and as few as 10^3 tumor cells added to 10^7 spleen cells sufficed to produce significant immunosuppression. It should be noted that immunosuppression occurred in the absence of any toxic effect of the tumor cells on the spleen cells.

Analysis of Tumor–Spleen Cell Interaction *In Vitro*

Having demonstrated that tumor cells are directly immunosuppressive, we next wanted to determine the basis for this immunosuppressive property.

Table 10-3 Changes in Responsiveness to sRBC of Spleen
Cells from C57Bl/6J following Inoculation
of Syngeneic, Chemically Induced Tumor

Day following tumor inoculation[a]	Antibody response (% control)
5	93
10	16
15	1
20	1

[a] At the times indicated, groups of mice were sacrificed and their spleens used to
prepare suspensions of cells, which were cultured with sRBC for 4 days, after
which the immune responsiveness of the spleen cells was assessed in terms of the
number of plaque-forming cells produced compared with the number produced in
cultures of spleen cells from normal nontumor-bearing mice.

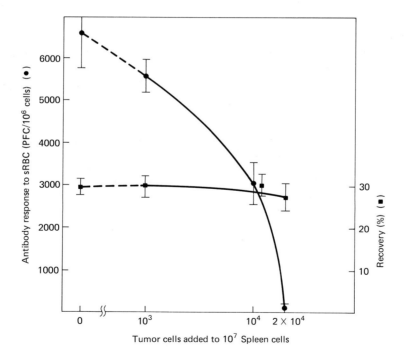

Figure 10-1. Demonstration of an immunosuppressive property of
syngeneic, methylcholanthrene-induced tumor cells (MC16). Tumor
cells were added to cultures of syngeneic C57Bl/6J spleen cells and
sRBC. After 4 days, the cultures were examined for plaque-forming
cells and viable spleen cells.

As a first step, mitomycin C-treated MC16 cells were tested for their ability to suppress the antibody response of syngeneic mouse spleen cells to sRBC. Treatment of the tumor cells with mitomycin C substantially reduced their immunosuppressive activity, the number of treated cells needed to produce the same degree of immunosuppression as viable untreated tumor cells being about 100 times greater (Fig. 10-2). It seems, therefore, that viability of tumor cells is an essential factor in tumor immunosuppression.

We next sought to determine whether tumor immunosuppression was the consequence of direct interaction of spleen cells with tumor cells or the reaction of spleen cells with some tumor-derived substance. Accordingly, a mixture of tumor and spleen cells or tumor cells alone were cultured *in vitro* for 24 hr prior to adding sRBC or sRBC plus spleen cells, respectively. Four days after the addition of sRBC, the cultures were assayed for 19 S antibody-forming cells and compared with base-line cultures comprising tumor cells, spleen cells, and sRBC added together at the start of the culture. The results are shown graphically in Figure 10-3. Increased immunosuppression by tumor cells was observed only when tumor and spleen cells were allowed to interact prior to the addition of antigenic sRBC. The possible involvement of tumor-derived immunosuppressive substances is, of course, not precluded by these results, if such substances are unstable or if they are secreted into the medium as a result of a tumor–spleen cell interaction.

Prostaglandins, particularly PGE$_2$, are known to affect the immune response

Figure 10-2. The viability of tumor cells as a factor in immunosuppression: ($\triangle$) Normal untreated and ($\bigcirc$) mitomycin C-treated MC16 tumor cells were added to cultures of syngeneic C57Bl/6J spleen cells and sRBC. After 4 days, the cultures were examined for plaque-forming cells.

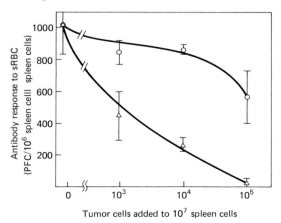

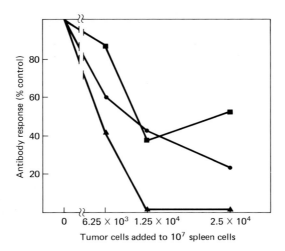

Figure 10-3. The interaction between tumor (MC16) and spleen cells (C57Bl/6J) as a factor in immunosuppression. Three sets of cultures were set up: (▲) tumor and spleen cells cultured for 24 hr prior to addition of sRBC, (●) tumor cells cultured for 24 hr prior to the addition of spleen cells, or (■) sRBC added at the start of the culture together with tumor and spleen cells. Cultures were examined for plaque-forming cells 4 days after the addition of sRBC.

(5), and they are reportedly produced in excess amount by certain tumor cells (2,8,9) so that tumor immunosuppression might conceivably be mediated by prostaglandins. For this reason, PGE₂ was tested for its influence on the response of spleen cells to sRBC. Spleen cells were exposed for 15 min to different concentrations of PGE₂, then sRBC was added, after which the cells were cultured for 4 days, and the antibody response was assessed. As shown in Table 10-4, PGE₂ proved to be immunosuppressive.

If, in fact, prostaglandins are mediators of immunosuppression by tumor cells, the expectation is that inhibitors of prostaglandin synthetase, such as indomethacin, would block tumor immunosuppression. It turns out that addition of indomethacin to cultures of tumor cells and spleen cells reduces immunosuppression by tumor cells, but indomethacin does not block it completely, since immunosuppression is still demonstrable in cultures containing relatively large numbers of tumor cells (Fig. 10-4). Whatever effect indomethacin has on tumor immunosuppression it is not a cytotoxic effect. The addition of indomethacin to cultures of tumor cells does not interfere with viability and proliferation of the tumor cells (Fig. 10-5).

In view of the positive effect of indomethacin in reducing tumor immunosuppression, indomethacin was administered intraperitoneally to tumor-bearing C57Bl/6J mice to test its possible effect on tumor growth. Treatment was

Table 10-4   Immunosuppression by Prostaglandin of
Spleen Cells from C57Bl/6J Mice

Prostaglandin (μg/ml culture)[a]	Antibody response to sRBC (% control)
0	100
0.0001	105
0.001	80
0.01	85
0.1	68
1.0	60
10.0	49

[a] PGE_2, in the amounts indicated, was added to cultures of spleen cells and sRBC, the addition of sRBC being delayed 15 min. After 4 days, the cultures were examined for plaque-forming cells as a measure of antibody response.

started on the day of tumor implantation and continued daily for periods of 10 or 14 days. Rate of tumor growth was significantly reduced as a result of indomethacin treatment (Fig. 10-6). Tumor growth, however, was not arrested even when the period of treatment was extended.

Suppression of cAMP Response during Tumorigenesis

In a study of early cellular events during the response of mice to sRBC, it was found that within 2 min following sRBC intravenous injection, there occurs a two- to three-fold increase in the cAMP level in the spleen (7). Since

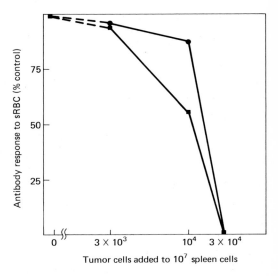

Figure 10-4. Testing of indomethacin for its ability to block immunosuppression by tumor cells. Here MC16 tumor cells were added to cultures of syngeneic C57Bl/6J spleen cells and sRBC: (●) indomethacin (5μg/ml) added to one set of cultures, (■) diluent added to second set. After 4 days, all cultures were examined for plaque-forming cells; the results are given as percent of plaque-forming cells in control cultures containing no tumor cells.

Antibody response to sRBC (% control)

Tumor cells added to 10^7 spleen cells

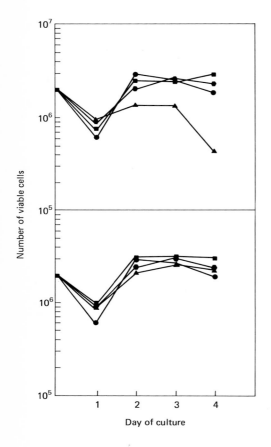

Figure 10-5. The effect of prostaglandin (PGE₂ and PGF2α) and indomethacin on the growth of MC16 tumor cells *in vitro*: Top (○) PGF₂ₐ (1.0 μg/ml), (●) control, (■) indomethacin (12.5 μg/ml), (▼) PGE₂ 1.0 μg/ml); Bottom (○) PGF2α (0.1 μg/ml), (●) control, (■) indomethacin (1.25 μg/ml), (▼) PGE₂ (0.1 μg/ml).

this early cAMP response to sRBC appears to be linked to antibody response, and since tumor cells are immunosuppressive, as shown above, the possible effect of tumorigenesis on the cAMP response to sRBC was studied. Groups of C57Bl/6J mice received implants of MC16 tumor. On day 6 after tumor implantation, growing tumors were excised from two of the groups as a check on the reversibility of any effect of tumorigenesis. Normal untreated mice served as controls. Beginning on day 6, and periodically thereafter, groups of mice were given saline or sRBC, and the spleen levels of cAMP were assayed 2 min later. From the results in Table 10-5, it is clear that tumorigenesis produced a progressive block in the cAMP response to sRBC. Spleen cells were also assayed for antibody response to sRBC in culture, and, as had already been observed (cf. Table 10-3), tumorigenesis also blocked antibody response. It is reassuring, however, that both effects of tumorigenesis, namely, blocks in the cAMP response and antibody response to sRBC, can be overcome by removal of the tumor.

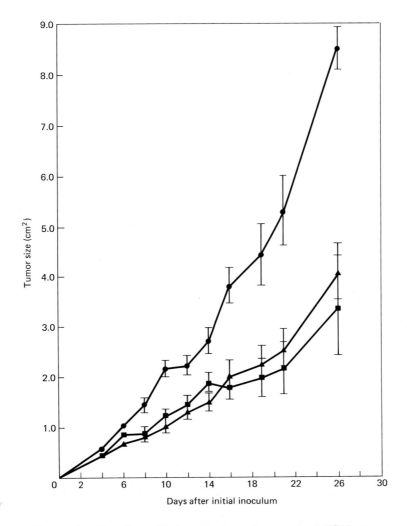

Figure 10-6. The effect of indomethacin on the growth of MC16 tumor cells in syngeneic C57Bl/6J mice. Tumor cells (10^6) were injected subcutaneously into three groups of mice (10 mice/group): One group (■) received indomethacin intraperitoneally (125μg/day throughout the first 10 days), a second group (▲) also received indomethacin but for a 14-day period, the third group (●) served as control and received diluent. Tumor size is expressed as (average diameter) squared.

Table 10-5   Effect of Syngeneic MC Tumor Cells on the Cyclic AMP
Response of C57Bl/6J Mice to sRBC

State of test mice[a]	Day after tumor implant	Antigen	cAMP (pmoles/mg protein)	Spleen cells (PFC/10^6) (4-day culture)
Normal	—	Saline	7.6	38
Normal	—	sRBC	23.1	432
Tumorous	6	Saline	15.3	—
Tumorous	6	sRBC	19.2	—
Tumorous	14	Saline	6.7	—
Tumorous	14	sRBC	6.2	—
Tumorous[b]	14	Saline	7.8	—
Tumorous[b]	14	sRBC	14.6	—
Tumorous	21	Saline	4.5	3
Tumorous	21	sRBC	6.8	10
Tumorous[b]	21	Saline	10.2	34
Tumorous[b]	21	sRBC	30.0	594

[a] All mice, except those in control groups, received subcutaneous implants of MC16 tumors. On the days indicated, normal and tumor-bearing mice received either sRBC or saline diluent, and 2 min thereafter, the mice were sacrificed and their spleens were assayed for cAMP, protein, and, in some instances, for responsiveness to sRBC in 4-day culture.

[b] The tumor was excised surgically on day 6 following implantation.

Discussion

Dramatic changes occur in the immunologic competence of mice soon after implantation of a syngeneic tumor. The mice become increasingly unresponsive to sRBC, in terms of antibody formation and changes in the spleen level of cAMP, as the tumor grows. This is presumptive evidence that tumor cells are immunosuppressive. There is, however, direct evidence, also, because the addition of tumor cells directly to cultures of normal syngeneic mouse spleen cells suppresses antibody formation to sRBC.

Immunosuppression by tumor cells is dose dependent, with 10^5 tumor cells in a culture of 10^7 spleen cells causing complete suppression. One tumor cell/10^3 spleen cells suffices to give significant suppression.

Immunosuppression by tumor cells appears to depend on direct interaction between tumor cells and immunocytes. There is evidence, for example, that such an interaction results in an increased level of cAMP, an important general regulator of cell activity (1). Conceivably, other regulatory substances in addition to cAMP might also be affected, the net result being in this case a block in the activation, differentiation, proliferation, or function of the cells involved in antibody formation. Alternatively, immunosuppression by tumor cells might

Immunotherapy of Cancer: Concepts and Problems

C. F. McKhann

Introduction

The ultimate goal of tumor immunology is effective immunization of the cancer patient against his own tumor. A variety of approaches have been tried, some on the basis of promising laboratory studies. For most physicians who attempted clinical immunotherapy, these trials have proved ambiguous in having met their minimal expectations, while not really living up to their hopes. A few clinical approaches have already been discarded, and among those currently in use there is no clear-cut panacea, but there is enough promise to justify more intensive study. These clinical trials carry with them the clear indication that better results will come only through better understanding of the mechanism of immunity and how it may be manipulated to better meet the needs of the cancer patient. The following pages will outline current approaches to immunotherapy, describe some of the recognized problems, and indicate some of the routes that new approaches to immunotherapy may be expected to take in the next few years.

Requirements for Immunotherapy

From a large number of experimental studies and also on the basis of some experience with human cancer, it is now possible to define some of the optimum requirements for immunotherapy. These are:

1. The tumor must be of proven antigenicity
2. Identical antigens should be involved when two allogeneic tumors are used for cross-immunization
3. Antigenicity should be maintained or increased through processing
4. Tumor cells should be free of "blocking" materials either in the form of an antibody or of antigen-antibody complexes
5. Injection of viable tumor cells should be avoided
6. The patient should be immunologically competent to respond to immunotherapy

Fundamental Aspects of Neoplasia,
edited by A. Arthur Gottlieb, Otto J. Plescia, and David H. L. Bishop.
© 1975 by Springer-Verlag New York Inc.

7. The tumor burden of the patient should be reduced to a minimum
8. Successful immunotherapy requires intensive immunization
9. Manipulation of the immune response should augment cellular immunity and minimize the production of (blocking) antibody
10. Clinical immunotherapy should be monitored by *in vitro* evaluation of the immune responses.

Methods of Immunotherapy

The approaches to immunotherapy fall into five general categories.

Prophylactic Immunization

This is a utopian goal, which will require that the specific antigen be identified and available in a safe form for immunization long before the patient actually develops the tumor. The antigen may assume the form of the agent responsible for the tumor, such as an oncogenic virus capable of provoking an immune response against its own capsid antigen. In an attenuated form, the virus could provide a route to preimmunization against the oncogenic agent itself. Prophylactic immunization may also be directed against tumor-specific antigens of malignant or premalignant tumor cells. When more is known about the etiology of some human tumors, preimmunization of populations at risk by means of attenuated virus or tumor antigen will become a real possibility.

Active, Nonspecific Immunization

This requires that the patient's own immune response be stimulated directly by means of an immunogen or a stimulant that is *not* antigenically related to the tumor itself. Here BCG is the prototype of a variety of microorganisms that have been found to nonspecifically "turn up" the immune capacity of the individual to react to other antigens, including antigenic tumors. In various studies, BCG has been given orally, subcutaneously, directly into lesions and intradermally by scarification, each route carrying its own spectrum of side reactions, ranging from minimal inconvenience to major reactions and even fatalities. Active nonspecific immunization can also be carried out by exposing lymphocytes from a tumor-bearing patient to a potent mitogen, such as PHA, *in vitro* and then returning the cells to the patient. Again, the stimulus has no antigenic relationship to the tumor.

Active Specific Immunotherapy

This form may use autologous or allogeneic tumor cells, antigenic extracts of these cells, or tumor cells that have been modified to render them more immunogenic (as with neuraminidase). These cells or extracts may be injected directly into the patient, or they may be used for *in vitro* immunization of lymphoid cells from the tumor-bearing patient, subsequently returning the lymphoid cells to the patient. In all cases when tumor cells are used, they are usually killed to render them incapable of growth and are often given as multiple injections, frequently in several locations to stimulate as much of the immune system as possible.

Adoptive Transfer of Immunity

This is an entirely different approach to immunotherapy, based on transferring immune capability from the "have's" to the "have not's." In this approach, adoptive transfer may be of the entire machinery for continuous maintenance of specific immunity, or one may transfer specific immunologic information that can then be utilized by the patient's own lymphocytes. In the first instance, cross-immunization of paired patients bearing identical tumors has been followed by the adoptive transfer of lymphoid cells back to the original tumor donor. Unfortunately, rapid immunization against the *normal* alloantigens present on both tumor and lymphoid cells almost always ensures the rapid demise of these transferred lymphocytes. The alternative approach is to extract from lymphocytes of a patient who has been "cured" of his tumor specific immunologic information in the form of transfer factor or an RNA extract and to deliver this information to the appropriate tumor-bearing patient, either by direct injection or by exposing his lymphocytes *in vitro*. In either case, the mediators of the transfer are nonantigenic in their own right and thus not subject to rapid destruction by the recipient.

Passive Transfer of Tumor-Specific Immunity

This entails the transfer of a serum factor, presumably an antibody, capable of relieving the tumor cell of any blockade imposed upon on it by circulating blocking factors in the serum of the patient. Such an "unblocking" antibody is usually found in an individual who has recently had his tumor removed.

Current Problems in Immunotherapy

Enhanced Tumor Growth

Our long-standing knowledge that experimental immunotherapy can result in enhanced tumor growth has raised the specter of this possibility in clinical trials. So far there are no proved instances of enhanced tumor growth as a result of clinical immunotherapy. Most clinicians working in this area, however, have encountered a few patients whose disease progressed rapidly enough following immunotherapy to make them mindful of this possibility. Immunotherapy of cancer can not be approached with a completely clear conscience until immunologic enhancement is understood to the point where it can be avoided.

In most early studies, the mediator of enhanced growth appeared to be circulating antibody. This led to the axiom that "cellular immunity is good and antibody production is bad." The multiple factors now known to be involved have weakened this simple analysis but have not done away with it altogether. A great deal of evidence now indicates that the blocking factors that appear to prevent the attacking lymphocyte from gaining access to the surface of the tumor cell are some form of antigen-antibody complex. What is not known is whether pure antibody, free of any antigen, is capable of blocking lymphocyte cytotoxicity, whether it is passive in the entire interaction, or whether, under some circumstances, it may even mediate cell destruction, either directly or through the activation of lymphocytes. A continuing gap in our knowledge is the relationship between *in vitro* "blocking" and enhancement of tumor growth *in vivo*.

Immune Capacity and Surveillance

The concept that immunologic surveillance may provide a primary defense mechanism against the establishment of aberrant clones of malignant cells was first voiced by Thomas and Burnet (1,4). Support for this concept in humans comes from the finding that patients with immunodeficiency diseases, or those whose immune mechanisms have been deliberately distorted by immunosuppressive therapy required for organ transplantation, have a significantly higher incidence of spontaneous malignancy than do normal, age-matched controls. The obvious implication of a surveillance mechanism is that it usually works well and that malignancy must result from failure at some level. Relatively few parameters of the overall immune response have been looked at critically. But, of those that have, the cellular immune capacity may be one of the most important. When measured by skin test delayed hypersensitivity and the response of lymphocytes to allogeneic cells and mitogens *in vitro*, it has been found that lymphocyte-mediated immune capacity can undergo profound lapses. A variety of virus infections, from the common cold through much more serious diseases, are frequently associated with loss of skin test responsiveness to antigens and failure of lymphocytes to be stimulated *in vitro* by allogeneic cells or appropriate mitogens. The stress of surgery in patients who are free of malignant disease gives similar evidence of a depressed immunoresponse. This may begin as early as one day *prior* to surgery, indicating the stress relationship. Ordinarily all of these measurable responses return to normal within 2 to 4 weeks of infection or surgery. The real relationship of these measurable indicators of cellular immune incompetence to the development of certain infections and of *de novo* malignancy are among the areas most urgently in need of study.

The possibility clearly exists that temporary "natural" lapses in an important compartment of immune resistance, cellular immunity, may open the door to the establishment of aberrant cells or clones of cells that could not become established under optimal circumstances.

Anatomically "privileged sites," including the anterior chamber of the eye and the meninges and brain, allow antigenic tumors to grow by retarding immunization and presenting some barrier between the tumor and the immune system. The common denominator appears to be the total absence of lymphatic drainage from these two areas. Neither area is a common site for spontaneous malignancy. Gittes (2), however, has noted that the prostate gland is also deficient in lymphatic drainage and postulates that this organ, too, is a privileged site, but one known to harbor a very *large* number of malignancies. Indeed, 40 percent of men in their 70s and 60 percent of men in their 80s have histologic evidence of cancer of the prostate. Gittes further postulates that antigen from the tumor gains access to the bloodstream, to induce what is primarily an antibody response, which may slow the growth of the tumor and prevent early metastases (2). Under some circumstances, such antibody may combine with tumor antigen or, in some other way, may convert to enhancing antibody, thence promoting rapid growth and dissemination of the tumor.

It must also be recognized that two of the most important conventional forms of therapy for cancer, irradiation and chemotherapy, are potent immunosuppressants. Studies on our own patients indicate that immunosuppression following both of these forms of therapy is profound. There have been reports of a rebound phenomenon in lymphocyte stimulation following chemotherapy, but, as Stratton (3) recently reported, 5,000 rads of irradiation was followed by depression of T cell numbers and function lasting more than 1 year after treatment. Although both of these forms of treatment have a great deal to offer patients, the day may come when the extent and timing of their use may take into account their interaction with the immune system.

Release of Soluble Antigen

The role that antibody may play in compromising the cellular immune response against tumors has long been recognized. More recently, it has become apparent that such an antibody may exert its influence by forming a complex with antigen and that antigen alone may also inhibit the interaction between immune lymphoid cells and tumor cells.

There is evidence that some tumors may produce large amounts of antigen, releasing it into the circulation. Such shedding of antigen can obviously provide a mechanism by which the tumor can satisfy the tumor-specific appetite of the entire immune response, including circularing antibody and lymphoid cells,

159

in lymph nodes, spleen, thymus, and bone marrow. This potential escape mechanism raises the important question of whether the specific immune response remains fully active in the presence of excessive production of antigen or whether it undergoes involution and suppression, developing a state of central tolerance. If the immune response continues at maximum activity, the problem is primarily one of trying to decrease production of antigen by the tumor or increase the rate at which antigen is disposed, thus cutting down on the overload. Alternatively, if the immune response backs away from maximum activity and a state of partial tolerance develops, the problem must be approached from the point of view of breaking the tolerance, as might be done by using slightly altered antigens or introducing nontolerant cells.

Recent studies from our laboratory indicate that some degree of immune suppression may occur in animals bearing large tumors. Lymph node cells from normal or preimmunized mice, or mice bearing small tumors, can be stimulated *in vitro* upon contact with cells of the same tumor. Lymph node cells from animals bearing large tumors, however, are incapable of further *in vitro* stimulation. They appear to have been maximally stimulated *in vivo* and to have entered a refractory phase. Stimulation and the induction of the refractory phase can be carried out *in vitro* by exposing lymphocytes to antigen extracts of tumors but, more importantly, by also exposing them to serum from animals bearing large tumors. The refractoriness is tumor specific, since the same cells can be stimulated upon exposure to other tumor cells or antigens. This same serum can be shown by other methods to contain free circulating antigen. It appears that circulating antigen, which indicates excessive production and shedding by the tumor beyond the point of saturation of the specific immune response, is associated with suppression of lymphocyte responsiveness to the same antigen *in vitro*.

Nonspecific Suppression of Immunity in Malignancy

It is relatively easy to explain in terms of known mechanisms how the specific immune response may be suppressed by the growing tumor. But, a wealth of clinical studies indicate that with many tumors the suppression goes far beyond that immediately related to the tumor. It was first noted that patients wih Hodgkin's disease show defective cellular immunity in that they respond poorly to skin test antigens and to lymphocyte stimulation *in vitro*. This finding has now been extended to many other tumors. Our own studies indicate that nonspecific immune deficiency, or anergy, as measured by these same parameters, can be observed in many patients with modest amounts of tumor as well as those individuals with extensive disease. Such anergy appears to be associated with a poor clinical prognosis.

However ill-defined the "cellular immunity" compartment may be, other aspects of immune resistance appear to function adequately, if not normally. Immunosuppression in connection with transplantation and studies of immunolodeficiency diseases have provided a profile of the clinical results of serious immunologic incapacity, characterized by bizarre virus and mycotic infections that are almost never seen in cancer patients. By comparison, even terminal cancer patients are not immunologic cripples. Again, it is not clear exactly which compartments are being measured by these assays or what their direct relationship to the patient's immunologic interaction with his tumor is; thus, the mechanism by which the tumor extends its inhibitory effect beyond immunologic activity directed specifically against the tumor is a new and important area for study.

Conclusions

The nature of "cancer" as a disease and the seemingly low risk of immunotherapy, coupled with a strong desire to add a new weapon to our anti-tumor arsenal, has brought immunotherapy to the point of clinical trials. These initial attempts have been gratifying in a few patients, but major efforts, and, we hope, the results that will justify them, still lie ahead. The machinery of the immune response is only partially understood, and our interpretation of its interaction with cancer is obliged to follow in line. This is clearly one area where today's clinical experience provides for tomorrow's laboratory protocol, in a cycle that will bear repetition several times.

REFERENCES

1. Burnet, F. M. Cancer: A biological approach. Br. Med. J., 1:779, 841, 1957.
2. Gittes, R. F. and McCullough, D. L. Occult carcinoma of the prostate—an oversight of immune surveillance? J. Urology, 112:241, 1974.
3. Stratton, J. T and B lymphocytes after thymic radiation in humans. Fed. Proc. 33:742, 1974.
4. Thomas, L. Discussion in Cellular and Humoral Aspects of Hypersensitivity States. New York, Harper & Row, 1961, p. 529.

12

Chemotherapy, Supportive Care, and Immunotherapy of Cancer—from Research Tools to Therapeutic Modalities

I. Djerassi, J. Sun Kim, and U. Suvansri

Introduction

The interdependence of basic studies and of practice is well illustrated in research on neoplastic growth and its clinical management. In recent years, all new fundamental information in this area has been scrutinized without delay for possible applications to the prevention or treatment of cancer. Massive efforts in applied research are often triggered by new basic information. In this fashion, cancer clinics around the world have become extensions of basic research laboratories, confirming, disproving, and, occasionally, even originating new basic concepts. Advanced clinical management of disseminated human neoplasms has become an inseparable mixture of research and practice, with its overall value usually depending on the extent and quality of the former. The research approaches of a few years ago are becoming accepted therapeutic modalities today. Chemotherapy and supportive care are eloquent examples in this respect. Some forms of immunotherapy are already following in their steps, whereas others continue to challenge basic scientists by their very inadequacy.

We will try in this presentation to illustrate the remarkable transition of research to practice in the field of cancer therapy by describing some of our personal experiences of this nature.

A number of "research tools" of concern to our group are in various stages of transition from investigation to practice. By reviewing them, we hope to justify the title of this chapter.

Chemotherapy: A Rational Approach for More Effective Use of Folic Acid Antagonists—The High Dose Pulse of Methotrexate

Our studies in this area started in 1962, with our intention being to explore, on the clinical level, the nature of resistance to folic acid antagonists. After their introduction by Sidney Farber in 1948, this class of anticancer drugs had performed less well than expected, with the notable exception of their effects

Fundamental Aspects of Neoplasia,
edited by A. Arthur Gottlieb, Otto J. Plescia, and David H. L. Bishop.
© 1975 by Springer-Verlag New York Inc.

Table 12-1 Effects of Continuous Massive Methotrexate Infusions in 10 Patients with Acute Lymphatic Leukemia

Patient	Age (years)	Initial white blood cells	Blasts (%)	Previous therapy	Duration of treatment (days)	Complete remission time (days)	Platelets transfused	Platelet concentrates used	Relapse at end of study
P.L.	14	4,400	98	MTX,[a] prednisone,[b] 6 MP,[b] hydroxyurea,[a] vincristine,[a] Cytoxan	42	165+ (off study)	86	525	No
S.R.	10½	1,600	95	MTX,[a] prednisone, vincristine	36	101	13	73	No
G.M.	3	26,500	85	MTX,[a] vincristine,[b] 6 MP,[b] prednisone,[b] hydroxyurea	50 (34 days to partial remission)	26	22	82	Yes
K.Z.	9½	3,000	40	MTX (i.m.),[a] prednisone 6 MP,[a] vincristine hydroxyurea[a]	25	20	4	21	Yes
M.B.	3	385,400	90	MTX[a] (continuous infusion), prednisone, vincristine	36	72	9	31	Yes

D.S.	7	1,150	98	MTX,[a] 6 MP,[a] prednisone[b]	31	74+ (off study)	8	35	No
M.C.	14	750	100	MTX (only 2 weeks), 6 MP,[a] prednisone[b]	16	97+ (off study)	30	210	No
J.G.	10½	110,000	98	6 MP, vincristine, prednisone, MTX[a]	25 (to partial)	128 (off treatment after 100 days)	11	61	No
T.W.	9½	5,000	10	MTX,[a] prednisone, 6 MP,[a] vincristine	20 (from partial relapse)	30+ (off study)	0	0	No
A.D.	3	4,500	13	MTX,[a] vincristine,[b] prednisone,[b] hydroxyurea[a]	12 (from partial relapse)	80 (died)	10	39	No

[a] Relapsed while receiving drug for maintenance.
[b] Failed to respond after adequate trial on first or subsequent treatments.

on chorioepithelioma. The limited scope of their clinical usefulness was due to the rapid emergence or initial presence of resistant cancer cell clones. The mechanism of action of antifolic acid agents (antifols) and of the resistance of cancer cells to this class of drugs has been the subject of extensive studies (1).

Consideration of these mechanisms led us to the hypothesis that resistance or response to folic acid antagonists is determined by the number of antifol molecules made available intracellularly for stoichiometric binding of dihydrofolic acid reductase. The means for saturating *in vivo* antifol-resistant cells with folic acid antagonists (methotrexate) was needed to test this hypothesis clinically. An approach to that end was suggested by a study we had carried out in the 50s, in which we tried to saturate human platelets with serotonin (5-hydroxytryptamine). Up to 100 times the expected limiting concentration of this compound in platelets was introduced by varying the concentration of serotonin in the medium and the time of incubation of the platelets with serotonin. The intracellular concentration of serotonin was a function of the product Ct (concentration times time). To reproduce these conditions for antifols in a patient, we devised and carefully explored the tolerance of patients to continuous infusions of methotrexate. Initially, the *concentration* of the drug in the blood and body fluids was kept rather low by infusing relatively small doses of the drug while the *time* of administration was prolonged. Ten children with acute lymphocytic leukemia, all resistant to folic acid antagonists (methotrexate), were thus treated with prolonged infusions of the same drug. All 10 children experienced hematologic remission (4). Resistance to folic acid antagonists could, therefore, be reversed. Increased tolerance to the drug, rather than absolute resistance to it, appeared to account for the therapeutic failures of this class of agents (Table 12-1). Subsequent studies indicated that similar effects with less toxicity could be achieved by increasing the concentration component in the Ct product at the expense of the time factor. Remissions were induced repeatedly in relapsing leukemia patients receiving methotrexate with the same drug used in different dose-schedules. As result of this work, dose-schedules of methotrexate pulses for remission maintenance treatment of children with acute leukemia were developed. These dose-schedules, which were eventually combined with other agents, resulted in a previously unattainable duration of remission and survival of the patients (3,10). The results in a series of patients with acute lymphocytic leukemia treated with high dose MTX and a combination of agents (BOMB) are shown in Table 12-2.

The same approach was utilized in studies of "inherent resistance" to folic acid antagonists characteristic of other tumors. Lymphosarcoma and reticulum cell sarcoma, notorious for their poor response to conventionally administered methotrexate (2.5 to 5 mg daily), responded extensively and consistently to high dose pulse methotrexate (12).

Table 12-2 MTX-BOMB Remission Maintenance in Acute Lymphocytic Leukemia

Patient	Date of diagnosis	Duration (months) of hematologic remission on protocol[a]	Total survival (months) as of 4/1/74[b]
N.B.	3/8/68	68	69
P.P.	10/10/68	67+	90+
R.L.	9/27/66	64+	65+
H.Z.	11/8/68	63+	64+
G.W.	4/6/68	62+	71+
C.P.	1/11/69	61+	62+
E.B.	2/19/69	60+ Median	61+ Median
L.L.	11/23/66	56+	87+
L.K.	5/1/69	42	43
R.O.	12/18/69	50+	51+
J.D.	12/31/69	50+	51+
P.N.	3/16/68	36	54
H.P.	7/8/69	28	29
J.C.	3/19/69	4	20

[a] Duration of single remission 5+ years 64 percent still in remission.

[b] Median survival 5+ years 64 percent alive.

[c] Vincristine, Daunomycin, 6-MP and Prednisone.

Citrovorum factor "rescue," given *after* the administration of methotrexate, which we had introduced earlier (3), was utilized more extensively in the studies of lymphosarcoma patients. The potential usefulness of folinic acid (citrovorum factor) "rescue" was suggested by animal studies carried out by Goldin in 1953 (13). Unfortunately, other studies in mice (2) as well as subsequent clinical trials had led to the conclusion that the toxicity of antifols could only be prevented if citrovorum factor is given just prior to or during the administration of the antifol in doses equimolar to the dose of the folic acid antagonist, thus preventing the antitumor effects of the latter as well. This conclusion did not agree with our interpretation of the information available on the mechanism of action of folinic acid as a co-enzyme required only at the time of DNA synthesis. Theoretically, folinic acid could protect from antifol toxicity when given after antifol administration and in doses independent of the dose of the inhibitor. Indeed, the above and subsequent clinical studies (9) demonstrated that these considerations were valid in humans.

The high dose pulse methotrexate, with or without citrovorum factor "rescue," was shown subsequently by this group and by others to have a wide scope of antitumor biologic activity. Reduction of tumor size, using a variety of dose-schedules of these agents, was observed by this group in neuroblastoma, breast cancer, melanoma, lung and pancreas cancer, and, jointly with Farber and Jaffe (16), in osteogenic sarcoma. Bertino reported its value in acute myelogenous leukemia and head and neck cancer. It must be noted that all these tumor tissues were historically known to be unresponsive to folic acid antagonists. The work with Sidney Farber and Norman Jaffe on osteogenic sarcoma signaled the transition of the high dose pulse methotrexate-citrovorum "rescue" to the status of a new therapeutic modality. Used by Jaffe as an adjuvant to surgery in osteogenic sarcoma, this chemotherapeutic maneuver has so far postponed the ever-present metastatic spread in this disease beyond the time of its usual appearance in the majority of the patients thus treated (17). Other investigators are using it as part of a combined drug regimen, prophylactic and therapeutic, for malignant tumors of the bone (J. Rosen at Sloan-Kettering Memorial Hospital, New York, Wilbur at Children's Hospital of Stanford, and Pratt at St. Jude, Memphis). The conceptual validity of the principles discussed above, concerning the acquired or inherent tumor resistance to folic acid antagonists, was thus demonstrated and established. While a specific dose-schedule of methotrexate-citrovorum (9) is being established as effective therapy for osteogenic sarcoma (16), similar regimens are being investigated and adapted for maximal effectiveness in other tumors.

Supportive Transfusions as Adjuvant to Chemotherapy

Platelet Transfusions

As early as 1948, the late Sidney Farber recognized the potential value of specialized transfusions aimed at temporarily replacing blood elements destroyed by the anti-cancer drug in cancer patients who were undergoing chemotherapy. In 1954 this author joined Farber and Klein in Boston in the study of platelet function, harvest, transfusion, and preservation. Platelet transfusions remained a highly experimental tool (8) until the 60s, when the conceptual validity of supportive transfusions was generally acknowledged. The arrest of hemorrhage in thrombocytopenic patients following platelet transfusions ceased to be an investigational phenomenon (14). The Platelet Task Force of the National Cancer Institute, under the direction of Gordon Zubrod, facilitated the transition of platelet transfusions from the experimental stages to their general acceptance as a *routine therapeutic modality*. The impact of platelet transfusions on chemotherapy research was substantial. They made possible not only the development of the high dose methotrexate pulse method in our clinic, but also early intensive drug combination regimens (VAMP, POMP, etc.), with subsequent major advances in the management of acute leukemia, Hodgkin's disease, lymphosarcoma, and other previously unresponsive malignancies.

Leukocyte Transfusions

Leukopenia and associated infections are a major obstacle to optimal chemo- and radiotherapy of malignancies. The clinical usefulness of platelet transfusions made replacement of granulocytes in a leukopenic patient conceptually acceptable. Unfortunately, the logistics of collection of adequate amounts of normal granulocytes from normal donors unduly postponed the actual testing, in animals and in patients, of the possibility of controlling infections by granulocyte replacement.

In 1970, our group described a new, conceptually different approach to harvesting of normal granulocytes (6). Instead of using the inefficient centrifugal sedimentation of granulocytes for their separation, a process based on their ability to stick to foreign surfaces was utilized to filter them out of extracorporeally circulated blood. The principles and the basic techniques for filtration-leukopheresis were subsequently described, and an apparatus for automated mechanical filtration-leukopheresis was constructed (Fig. 12-1), increasing even further the efficiency of this process. An average of 10^{11} granulocytes can thus be collected from one normal human donor in a single leukocyte donation.

Intensive clinical studies are being carried out at major centers to demonstrate the effectiveness of granulocyte transfusions for the control of otherwise intractable infections in leukopenic patients. Preliminary information gathered at this center seems to indicate that granulocyte transfusions will indeed enlarge the scope of currently available chemotherapeutic approaches (Table 12-3) (11). It is very likely, therefore, that over the next few years granulocyte transfusions may become a standard therapeutic modality.

Clinical Immunotherapy of Cancer—A Testing Ground for Laboratory and Theoretical Considerations

Immunotherapy of cancer, from Cooley's work with bacterial toxins at the turn of this century to the early 60s, has largely been regarded as an investigational exercise. The clarification of the basic mechanisms of cellular immunity by Robert Good and the demonstration by Edmund Klein of the therapeutic value of immunotherapy in cancer of the skin were followed by a surge of interest and research efforts in this area. Important advances in the use of immunotherapeutic approaches to the management of melanoma and sarcomas were reported by Morton. Fudenberg is making exciting observations in his use of transfer factor in osteosarcoma. George Mathé promoted the clinical use of BCG as a nonspecific immunostimulant, following up on the pioneering work of Lloyd Old and others. But despite widespread interest and many studies, the

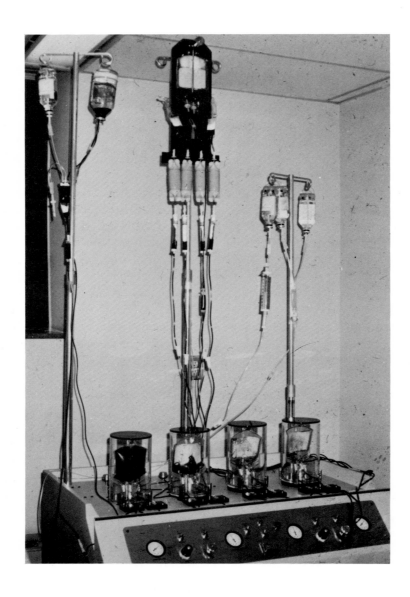

Figure 12-1. Apparatus for automated mechanical filtration–
leukopheresis using air pressure for blood propulsion.

indications for immunotherapy of cancer at this state of our knowledge remain largely "theoretical."

Recognition of the loss of cellular immune responsiveness with advancing neoplasia in man has led to widespread efforts to use specific (tumor cell) or nonspecific (BCG, *C. parvum*) immunostimulation of the patient in combination with other established therapeutic modalities. Surgery and/or chemotherapy are widely studied in combination with immunostimulation, the latter usually termed immunotherapy. Although the present authors make no exception to the rule (see below), we generally see clinical studies in the area of immunotherapy as a testing of concepts derived from fundamental, animal, or *in vitro* work. Studies of this nature, oriented to test, in man, basic concepts which, despite their wide acceptance, have yet to be proved or exploited at the clinical level are described below:

Effects of Monocyte Instillation in Human Tumors

Blood monocytes were recently identified as the circulating form of tissue macrophages. The latter, on the other hand, were recognized as a major arm of antitumor cellular immunity (19). Stimulated by specific lymphocyte-released materials (lymphokines), tissue macrophages allegedly actively attack and destroy malignant cells.

A method for the separation and concentration of large numbers (up to 5×10^9 cells) of human monocytes was developed by our group, utilizing the filtration–leukopheresis method to harvest granulocytes and monocytes and the Ficoll–Hypaque gradient centrifugation technique to separate them from granulocytes. The monocytes thus collected are morphologically intact, and their function is sufficiently preserved so that they exhibit phagocytosis. The intradermal injection of concentrated human monocytes (0.5×10^8 cells) was studied in patients with neoplastic diseases. Invariably, an intense red discoloration of the skin appeared, often within 15 min, at the site of the injection, reaching a maximal intensity in 24 hr and usually fading by 48 hr without leaving any sign of damage to normal skin. This monocyte skin reaction (MSK) was equally intense in anergic patients as well as in patients with competent cellular immunity (determined by skin testing to PPD, mumps, and candida antigens).

A study of the effects of intratumor injections of human monocytes was carried out jointly with Edmund Klein on patients in our institution as well as at the Roswell Park Memorial Institute in Buffalo. Metastatic lesions on the patients' skin, originating from cancers of the breast and colon, melanoma, reticulum cell sarcoma, and mycosis fungoides, were injected with fresh, viable, normal human monocytes. Detectable reduction of the injected tumors was

Table 12-3   White Blood Cell Transfusions in Patients with Acute Leukemia

Patient	Leukopenia (days)	MTX[a]	Cells/m² (×10^11)	Infection site	Organism	Outcome (infection)	Outcome (relapse)
J.P.	39	35	0.23	Fever, cellulitis of mandible Skin infection (hands)	*Candida* NP *Klebsiella* *E. coli* NP *Candida*	Recovered	Remission
C.M.	31	12	0.35	Pneumonia, fever	NP *Staph. aureus*	Recovered	Remission
	30	30	0.36	Oral ulcers (mild fever)	Due to MTX toxicity (NP culture)	Recovered	Remission
D.D.	18	17	0.21	Fever (blastic crisis)	Unknown	Recovered	Remission
N.B.	12	12	0.40	Fever, Gram-negative shock	Blood culture *Pseudomonas*	Failed	
C.U.	24	23	0.40	Fever, jaundice, hepatitis	NP *Staph. aureus*	Improved	Remission
J.C.	68	62	0.41	Fever, hemorrhagic cystitis	Unknown (aspergillosis at post mortem)	Improved	Failed
S.WI.	101	47	0.36	Oral ulcers	*Strepococcus*	Recovered	Partial
	14	7	0.37	Oral ulcer and cellulitis	*Pseudomonas*	Recovered	Remission

				Symptoms	Organism		
S.WE.	65	54	0.40	Oral ulcers	E. coli	Recovered	Remission
G.S.	43	20	0.23	Fever, sore throat	Pseudomonas Monilia	Recovered	Remission
J.F.	31	28	0.21	Fever, pneumonia	Staph. aureus septicemia	Recovered	Remission
L.K.	61	54	0.55	Fever, pneumonia	E. coli sepsis (NP enterococci candida)	Recovered	Remission
J.G.	36	36	0.38	Fever, pneumonia	Unknown	Improved	Failed
B.L.	48	16	0.58	Fever	Salmonella sepsis	Failed	Failed
R.O.	57	45	0.38	Fever, Gram-negative sepsis	E. coli Klebsiella Pseudomonas	Recovered	Remission
R.B.	58	53	0.28	Oral ulcers (fever)	(NP candida Strepococcus)	Recovered	Failed
L.M.	20	10	0.35	Septic fever	Pseudomonas NP Klebsiella Pseudomonas in urine	Recovered	Remission
	7	7	0.19	Vaginal discharge	Pseudomonas Candida	Recovered	
				Oral ulcers (fever)	(NP Pseudomonas)	Recovered	

a Number of transfusions.

usually noticeable within 24 hr in most (8 of 10) patients (Fig. 12-2). Injection of a variety of control materials, including plasma and "buffy coat" cells, was without effect. It should be noted that regrowth of the tumors was usually observed in 3 to 5 days. The direct demonstration of the effects of human monocytes (or monocyte cellular components ?) on human malignant tumors without a concomitant effect on the normal surrounding tissues, has a number of interesting implications concerning the mode of action of tissue macrophages and their specificity. Intensive studies, of a basic laboratory nature, were initiated in both institutions as a result of these clinical observations.

Transfusions of Human Monocytes

In the course of the chemotherapy of patients with acute leukemia or with solid tumors, exceptionally large amounts of granulocytes, obtained by filtration–leukopheresis, were transfused to these patients in an attempt to abbreviate their prolonged leukopenia and chronic infections. In the course of these transfusions, large amounts of normal monocytes were also given, since the filtered granulocyte concentrates contain an average of 5 percent monocytes. It was noted that antitumor effects exceeding the expected results from chemotherapy alone occurred in these patients (7). Subsequent studies on transfusions of large amounts of purified monocytes (1.5 to 5×10^9 cells) were carried

Figure 12-2. Effects of intratumor (breast cancer) injection of normal human monocyte concentrates. Left, before injection; right, 24 hours after injection.

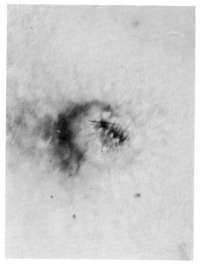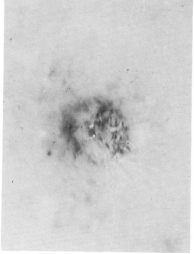

out. A frequent association of febrile reactions with these transfusions was seen. One patient with advanced cancer of the pancreas, with ascites and massive edema of the legs, was given monocyte transfusions without concomitant chemotherapy. Substantial improvement in the general condition of the patient, with a reduction of her ascites, followed.

Combination of Chemotherapy and Immunotherapy

Adjuvant immunotherapy, consisting of intradermal BCG and monocyte transfusions whenever available, was initiated in advanced cancer patients, who were also receiving intermittent chemotherapy. Seven of seven patients with inoperable cancer of the pancreas, who received "immunotherapy" as above during the intervals between pulses of high dose methotrexate (up to 100 mg/kg) followed by citrovorum factor, have so far improved and have survived beyond anticipation (Table 12-4). Although this is indeed encouraging, as far as treatment of pancreatic cancer is concerned, the contribution of the immunotherapy component of this treatment regimen cannot be evaluated objectively at this time. Controlled studies aimed at comparing the effects

Table 12-4   Survival of Patients with Inoperable Pancreatic Cancer on MTX–Citrovorum Factor Rescue

Patient	Tissue diagnosis	Location	Date MTX started[a]	Survival (months)
Sh.	Carcinoma of pancreas	Head	5/2/73	18+
Kl.	Adenocarcinoma of pancreas	Body	5/2/73 (9)	12[b]
Gor.	Carcinoma of pancreas metastasis,liver, peritoneum	Body	3/9/73 (4)	12
Sus.	Poorly differentiated carcinoma of pancreas, pleural metastasis	Tail	6/16/73 (11)	12+
Hart.	Well-differentiated adenocarcinoma of pancreas, inoperable	Head	July, 1973 (9)	10+
Ros.	Carcinoma of pancreas metastatic to stomach and duodenum	Tail	11/12/73 (4)	8½+
Lip.	Carcinoma of pancreas liver metastasis	Head	11/26/73 (4)	5+

[a] Numbers in parentheses are times of MTX administration.

[b] Drug-related death.

of high dose pulse methotrexate–citrovorum "rescue," used alone or in combination with immunostimulation, are needed for this purpose. Studies of this nature are currently in progress.

Clinical Therapeutic Evaluation of the "Blocking Factor" Concept

We mentioned in the introduction to this chapter that clinical research in the course of treatment of cancer often serves as a testing ground for important basic concepts. This was, in part, the case in the observations we described above, as they relate to inoculation of monocytes into tumors and, to some extent, to monocyte transfusions and adjuvant immunostimulation.

A clinical therapeutic trial that was clearly a test of basic scientific concepts was recently undertaken in our laboratories. The cellular immunosuppressive effects of the so-called blocking antibodies or blocking antibody–antigen complex or blocking factor have been emphasized as a major obstacle to cancer control by the patient's own immune defenses (15). The validity of this widely accepted concept could be tested in humans by removing the blocking factor for a long enough period to allow at least a temporary return of the patient's own immunocompetence against his tumor. Theoretically, this could be done by total plasma exchange. This approach, however, has always been considered impractical. Simple replacement of the patient's plasma with normal plasma would not be an adequate trial, since blocking antibodies and/or blocking factor would be replaced quickly by the patient. Continued daily plasma exchanges for long periods of time could theoretically provide an adequate trial of this concept, had such exchanges not been considered technically impossible. Indeed, an unusual concentration of facilities in one single center would be needed to make such a study feasible. Such facilities include the simultaneous presence of complicated apparatus and skilled personnel, adequate patients for the study, and unlimited supplies of normal plasma. In January of 1974, all these requirements were present at this institution.

A patient with metastatic melanoma, a 47-year-old male, in good general condition with recurring melanoma involving the inguinal lymph nodes and soft tissues along a previous surgical excision, but without internal organ involvement, had just started to escape control by high dose methotrexate–citrovorum pulses. The multiple deep lesions in the right inguinal area enlarged, despite an 18-g infusion of methotrexate. The size and position of the lesions could be well outlined by palpation as well as by direct visual observation. Daily plasma exchanges were initiated, using the NCI–IBM continuous flow centrifuge. An arterial-venous shunt, similar to the one in use for chronic renal dialysis, was placed on the patient's left wrist under local anesthesia. The arterial cannula was connected daily to the input line of the continuous flow centrifuge, while the venous cannula was attached to the return line after modifying the latter to include a vented blood receptacle similar to the return system we devised for filtration–leukopheresis. In this fashion, all blood elements were returned to the patient under the hydrostatic pressure of the atmosphere. The patient was heparinized every day for the procedure with 15,000 units of heparin sodium initially and 5,000 units every 3 hours during the procedure. The patient's plasma, separated in the centrifuge bowl, was collected separately in plastic bags placed on a portable scale. Normal plasma was introduced into the return line at the rate of removal of the patient's plasma. The normal plasma, joining the patient's red blood cells, white blood cells, and platelets, was mixed with the latter in a high vented receptacle from which the reconstituted blood was returned to the patient by gravity via the venous cannula. The normal plasma used was frozen fresh after collection in acid citrate dextrose solution by plasmapheresis of normal donors. Adequate serum samples were obtained from the patient each morning prior to heparinization.

During the first 2 days of plasma exchange, a total of 4,000 ml of plasma were replaced. Subsequently, an average of 8,000 ml/day were removed and replaced. This patient, who had been transfused extensively during the 14 months of chemotherapy that preceded this study, had rather severe allergic reactions to the plasma during the first 2 days, including urticarial rashes, chills, and fever. No reactions occurred, however, after the 3rd day of plasma exchange. After 6 consecutive days of plasma exchange, at an average of over 90 percent efficiency, the series was interrupted temporarily to assess its safety. During the first 3 days of plasma exchange, the platelet count of the patient dropped from 170,000 to 80,000/mm³. The leukocyte count remained unchanged. Platelet transfusions were then started daily, to maintain his platelet count at above 100,000/mm³. Two days after the first series of plasma exchange was stopped, a noticeable but minimal reduction in the size of some of his lesions was observed. No further change occurred up to day 7, when the daily plasma exchanges were renewed. But 5 days later, or after a total of 11 exchanges, a definite decrease in the size of most of his lesions could be observed (Fig. 12-3). The plasma exchanges were continued for a total of 18 days, with small but definite further decreases in the size of the lesions. At this point, the plasma exchanges were stopped. A month later the patient was seen again, and at that time the lesions had increased to slightly more than their original size. A series of 11 daily plasma exchanges was again carried out. A measurable decrease in the size of the lesions occurred by the 4th day, involving, again, the periphery of the lesion. No further change was observed until the 11th day, when the exchanges were again stopped. A third series of daily plasma exchanges was carried out a month later. At that time, the local

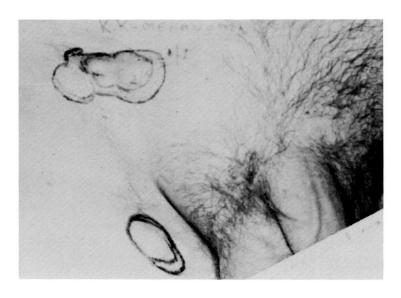

Figure 12-3. Size of melanoma lesions before (outside lines) and after (sinde lines) eleven daily plasma exchanges.

lesions had grown considerably beyond their original size but no other spread of the disease was found by extensive radiologic and scanning procedures. After 12 daily plasma exchanges only a minimal and questionable decrease of the lesions was observed, and the study was accordingly terminated.

During this clinical experiment we had the privilege of the assistance and collaboration of Lloyd Old, Edmund Klein, Karl E. Hellström, and Ronald Herberman. Serum and lymphocyte samples of the patient were supplied to the above investigators for studies of lymphocytic cytotoxicity and blocking factor levels. Additional testing on stored samples is in progress at the time of this writing.

It should be noted that just prior to starting this study this patient had strongly positive skin reactions to PPD, mumps, and candida antigens. These reactions remained unchanged throughout the 1st and the 2nd periods of plasmapheresis, but they were considerably weakened at the start of and by the end of the 3rd period of the experiment.

The apparent declining response as a result of the consecutive series of plasma exchanges complicates the interpretation of these observations. The initial clear-cut decrease in the size of the observable lesions could have been due to: (a) removal of the blocking system with a temporary reactivation of the cellular immune response, (b) the administration to the patient of factors (deblocking factor?) or blood components (complement?), as suggested by

Old's work (18), present in the normal plasma used for the exchange, or (c) an indirect stimulation of the patient's cellular immune response resulting from nonspecific stimuli (such as the heparinization, vasomotor changes, stress, or other unknown effects of the procedure itself). The declining effectiveness of the same procedure during the subsequent two time periods, however, seriously weakens the case for either one of the first two possibilities. The removal of blocking factor, or the administration of a normal blood component, if instrumental, were constant throughout the study. It is apparent, therefore, that further and more detailed studies of this nature are required, and those are accordingly in progress.

REFERENCES

1. Bertino, J. R., Donohue, D. M., Simmons, B., Gabrio, B. W., Silber, R., and Huennekens, F. M. The "induction" of dihydrofolic reductase activity in leukocytes and erythrocytes of patients treated with amethopterin. J. Clin. Invest., 42:466, 1963.

2. Burchenal, J. H., Babcock, G. M., Broquist, H. P., and Jukes, T. H. Prevention of chemotherapeutic effect of 4-amino-N^{10} methylpteroylglutamic acid on mouse leukemia by citrovorum factor. Proc. Soc. Exp. Biol. Med., 74:735, 1950.

3. Djerassi, I., Abir, E., Royer, G., and Treat, C. Long-term remissions in childhood acute leukemia. Use of infrequent infusions of methotrexate; supportive roles of platelet transfusions and citrovorum factor. Clin. Pediatr. (Phila.), 5:502, 1966.

4. Djerassi, I., Farber, S., Abir, E., and Neikirk, W. Continuous infusion of methotrexate in children with acute leukemia. Cancer, 20:233, 1967.

5. Djerassi, I., Kim, J. S., Ciesielka, W., Chaimongkol, B., and Suvansri, U. Separation and concentration of transfusable amounts of normal human monocytes. Transfusion, 15:353, 1973.

6. Djerassi, I., Kim, J. S., Mitrakul, C., Suvansri, U., and Ciesielka, W. Filtration–leukopheresis for separation and concentration of transfusable amounts of normal human granulocytes. J. Med. (Basel), 1:358, 1970.

7. Djerassi, I., Kim, J. S., and Suvansri, U. Harvesting of human monocytes (macrophages) as by-product of filtration–leukopheresis. Proc. AACR, 14:103, 1973.

8. Djerassi, I., Klein, E., Farber, S., and Toch, R. Transfusion of platelet concentrates to thrombocytopenic patients. Proc. VIIth Cong. Internat'l Soc. Blood Transfusions, Rome, 1958. Publisher, S. Karger, Basel, 1959, p. 1012.

9. Djerassi, I., Rominger, C. J., Kim, J. S., Turchi, J. Suvansri, U., and Hughes, D. Phase I study of high doses of methotrexate with citrovorum factor in patients with lung cancer. Cancer, 30:22, 1972.

10. Djerassi, I., Suvansri, I., and Kim, J. S. Long remissions in acute lymphocytic leukemia: Pulse methotrexate and a 4 drug combination. Proc. AACR, 13:94, 1972.

11. Djerassi, I., Suvansri, U., and Kim, J. S. Clinical effects of massive transfusion of normal granulocytes separated by filtration–leukopheresis. Presented at 25th Annual AABB Meeting, Washington, D.C., 1972.

12. Djerassi, I., Treat, C., Royer, G., and Carim, H. Management of childhood lympho-sarcoma and reticulum cell sarcoma with high dose intermittent methotrexate and citrovorum factor. Proc. AACR 9:18, 1968.

13. Goldin, A., Mantel, N., Venditti, J. M., and Greenhouse, S. W. An analysis of dose response for animals treated with aminopterin and citrovorum factor. J. Natl. Cancer Inst., 13:1463, 1953.

14. Greenwalt, T. et al. The clinical application of platelet transfusions. Transfusion, 6:62, 1966.

15. Hellström, I., Hellström, K. E., Evans, C. A., Heppner, G. H., Pierce, G. E., and Young, J. P. S. Serum-mediated protection of neoplastic cells from inhibition by lymphocytes immune to their tumor specific antigens. Proc. Natl. Acad. Sci. USA, 62:362, 1969.

16. Jaffe, N., Farber, S., Traggis, D., Geiser, C., Das, L., Kim, B., Frauenberger, G., and Djerassi, I. Favorable response of metastatic osteogenic sarcoma to pulse high dose methotrexate-citrovorum administration (HDMC). Proc. AACR, 13:27, 1972.

17. Jaffe, N., Traggis, D., Andonian, S., Chan, D., Sallan, S., Kim, T., and Frei, E., III. "Adjuvant" high dose methotrexate and citrovorum rescue (HDMC) following primary treatment of osteogenic sarcoma. Proc. AACR, 15:132, 1974.

18. Kassel, R. L., Old, L. J., Carswell, E. Z., Fiore, N. C., and Hardy, W. D., Jr. Serum-mediated leukemia cell destruction in AKR mice. Role of complement in the phenomenon. J. Exp. Med., 138:925, 1973.

19. LoBuglio, A. F. The monocyte: New concepts of function. New Engl. J. Med., 288:212, 1973.

Immunologic and Clinical Responses to Active Immunotherapy of Malignant Melanoma

D. L. Morton, S. H. Golub, H. L. Sulit, R. K. Gupta, F. R. Eilber, E. C. Holmes, and F. C. Sparks

Introduction

During the past seven years, evidence of the importance of the immune system in malignant melanoma has accumulated from numerous sources. Morton and Malmgren's initial description of tumor-associated antigens in human malignant melanomas using immunofluorescent techniques (11) was soon confirmed and extended by a number of independent investigators using a variety of immunologic techniques (8,10,14,16). The evidence to date implies that malignant melanomas contain tumor-specific antigens, which elicit the production of circulating humoral antibodies and cytotoxic lymphocytes in patients with melanoma.

Furthermore, there appears to be a correlation between the clinical status of the melanoma patients and the incidence of anti-melanoma antibodies in their sera. Patients with a localized melanoma are more likely to have antibody in their sera than those patients with disseminated disease. Also, the serum antibodies, in some patients who were observed frequently throughout their clinical course, disappeared as the disease progressed (10,12).

Evidence that manipulation of the immune system can favorably affect the clinical course of patients with malignant melanoma was suggested by our preliminary studies with BCG immunotherapy of malignant melanoma, reported in 1970 (9,10). A series of eight patients, with intradermal or subcutaneous metastases, were treated by intralesional injections of BCG vaccine, a powerful, nonspecific stimulant of the immune system. Approximately 90 percent of the melanoma nodules directly injected with BCG regressed in the patients who were immunologically competent, as measured by their ability to display delayed cutaneous hypersensitivity to dinitrochlorobenzene (DNCB) or tuberculin. Moreover, the nodules at sites distant from the BCG inoculation also regressed in approximately 20 percent of the patients who were immunologically competent.

Fundamental Aspects of Neoplasia,
edited by A. Arthur Gottlieb, Otto J. Plescia, and David H. L. Bishop.
© 1975 by Springer-Verlag New York Inc.

These observations of the effectiveness of immunotherapy in malignant melanoma by intralesional injections of BCG were soon confirmed by a number of investigators including Nathanson (15), Pinsky (17), and Siegler (18). The complete regression rates in all of these series were remarkably constant at 15 to 25 percent.

During the past 7 years, we have treated 151 melanoma patients by active specific or nonspecific immunotherapy. This chapter will summarize our observations on the clinical and immunologic response to immunotherapy in these patients.

Methods

The patients included in this study were seen by the authors in the Surgery Branch of the National Cancer Institute, from 1967 to 1970, or by clinicians in the Division of Oncology, Department of Surgery, UCLA School of Medicine, from 1971 to 1974. The patients selected for immunotherapy had documented recurrent melanoma, known residual disease, or a high risk of recurrence. All patients gave informed consent for experimental immunotherapy.

Each patient was extensively evaluated to establish the stage of the disease as thoroughly as possible before immunotherapy was started. This evaluation included a complete history and physical examination, liver function tests, X-ray films of the chest, metastatic bone series, and radioisotopic scans of the bone, brain, and liver. X-ray films of the chest and liver function tests were obtained at 3-month intervals, and repeat liver scans at 6-month intervals, or more frequently, as the clinical situation dictated.

Immunologic Evaluation

Skin testing. Immunologic evaluations of all patients were carried out by skin testing prior to immunotherapy. Each patient was sensitized using the method of Eilber and Morton by applying 2,000 μg of DNCB, dissolved in 0.1 ml of acetone, topically to the medial aspect of the arm (4). A challenge dose of 100 μg of DNCB was applied on the day of sensitization, and doses of 100, 50, and 25 μg were applied to the ipsilateral forearm 14 days after sensitization. After an additional 48 hr, the skin tests were examined and graded. Reactions were quantitated by a hypersensitivity score determined by the smallest amount of DNCB that elicited a positive hypersensitivity over one-half of the area of the test site. The patient was considered DNCB positive if the delayed hypersensitivity reaction was present at the 100-μg site.

At the time of DNCB challenge, each patient was also tested for delayed cutaneous hypersensitivity to four common microbial recall antigens. The antigens were mumps (Lilly, 2 units), PPD (Connaught, 5 units intermediate strength), Varidase (Lederle, 10 units), and Monilia antigen (Hollister-Stier, 2 units). All antigens were applied as 0.1 ml intradermal injections in the forearm contralateral to the DNCB test. A response of greater than 5 mm of induration was considered positive.

In vitro studies. Humoral anti-melanoma antibody levels of patients' serial serum samples were monitored by the complement-fixation test of Eilber and Morton (5), which had been modified to a microtechnique as described by Colombani et al. (2). Human umbilical cord serum (fresh) was used as the source of complement. All appropriate complement-fixation test controls were included with each test. Antigens were prepared from allogeneic melanoma (line M.D.) and fibroblast cell lines. The cells were harvested, washed three times with 20 volumes of veronal-buffered saline (pH 7.2), and suspended in the buffer (20 percent v/v). The suspension was frozen ($-180°C$) and thawed ($37°C$) twice, sonicated, and stored at $-180°C$. Melanoma antigen was used at a 1:64 dilution; normal fibroblast was used at a 1:6 dilution.

Experiments on cell-mediated reactions were performed with Ficoll–Isopaque purified lymphocytes from heparinized peripheral blood samples. All lymphocyte samples were stored by a freezing process that maintained full activity in the assays employed, and the samples were tested on one occasion after collection of all the samples. This approach was utilized in order to minimize experimental variation. Details of the methods of preparation, freezing, and testing the lymphocytes were described elsewhere in detail by Golub et al. (6).

Two assays were used to monitor the lymphocyte-mediated reactions of the patient: lymphocyte blastogenesis and lymphocyte-mediated cytotoxicity. For the blastogenesis assay, the microtest described in detail by Thurman *et al.* (20) was employed. Lymphocytes were placed in the wells of a Microtest II Falcon Plastics plate in 0.1-ml aliquots, at a concentration of 2×10^5/well. Stimulants were added in an additional 0.1 ml; the plate was then incubated for five days, pulsed with 0.5 μc of [^{3}H]thymidine well, and harvested on day 6. The stimulants employed were Concanavalin A (Miles, 1 μg/well), PPD (Parke-Davis, 1 μg/well), and pooled allogeneic normal lymphocytes for mixed lymphocyte culture (MLC) testing. The MLC stimulator pool was derived from 16 normal donors, representing over 20 HL-A specificities and was mitomycin-treated and added at a ratio of 1:2 responder:stimulator cells in the assay. Data in all the blastogenesis assays were expressed as average $\log_{10}$ of quadruplicate samples.

For investigations of lymphocyte-mediated cytotoxicity, we utilized the microcytotoxicity assay described by Cohen et al. (1). In this test, target tumor cells were labeled with ^{125}I-iododeoxyuridine (IDU), exposed to lymphocytes from the test subject, and the dead target cells were then removed by washing. The counts per minute (cpm) retained thereby reflected the number of surviving target cells. Target cells employed in our assays were several melanoma-derived lines established in culture by Hector L. Sulit (the UCLA Division of Oncology). Cytotoxicity was assessed in the presence of the patient's own serum or in the presence of normal pooled AB serum. Cytotoxicity was expressed as a survival fraction (SF) derived by the formula:

$$SF = \frac{\text{average cpm retained in wells with lymphocytes}}{\text{average cpm retained in wells in absence of lymphocytes}}$$

Thus, a lower figure represents a higher degree of cytotoxicity.

Immunotherapy

The method of BCG administration, by intratumor injection, has been previously described (11). Briefly, direct injection of intracutaneous and subcutaneous malignant melanoma nodules was performed, using 0.1 to 0.5 ml of Glaxo strain BCG for each lesion.

Systemic immunotherapy was begun for patients with Stage II melanoma from 3 to 6 weeks following the operative procedure and involved (a) BCG alone (Tice strain, Chicago Research Laboratories) given by the tine technique adjacent to each axilla and groin at weekly intervals for 1 year, biweekly for 6 months, and then monthly thereafter or (b) BCG plus allogeneic melanoma cells (24 of 67 Stage II patients). In the latter procedure, the BCG was given by the tine technique and 1×10^8 autologous irradiated or allogeneic tissue culture melanoma cells were injected separately at each time interval.

The BCG was administered alone or as an adjuvant mixed with tumor cell vaccine to patients with Stage III disease following resection of gross disease at distant metastatic sites. The surgical procedures employed included multiple pulmonary resections (7 patients), small bowel resections (4 patients), splenectomy (1 patient), lymphadenectomy at a site distant from the draining lymph nodes (10 patients), resection of a cerebral metastasis (1 patient), and excision of distant bulky subcutaneous tumor nodules (16 patients). Surgical procedures in these patients were palliative and designed to lower the tumor burden to make immunotherapy more effective.

Recurrence and survival rates were analyzed by the actuarial life table method in order to include all patients treated to date (3). The horizontal axis on these graphs represents the proportion of patients free of recurrence or who survived at each point in time. The number of patients who were free of recurrence or who survived versus the number of patients at risk is given on the graphs at each point.

Results

Immunologic Response to Immunotherapy

Analyses of the data from *in vitro* assays of the immunologic response to immunotherapy and their correlation with clinical course are not complete at the present time. But, sufficient data have been accumulated to draw some preliminary conclusions.

Serial skin testing reveals that most patients become tuberculin positive within 3 weeks after the initiation of BCG therapy, regardless of the mode of administration. The response to tuberculin and DNCB following immunotherapy tends to correlate with the clinical course in most patients. For example, patients who initially respond to these antigens often respond less well or become anergic with the development of recurrent disease and increasing tumor burden. Conversely, patients who are weak responders initially usually react more strongly with successful control of their disease following immunotherapy.

The results of the *in vitro* assays of the immune response to immunotherapy have not correlated with the clinical course in all patients. Interpretation of the results of these assays are further complicated by the responses to foreign HL-A antigens elicited in patients immunized with allogeneic melanoma cell lines. Such allograft responses can be confused with true, melanoma-specific response.

The data available at the present time can best be summarized by giving examples of results from *in vitro* assays of two patients:

G.M., a 56-year-old white male, had an excisional biopsy in 1965 of a benign pigmented lesion of the right anterior chest wall. A diagnosis of malignant melanoma could not be made. In January of 1973, he developed palpable axillary lymph nodes, and underwent a bilateral axillary node dissection. In the right axilla, 21 of 32 lymph nodes excised contained melanoma; no tumor was found in the left axillary nodes. Postoperatively, he received weekly immunotherapy with BCG, plus an allogeneic tumor cell vaccine.

He remained free of disease until August 1973, when he developed painless hematuria. Histopathologic examination of a small amount of tissue passed per urethra revealed metastatic malignant melanoma and cystoscopy revealed melanoma nodules in the bladder. One ampoule of BCG was injected into the base of the mass and into the pigmented tumor, through a cystoscopic needle.

Seven days after the injection, the patient again underwent cystoscopy. At this time, the previously described lesion was completely absent; in its place there was a 2-mm area of inflammation. Several biopsies proved this new area to be active granulomatous inflammation. No tumor was found. Exploratory laparotomy subsequently revealed no evidence of intra-abdominal metastatic tumor, and a segmental bladder resection was performed. The mass was very firm and involved all layers of the bladder wall. Histopathologic examination revealed granulomatous inflammation consistent with BCG treatment. No tumor was found. The patient has remained free of disease for 9 months.

The results of the complement-fixation studies on serial serum samples from this patient are summarized in Figure 13-1. Sera were tested against an allogeneic melanoma cell line from tissue culture and its normal fibroblast control, which differed from the melanoma cell line with which the patient had been immunized.

Following node dissection, the anti-melanoma antibody titer declined progressively for 8 weeks. But 4 weeks after the initiation of BCG therapy, the antibody level increased sharply (eightfold) and remained at this level for about 11 weeks. During the next 2 months, the antibody level rapidly declined; the bladder lesion was also noted at this time. Intralesional BCG therapy restored a high antibody level. None of the serum samples reacted against the

Figure 13-1. Humoral anti-melanoma antibody titers in serial serum samples from patient G.M. Serum samples were tested for complement-fixing antibodies (●) against an antigen derived from a melanoma tissue culture cell line and (○) against an antigen extracted from a tissue culture of normal skin from a melanoma patient.

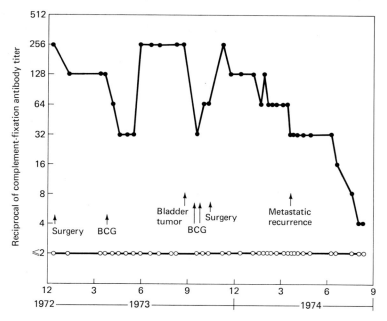

normal fibroblast antigen, which was used at a concentration 10 times that of the melanoma antigen. Thus, it is unlikely that the antibody being measured was directed against normal HL-A antigens in the melanoma cell line used as the source of the melanoma antigen.

The results of the blastogenesis assays are summarized in Figure 13-2. The response to the mitogen ConA was quite stable, with a slight trend toward greater incorporation after treatment. The response of the patient's lymphocytes in MLC, or in the unstimulated control cultures, fluctuated somewhat around the time of the intralesional BCG therapy, and a slight trend toward decreased values was observed. Additional studies with the mitogens phytohemagglutinin and pokeweed mitogen (not depicted in Fig. 13-2) also showed a very stable pattern over this time period. The only stimulant that displayed any notable change over the period of testing was PPD. The response to PPD showed a clear conversion from unresponsive, prior to treatment, to a strong positive blastogenesis response, several weeks after therapy. The response to streptokinase–streptodornase (not shown) remained negative throughout this period, indicating the specificity of the response to PPD.

Lymphocyte samples were tested for cytotoxicity against MLA 14 melanoma cells in the presence of the patient's serum (taken on the same date as the lymphocyte samples), and were separately tested for cytotoxicity in the presence of normal serum. These results are depicted in Figure 13-3. The lymphocytes were clearly cytotoxic against melanoma cells, as typified by the activity against MLA 14 target cells. Cytotoxicity in normal serum and in the patient's serum was usually the same, except for some decreased activity on the same sample drawn prior to therapy. This suggests that the serum may have contained some "blocking factor" at the time that the tumor was growing progressively. The cytotoxicity against MLA 14 showed a slight decline during therapy, with a sharp increase after the completion of therapy while the tumor was regressing,

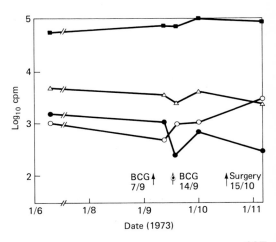

Figure 13-2. Serial blastogenesis studies with lymphocytes from patient G.M. as follows: (●) control lymphocytes not stimulated *in vitro*; experimental samples stimulated with (■) 1 μg/ culture of ConA, (○) 1 μg/culture of PPD, or (△) in MLC with mitomycin C-treated allogeneic lymphocytes.

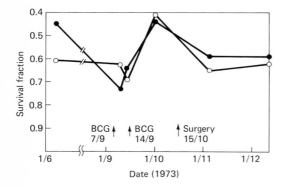

Figure 13-3. Serial cytotoxicity studies with lymphocytes from patient G.M. Lymphocytes were tested for cytotoxic affect on a melanoma target cell in the presence of (●) pooled normal serum or (○) G.M. serum.

and, finally, a return to pre-therapy levels. Activity against two other melanoma-derived target cells was quite similar to the pattern seen with MLA 14.

The cell-mediated immune response of another patient to immunotherapy with BCG alone is summarized in Figures 13-4 and 13-5. This patient (R.C.), a 28-year-old male with melanoma metastatic to the regional lymph nodes, had been placed on weekly BCG adjuvant immunotherapy following lymphadenectomy. The lymphocyte samples included one drawn just prior to surgery, two samples from the postoperative period, and five samples taken at intervals during BCG therapy. All samples were frozen and tested on the one occasion. Blastogenesis was tested with stimulation induced by ConA, PWM, PHA, PPD, and MLC with pooled allogeneic lymphocytes. Data are presented as log_{10} cpm of incorporated [^{3}H]thymidine. During the immediate postoperative period, the patient's lymphocytes showed some loss of responsiveness to mitogens; the decline in ConA and PWM response was more dramatic than to PHA. All responses recovered to the approximate preoperative levels 3 weeks postsurgery, when the patient was placed on BCG therapy. Prior to the initiation of BCG therapy, none of the samples were reactive to PPD; after the initiation of immunotherapy, however, the *in vitro* response to this antigen changed to positive. The response to PPD remained much weaker than the response to the mitogens, and MLC response was slightly depressed at the beginning of BCG therapy, but soon returned to preoperation levels.

In another experiment (Fig. 13-5), the same lymphocyte samples were tested for cytotoxicity against an allogeneic melanoma cell line (MLA 10) and a skin fibroblast line from the same tumor cell donor (MLA 10F). When the lymphocytes were tested in the presence of normal serum, significant cytotoxicity was observed against the tumor cell line but not against the normal fibroblasts. Cytotoxicity decreased slightly in the postoperative period and again after the start of the BCG therapy, but it was difficult to determine if these

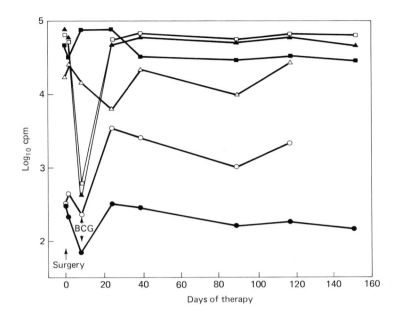

Figure 13-4. Retrospective blastogenesis study of lymphocytes from patient R.C. All samples collected over about a 5-month period were tested in one experiment. Samples were tested for responses to (■) ConA, (×) PWM, (+) PHA, (○) PPD, and (△) in MLC; (●) control indicates lymphocytes cultured in the absence of any added stimulant. Results are expressed as average $\log_{10}$ cpm of [³H]thymidine incorporated.

slight changes were biologically significant. Samples of the patient's serum, drawn at the same time as the lymphocytes, did not appear to show any significant blocking effect. There was a slight indication of some blocking activity in the first serum sample taken prior to resection of the tumor. Studies with other patients' sera, however, have shown significant blocking effects in this assay.

Immunotherapy by Intratumor Injections

Forty-five patients were treated with intratumor injections of BCG vaccine for their metastatic disease. The results are summarized in Table 13-1.

Patients with intradermal metastases who were treated with intratumor injections of BCG were most likely to respond to treatment. Table 13-1 gives the results in 36 patients treated during the past 7 years. In this time, 14 patients had in-transit metastases in the same extremity as the primary region, and 22 patients had distant metastases beyond the primary region. A total of

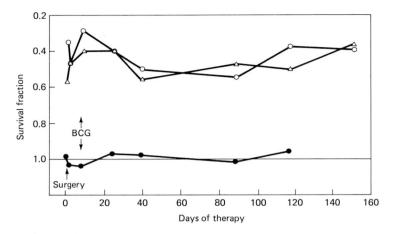

Figure 13-5. Retrospective cytotoxity study of lymphocytes from patient R.C. Lymphocytes were tested against an allogeneic melanoma target cell, MLA 10, in the presence of (○) normal pooled human AB serum or (△) patient R.C.'s serum from the same date as the lymphocyte sample; (●) lymphocytes tested in normal serum against normal skin fibroblasts, MLA 10F, from the same donor as the tumor target cell line.

754 melanoma nodules were injected in these 36 patients and 684, or 91 percent, of the injected lesions underwent complete regression. In addition, in 6 of these 36 patients, or 17 percent, there was regression of uninjected melanoma nodules. A total of 22 uninjected nodules regressed in these 6 patients. Following BCG immunotherapy, 11 of the 36 patients, or 31 percent, remained free of disease in a 6- to 74-month period.

We could correlate three factors with response to BCG immunotherapy: (a) the location of the metastases, (b) the amount of tumor present, and (c) the

Table 13-1 Results of Intratumor Injections of BCG[a]

Location of metastases	Intracutaneous[b]	Subcutaneous and/or visceral[b]
Number of patients	36	9
Proportion of directly injected metastatic lesions regressing	684/754 (91%)	8/26 (31%)
Patients with regression of uninjected nodules	6/36 (17%)	0/9 (0%)
No evidence of disease	11/36 (31%)	0/9 (0%)

[a] Follow-up from 6 to 74 months.

[b] Numbers in parentheses are percentages.

190

immunocompetence of the patient. Patients with subcutaneous or visceral metastatic lesions had a poor response to BCG immunotherapy. The results in nine of these patients are summarized in Table 13-1. Only 31 percent of the 26 lesions directly injected with BCG regressed. Complete regression of uninjected lesions has not been observed in patients with subcutaneous or visceral disease, and no patient has remained completely free of disease. One patient with liver metastases, however, appeared to have a temporary remission following injection of BCG into subcutaneous metastatic nodules in the neck. This 3-month remission was manifested by weight gain, improved performance status, decrease in the size of liver metastases as measured by liver scan, and improvement in liver function tests.

The immunocompetence of the melanoma patient, as judged by delayed cutaneous hypersensitivity to DNCB at the time of initial testing, or the development of a positive tuberculin reaction and acquisition of a positive response to DNCB following immunotherapy, correlated well with response to BCG immunotherapy. Most patients whose lesions regressed upon direct injection with BCG and all of those whose non-injected lesions regressed were immunocompetent upon initial testing. Also, all of the few patients whose lesions regressed upon direct injection, and who were initially DNCB negative, converted to positive following intralesional BCG.

Sequential biopsies of tumor nodules were obtained in many patients for histopathologic studies following immunotherapy. Prior to immunotherapy, biopsy usually showed minimal mononuclear collections adjacent to the melanoma nodule but no infiltration among the tumor cells themselves. After BCG injection, an intense lymphocytic and mononuclear infiltration usually occurred within 3 to 4 weeks, with destruction of all viable melanoma cells within the melanoma nodule. Serial biopsies of uninjected melanoma nodules following BCG immunotherapy at distant sites frequently showed an increasing mononuclear infiltrate.

BCG Immunotherapy as an Adjunct to Surgical Resection in Patients with Stage III Disseminated Malignant Melanoma

As a result of the experience summarized above, we concluded that BCG administered by intratumor injection did have immunotherapeutic activity in patients with advanced disease when the amount of tumor in any one site was small and when the disease was limited to the skin. But BCG clearly had little immunotherapeutic activity in patients with bulky disease or in patients with visceral metastases. Therefore, we investigated the possibility of resecting the large visceral and subcutaneous metastases and providing postoperative adjunctive immunotherapy with BCG alone or BCG with autologous irradiated tumor cells or cultured allogeneic melanoma cells.

Thirty-nine patients have now been treated in this manner. The results, summarized in Figures 13-6 and 13-7, compare the number of patients free of disease and their survival rates to a similar group of patients reported from M. D. Anderson Hospital (7). Although this comparison may be questioned, the results of such treatment in patients with Stage III disease are surprisingly good. Almost 40 percent of these patients are free of disease at 2 years.

Similarly, the survival rates in this group of Stage III melanoma patients who received immunotherapy are higher on the curve at all points than those in other series (9). It is obvious that the majority of these patients were followed for less than 2 years, and, therefore, no statistical analysis of survival rates can be made. Furthermore, the use of historic controls for survival may become invalid because improvement in chemotherapy may prolong survival in patients with recurrent disease. Nevertheless, the fact that the life table curve for both recurrence and survival remains higher at every point in time in immunotherapy patients suggests that adjunctive immunotherapy has helped these patients.

When the different immunotherapy groups were analyzed, no differences were noted between those who received BCG alone or BCG in tumor cell vaccine. But, the number of patients treated with allogeneic tumor cell vaccine was small, compared to the total number of patients treated. Thus, it is not possible at this time to state definitely whether the addition of allogeneic

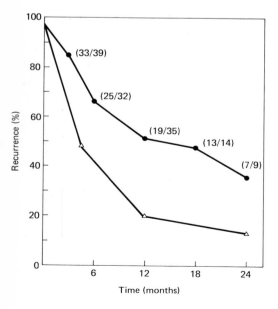

Figure 13-6. Recurrence rate: Stage III melanoma. Percentage of patients free of recurrent melanoma following surgical resection of all gross disease and postoperative adjuvant immunotherapy. Numbers in parentheses indicate number of patients who remained free of disease to number of patients at risk of recurrence during that time interval; (●) UCLA immunotherapy (39 patients), (△) M. D. Anderson Hospital (24 patients).

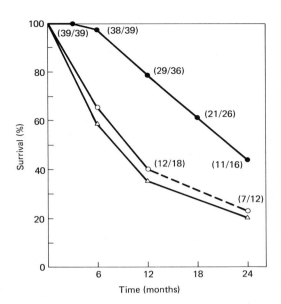

Figure 13-7. Survival rate: Stage III melanoma. Percentage of patients surviving after surgical resection of all gross disease and postoperative adjuvant immunotherapy. Numbers in parentheses indicate number of patients surviving to number of patients at risk of dying during that time interval; (●) UCLA immunotherapy (39 patients), (○) Ellis Fischel (30 patients), (△) M. D. Anderson Hospital (24 patients).

melanoma cells to BCG alters either the recurrence rate or the survival rate, compared to treatment with BCG alone.

BCG Immunotherapy as an Adjunct to Surgery in Patients with Stage II Malignant Melanoma

Having demonstrated the effectiveness of BCG immunotherapy in patients with advanced malignant melanoma, in 1970 we began to investigate its possible usefulness as an adjunct to primary surgery for regional melanoma. Patients who had metastases to regional nodes were given immunotherapy following regional lymphadenectomy with BCG alone or BCG mixed with allogeneic melanoma cells. This study began as a nonrandomized Phase I trial to determine if BCG could be administered in this manner with an acceptable toxicity and to look for evidence of therapeutic effect. The results are depicted in Figure 13-8. The overall tumor-free rate for the entire group of 67 patients is lower at all points in time when compared to 34 patients seen at UCLA during the same time interval who did not receive BCG immunotherapy. Although this was not a strictly randomized protocol, patients were not selected for immunotherapy on any basis except distance from UCLA and their willingness to participate in an investigational protocol. Note that the recurrence rate is also lower in the BCG immunotherapy group than is that of a comparable group of patients treated by surgery alone, reported from the M. D. Anderson Hospital (7).

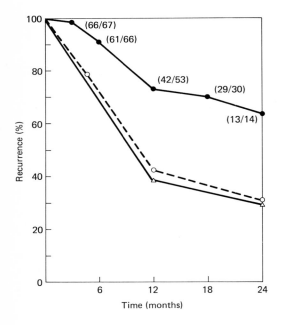

Figure 13-8. Recurrence rate: Stage II melanoma. Percentage of patients free of recurrent melanoma following regional lymphadenectomy alone or lymphadenectomy with postoperative immunotherapy. Numbers in parentheses indicate number of patients who remained free of disease to number of patients at risk of developing recurrence during that time interval; (●) UCLA immunotherapy (67 patients), (○) UCLA simultaneous controls (34 patients), (△) M. D. Anderson Hospital (54 patients).

Complications of BCG Immunotherapy

We have summarized the complications of BCG immunotherapy in cancer patients in an earlier publication (19). Nevertheless, these complications should be restated to emphasize the potential danger of this type of therapy. Intratumor injection with BCG frequently resulted in fever, chills, localized abscesses, and sinuses that drained for long periods (up to 3 months). Regional lymphadenitis was frequent. Occasionally a systemic infection occurred with an associated granulomatous hepatitis. Although not observed in our series, fatal anaphylactoid reactions have been reported following repeated administrations of large doses of BCG vaccine. Because of these complications, we recommended much smaller doses of BCG for those patients who had been previously sensitized to BCG or who are known to be tuberculin positive. Pretreatment with antihistamines and aspirin, prior to and for several days following the intralesional injections, appeared to decrease toxicity. Symptoms that persisted despite this regimen were treated with Isoniazid (300 mg daily). Patients who had marked malaise and an influenza-like syndrome following BCG therapy generally responded quickly to Isoniazid. By careful adherence to these principles of management, we did decrease toxicity following repeated intratumor injections of BCG.

In contrast to intratumor injections with BCG vaccine, the administration of BCG by the intradermal multiple puncture tine technique alone or of BCG mixed with tumor cell vaccine was usually tolerated very well with a low incidence of hepatic dysfunction and only mild fever and malaise for short periods following vaccination. No instances of anaphylactoid reactions or marked toxicity have been associated with this method of administration. Some patients, however, developed hyperplasia of the regional lymph nodes draining the vaccination sites, which required biopsy to differentiate the hyperplasia from metastatic melanoma.

Enhancement of tumor growth is another possible complication of BCG immunotherapy. Enhancement has clearly been demonstrated in some animal tumor host systems in which large doses of BCG are administered prior to or shortly after tumor transplantation. Furthermore, repeated administration of BCG has been shown to depress cellular immunity in both man (Klein, personal communication) and animals, as measured by delayed cutaneous hypersensitivity reactions to certain common skin test antigens. The conditions for BCG enhancement of tumor growth and immunosuppression vary somewhat with different tumor host systems, but they appear to be dose dependent. For these reasons, caution must be exercised in clinical trials in which large doses of BCG are administered repeatedly for long periods. Therefore, careful monitoring of the immune response should be carried out simultaneously so that any immunosuppressive effects can be detected at once in these patients.

Discussion

We must await further studies of the immune response to immunotherapy to better define the *in vitro* immune assays that are the most useful in monitoring response to immunotherapy. But, these studies do provide some confirmation of the effectiveness of BCG immunotherapy. The blastogenesis data indicate no general, or nonspecific, alteration in immunocompetence during the period of treatment. This is consistent with our findings in a number of other melanoma patients in whom BCG immunotherapy was not generally associated with dramatic alterations in responsiveness to mitogens (Golub and Morton; unpublished data). Patient response to PPD did improve after intralesional therapy, however. It was somewhat surprising that one of our patients (G.M.) was unresponsive to PPD *in vitro* before intralesional therapy even though he had received previous BCG doses and was clearly responsive to PPD by delayed cutaneous hypersensitivity. The improvement in *in vitro* response to PPD may be related to the different route of administration.

The cytotoxicity studies suggest some fluctuations of cytotoxic activity during the period of intralesional therapy. A transient decline in activity was also seen in the number of T lymphocytes, as determined by spontaneous sheep cell rosettes. Whether these fluctuations are relevant to the BCG-induced regression

195

is difficult to determine. The low to nonexistent levels of blocking factors suggest a limited tumor burden in this patient, and the blocking factors, cytotoxicity, and blastogenic responses did not seem to be adversely affected by the therapy. In general, cell-mediated reactions do not indicate any major systemic effects resulting from BCG therapy alone.

The complement-fixation studies, however, showed a definite correlation between BCG therapy and anti-melanoma antibody level. After a lag of 2 to 4 weeks after the start of BCG therapy, the antibody level increased significantly. Similar rises in antibody levels after BCG therapy have been observed in other cancer patients. (Gupta and Morton, unpublished). During the period when the antibody levels were highest (1:256), the patient was free of clinically detectable disease, and his blocking factors, cytotoxicity, and blastogenic responses were not adversely affected by the therapy. This suggests that humoral anti-melanoma antibodies were of a protective, rather than an enhancing, nature. Furthermore, recurrence of the disease in the bladder was associated with a sharp decline in the antibody titer (Fig. 13-5). Intralesional injection of BCG again elevated the antibody level. In view of these results, it appears that the complement-fixation test may be a useful technique in assessing the humoral immune responses to local immunotherapy.

The results of BCG immunotherapy in patients in advanced stages of malignant melanoma are encouraging. Direct injection of BCG into intradermal metastasis of malignant melanoma appears to be a highly effective means of therapy, with 90 percent of the directly injected lesions destroyed and with 17 percent of the patients so treated showing a regression of uninjected nodules. This phenomenon was observed in patients with both regional and disseminated malignant melanomas. The fact that 32 percent of the patients remained free of recurrence for periods up to 6 years following initiation of immunotherapy is encouraging. These results indicate that there is not only a local effect with direct BCG injection into intracutaneous nodules but that, in some patients, a systemic effect is also achieved.

Patients with subcutaneous or visceral metastases did not respond as well as those with intradermal metastases. Temporary regression was noted in only 31 percent of the subcutaneous metastases injected with BCG, and all the patients in this group subsequently developed progressive disease. Rarely was there evidence of regression of uninjected or grossly visible visceral metastases in these patients. In general, patients with large bulky lesions or visceral metastases did not benefit significantly from the BCG immunotherapy alone. These disappointing results in this group of patients occurred early in our experience; more recently, we placed these patients on BCG immunotherapy following palliative surgical therapy to reduce tumor burden.

The reason for the differences in response between these two types of patients is not completely clear at this time. There are several possible explanations that deserve consideration, however. First, there may be some basic biologic differences between the behavior of malignant melanoma metastatic to skin and that involving the visceral organs, because it has been observed that response to chemotherapy is frequently better in patients with intradermal disease. But, these differences may be more quantitative than qualitative because patients who present intracutaneous disease almost invariably develop visceral metastases within the first year and eventually die of their disease. Thus, almost all of those patients with intradermal metastases who were treated with immunotherapy probably had microscopic subclinical metastatic lesions in their lungs and liver, which were not clinically detectable at the time of initial presentation, and which then regressed following intratumoral injections of BCG into their intracutaneous metastases.

Another possible explanation for the differences in response rate between these two groups of patients may relate to the immunocompetence of the host, since patients who are immunocompetent as judged by their ability to be sensitized to DNCB generally are more likely to respond to intratumor administration of BCG. There is increasing evidence that the lack of immunocompetence in melanoma patients is primarily a manifestation of tumor burden. This is compatible with the observation that the patients who are most frequently anergic, as judged by the hypersensitivity parameters, are those who have visceral and subcutaneous metastatic lesions. Therefore, it is not surprising that these patients did not respond as well to intratumor injections of BCG vaccine.

The correlation of nonspecific immunocompetence to tumor regression offers a clue to the mechanism of tumor regression in these patients. It would appear that BCG had no direct antitumor effect, since it did not cause tumor regression in patients who remained tuberculin negative following BCG therapy. Those patients who became tuberculin positive following BCG therapy, however, usually had regression of their melanoma nodules following direct injection of the nodules. This suggests that the antitumor effect was nonspecific, resulting from the induction of a delayed hypersensitivity reaction within the melanoma nodule. It is possible that the melanoma cells were destroyed by the immunologic reaction against the BCG-associated antigens as a result of an intense infiltration by lymphocytes and monocytes.

It is our opinion that intralesional BCG immunotherapy is the treatment of choice for patients with metastatic malignant melanoma limited to the skin. Up to 36 percent of these patients will have their disease controlled by this therapy alone, with much less toxicity than that associated with chemotherapy or regional perfusion for extremity lesions. Although heat perfusion for extremity melanomas may be equally effective, we reserve it for patients who fail to respond to intralesional BCG. Chemotherapy with imidazole carboximide alone or in combination with other chemotherapeutic agents has not had nearly the quality or frequency of complete responses that we have seen with intra-lesional BCG in this group of patients.

Attempts to improve the effectiveness of systemic BCG immunotherapy in Stage III melanoma patients with visceral metastases and large bulky sub-cutaneous metastases by lowering tumor burden with surgical resection fol-lowed by adjuvant immunotherapy with BCG alone, or BCG and autologous or allogeneic tumor cell vaccine, have been only partially effective. Clearly, some patients have benefited from this therapy program, but most patients have proceeded to recurrence and death. As a result, we believe that these patients should be managed by a combination of surgery to reduce tumor burden, chemotherapy to further lower tumor burden, and adjuvant immuno-therapy to maintain remission. It is hoped that this new combined modality approach will be more effective than the use of any single modality alone.

The most exciting area for future development concerns the possible use of BCG immunotherapy as an adjunct to the definitive surgical treatment of patients with Stage II malignant melanoma and a poor prognosis because of metastasis to the regional nodes. The natural history of this disease is such that, despite the surgical removal of all gross metastatic disease in the regional nodes, 60 to 70 percent of these patients have a recurrence of their disease within 2 years. Thus, patients with malignant melanoma and regional meta-stasis, in the majority of cases, have a local and regional manifestation of a systemic illness. Therefore, these patients are an ideal group in which to test the effectiveness of postsurgical immunotherapy based upon the principles of immune destruction of a limited number of subclinical metastases.

Our early results, using BCG immunotherapy as an adjunct to primary surgical therapy, are most encouraging and support the logic of this principle. Our results and those of others (7) suggest that the recurrence rate is lower and the survival rate greater for patients with Stage II melanoma treated with adjunctive BCG immunotherapy. The preliminary nature of these findings, however, must be stressed, since the length of follow-up evaluation of these patients is not sufficient to make a definite statistical statement concerning its effectiveness. Additionally, it must be pointed out that these patients were not chosen at random and therefore it is possible that an unknown bias intro-duced into their selection may have influenced the results. With our present knowledge, however, it does appear that BCG immunotherapy may be comple-mentary to surgery but only continued follow-ups of these patients can prove this hypothesis. We are now randomizing patients into properly stratified and prospective clinical trials to compare no additional therapy after surgery with postoperative adjuvant immunotherapy using BCG alone or BCG with allogeneic tumor cell vaccine.

Summary

We have studied 150 patients with malignant melanoma who have been treated with BCG immunotherapy alone or as an adjunct to surgical therapy. *In vitro* monitoring of the response to active immunotherapy was undertaken, utilizing a variety of assays for cell-mediated and humoral immunity. Lymphocyte blastogenesis studies revealed no significant alteration in general immunocompetence secondary to the therapy, except for an increased responsiveness to PPD. There was no evidence of the presence of blocking factors following immunotherapy, and cytotoxicity against allogeneic melanoma cells sharply increased after intralesional injection with BCG. Humoral anti-melanoma antibody levels, determined by complement fixation, usually rose immediately following immunotherapy, but fell with recurrence of disease despite continued immunotherapy.

We found that BCG immunotherapy as a single therapeutic modality administered by intratumor injections was extremely effective in patients with metastatic melanoma limited to the skin. Direct injection of intradermal metastases resulted in a 90 percent regression rate in the injected lesion, and 17 percent of the patients had regression of uninjected lesions at distant sites. Approximately 25 percent of these patients remained free of disease for periods of 1 to 6 years. Direct injections of BCG into nodules of patients with subcutaneous or visceral metastases resulted in a lower incidence of local control and no long-term survivors. Lack of response was associated with large tumor burden, lack of immune competence, and clinically detectable metastases to the lungs, liver, or brain. Attempts to improve the results of immunotherapy in these patients by palliative surgical resection of large metastatic lesions to lower tumor burden followed by BCG immunotherapy significantly improved the response, although many patients still developed recurrent disease.

Early results of a clinical trial, combining BCG immunotherapy with regional lymphadenectomy in patients with malignant melanoma metastatic to regional lymph nodes, have been encouraging. We report some very promising but non-definitive data, which suggest that postoperative adjuvant immunotherapy in selected patients appears to decrease the recurrence rate and increase survival rates in patients with this disease. Further controlled clinical trials are necessary to definitively elucidate the role of BCG immunotherapy in melanoma, however. Since BCG is only one of a number of potential immunologic adjuvants, we hope that even more effective adjunctive immunotherapy will be possible as further knowledge of the interatcions of cellular and humoral immunity is acquired.

ACKNOWLEDGMENTS

These investigations are supported by USPHS Grants CA 12582, CA 05252, CA 12285, NIH 0732001 CB 43852, and grants from the California Institute for Cancer Research, and the Surgical Services, Sepulveda VA Hospital.

REFERENCES

1. Cohen, A. M., Burdick, J. F., and Ketcham, A. S. Cell-mediated cytotoxicity: An assay using ^{125}I-Iododeoxyuridine labeled target cells. J. Immunol. 107:895, 1971.
2. Colombani, J., D'Amero, J., Gibb, B., Smith, G., and Svejgaard, A. International agreement on a microtechnique of platelet complement fixation (Pl. C. Fix.). Transplant. Proc., 3:121, 1971.
3. Cutler, S. J. and Ederer, F. Maximum utilization of the life table method in analyzing survival. J. Chronic Dis., 8:699, 1958.
4. Eilber, F. R. and Morton, D. L. Impaired immunologic reactivity and recurrence following cancer surgery. Cancer, 25:362, 1970.
5. Eilber, F. R. and Morton, D. L. Sarcoma-specific antigens: Detection by complement fixation with serum from sarcoma patients. J. Natl. Cancer Inst., 44: 651, 1970.
6. Golub, S. H., Sulit, H. L., and Morton, D. L. The use of viable frozen lymphocytes for studies in human tumor immunology. Transplant, 19:195, 1975.
7. Gutterman, J. U., Mavligit, G. McBride, C., Frei, E., III, Freireich, E. J., and Hersh, E. M. Active immunotherapy with BCG for recurrent malignant melanoma. Lancet, I:1208, 1973.
8. Hellström, I., Hellström, K. E., Sjogren, H. O., and Warner, G. A. Demonstration of cell-mediated immunity to human neoplasms of various histological types. Int. J. Cancer, 7:1, 1971.
9. Knutson, C. O., Hori, J. M., and Spratt, Jr., J. S. Melanoma. *In* Current Problems in Surgery. Chicago, Year Book Medical Publishers, 1971, pp. 1–55.
10. Lewis, M. G., Ikonopisov, R. L., Nairn, R. C., and Alexander, P. Tumor-specific antibodies in human malignant melanoma and their relationship to the extent of the disease. Br. Med. J., 1:547, 1969.
11. Morton, D. L., Malmgren, R. A., Holmes, E. C., and Ketcham, A. S. Demonstration of antibodies against human malignant melanoma by immunofluorescence. Surgery, 64:233, 1968.
12. Morton, D. L., Eilber, F. R., Malmgren, R. A., et al. Immunologic factors which influence response to immunotherapy in malignant melanoma. Surgery, 68:158, 1970.

13. Morton, D. L., Eilber, F. R., Joseph, W. L., et al. Immunologic factors in human sarcomas and melanomas: A rational basis for immunotherapy. Ann. Surg., 172:740, 1970.

14. Muna, N. M., Marcus, S., and Smart, C. Detection by immunofluorescence of antibodies specific for human malignant melanoma cells. Cancer, 23:88, 1969.

15. Nathanson, L. Regression of intradermal malignant melanoma after intralesional injection of BCG. Cancer Chemother. Rep., 56: 659, 1972.

16. Oettgen, H. F., Aoki, T., Old, L. J., Boyse, E. A., DeHarven, E., and Mills, G. M. Suspension culture of a pigment-producing cell line derived from a human malignant melanoma. J. Natl. Cancer Inst., 41:827, 1968.

17. Pinsky, C., Hisschant, G., and Oettgen, H. Treatment of malignant melanoma by intralesional injection of BCG. Proc. Am. Assoc. Cancer Res., 13:21, 1972.

18. Seigler, H. F., Shingleton, W. W., Metzgar, R. S., Buckley, C. E., Bergoc, P. M., Miller, D. S., Fetter, B. F., and Pauf, M. G., Nonspecific and specific immunotherapy in patients with melanoma. Surgery, 72:162, 1972.

19. Sparks, F. C., Silverstein, M. J., Hunt, J. S., Haskell, C. M., Pilch, Y. M., and Morton D. L. Complications of BCG immunotherapy in patients with cancer. New Engl. J. Med., 289:827, 1973.

20. Thurman, G. B., Strong, D. M., Ahmed, A., Green, S. S., Sell, K. W., Hartzman, R. J., and Bach, F. H. Human mixed lymphocyte cultures. Evaluation of a microculture technique utilizing the multiple automated sample harvester (MASH). Clin. Exp. Immunol., 15:289, 1973.

Viral Etiology of Human Osteosarcoma: Evidence Based on Response to Tumor-Specific Transfer Factor and on Immunoepidemiologic Studies

H. H. Fudenberg, V. S. Byers, and A. S. Levin

Introduction

On the basis of clinical observations more than a dozen years ago, we suggested that genetically determined immunologic deficiency was responsible for both "autoimmunity" and at least certain forms of neoplasia (6). We then studied patients with "acquired" (adult onset) agammaglobulinemia and infantile X-linked agammaglobulinemia and their first-degree relatives. A high incidence of "autoantibodies" (7), and of malignancy (Fudenberg, unpublished observations), was present in first-degree relatives of patients with "acquired" agammaglobulinemia (now termed "common variable immunodeficiency"), but not in first-degree relatives of infantile X-linked agammaglobulinemia patients.

Later, after delineation of the separate T and B systems for cellular and humoral immunity, respectively (2), our observation of a patient with long-standing thymoma, agammaglobulinemia, and rheumatoid arthritis (8), coupled with our observations that "acquired" agammaglobulinemia (Ac–aIg) is genetically determined (24), and that (Ac–aIg) patients late in the course of their disease develop deficient cellular immunity (4), led us to suggest that genetic defects in cellular immunity were responsible for the high incidence of neoplasia in such patients (9). We further postulated, having observed patients with recurrent staphylococcal infection with immune defects restricted only to staphylococci (3), that genetically determined defects in cellular immunity restricted to *only* one antigen ("selective defetcs") were a neecssary but not sufficient cause for human malignancy, at least those forms presumably associated with viral rather than chemical carcinogenesis (10).

Our experiments in neonatally thymectomized mice of the RF/Un strain produced results consistent with this concept, in that these animals developed renal disease indistinguishable from that of the NZB/W strain, and from that

Fundamental Aspects of Neoplasia,
edited by A. Arthur Gottlieb, Otto J. Plescia, and David H. L. Bishop.
© 1975 by Springer-Verlag New York Inc.

of patients with lupus (18). Of those animals surviving the disease, a significant percentage developed malignancy (19). Continuous administration of interferon-inducing agents prevented renal disease and the malignancies (20). Consequently, we stated in 1966 that "predisposition to autoimmune diseases (and to neoplasia) merely reflects genetically determined selective immune defects to one or another microorganism" (11), presumably a virus (12), and, in 1968, that such genetic predisposition involves defective cellular immunity for one or another virus (12,20), since the T cell system is responsible for protection against most viruses and the B cell system against most bacteria (13) (especially such classic microorganisms as *Pneumococcus, Meningococcus*, and *Streptococcus*).

To our knowledge, direct proof that viruses cause human tumors is lacking despite the strong inferential evidence (e.g., reverse transcriptase associated with certain human tumors) (17). In view of the strong evidence for the viral etiology of osteosarcoma (OS) in mice and other species (5,30), and reports of familial clustering of this tumor in humans (21), this seemed to be the best tumor to use in a search for evidence of a viral etiology of these tumors by immunologic means. Two immunologic approaches were used: (a) stimulation of human OS patients with OS-specific transfer factor and (b) epidemiologic studies of patient contacts in a search for T cell-mediated immunity to OS. Transfer factor directly or indirectly (perhaps via macrophages), affects the function of T lymphocytes (26–28,32), which (as stated above) protect us against infection from most viruses, but does not affect B cell function. Thus, demonstration of the efficacy of OS-specific transfer factor, either *in vivo* or *in vitro*, in patients with OS would provide evidence that any infectious microorganism involved in the etiology of this human tumor would be viral rather than bacterial.

Further, nonspecific transfer factor was shown by us to be useful in prophylaxis and treatment of generalized T cell immunodeficiency (26–28,32), and *Candida*-specific transfer factor therapy has proved dramatic in certain patients with chronic mucocutaneous candidiasis (14,28,31), one form of which is presumably associated with familial genetic defects in T cell function (e.g., auto-antibodies) (34). It therefore seemed reasonable for us to attempt to treat OS patients, after removal of the primary tumor by amputation, with OS-specific transfer factor. We chose this tumor as a starting point because the life expectancy of such patients is very short (approximately 85 percent die within 18 months despite irradiation or hormonal therapy or conventional chemotherapy) (23), the spontaneous remission rate is less than 1 percent, thus eliminating the need for a large number of control patients and because of the animal and human familial evidence cited earlier.

Before initiating the epidemiologic studies, to be described, and the transfer factor therapy, it was necessary to have a quantitative assay for T cell function. A test, the "active T rosette-forming cell test," was devised (35), and studies showed a significant reduction of "active" rosette-forming cells (E-Tₐ) in both cancer and viral disease without a reduction of B cells (36). We further identified T cells as the cells that destroy at least certain human tumor cells *in vitro*, using both the Hellström technique (32) and photomicrographs of tumors infiltrated with human lymphocytes, classified as B or T on the basis of membrane immunofluorescence and their ability to form rosettes with sheep red blood cells.

Methods

Epidemiologic Studies

Patients with OS, hypernephroma, and other tumors of presumably viral origin, as well as their close contacts (first-degree relatives; guardians; household contacts; and spouse, in one patient over 20), were tested for the ability of their lymphocytes to kill tumor cells of given types. The cell lines were cultured *in vitro*, the 12th to 20th passages being used,* and the tumor cell suspensions were free of contaminating fibroblasts. At least three different tumor lines were used for each test; the control cells used were (a) matching fibroblasts and (b) cell lines from other types of tumors. Killing was measured by ^{51}chromium release from the labeled cells after addition of donor lymphocytes in standard media, standard lymphocyte/target cell ratios, and 3-hour incubations. (The method is illustrated diagrammatically in Figure 14-1.) A cytotoxicity index was computed, using water lysis as 100 percent chromium release and spontaneous lysis (background) as 0 percent release (29).

Transfer Factor Therapy

Dialyzable transfer factor (TFd) was prepared by a modification of Lawrence's method (25). Factor obtained from 10^9 leukocytes was termed "one unit" of TFd, with TFd preparations made from the leukocytes of two types of donors: (a) those with high (50 to 95 percent) cytotoxicity indices against OS lines and (b) from individuals without such reactivity who were strongly positive for PPD, coccidiomycosis, or antigens measurable by routine methods of cellular immunology ("nonspecific TF"). Control subjects received no TF, test subjects received injections of either OS-specific (OS-TFd), nonspecific (NS-TFd), TFd or courses involving several injections of the specific TF, then NS-TF, or, conversely, NS-TF, followed by OSS-TFd.

* There is no difference in results using the lowest, the highest, and intermediate passage levels; thus excluding genetic drift.

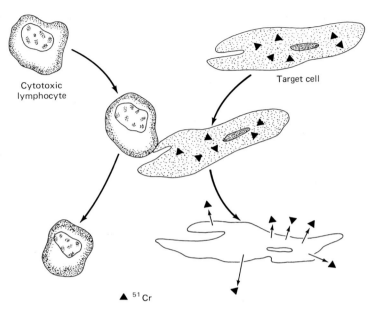

Figure 14-1. Schematic representation of the lymphocyte-mediated cytotoxicity text.

Patients were monitored by cytotoxicity index, by active and total T cells, and by monthly chest tomograms.

Results

Epidemiologic Studies

The cytotoxicity index results in any single individual were remarkably constant over long time periods; for example, the index in one individual studied periodically over a 16-month period varied from 68 to 72 (29). Results in replicate cultures done simultaneously were almost indistinguishable. Approximately 20 percent of the close contacts of OS patients had cellular immunity to osteosarcoma (but not fibrosarcoma, rhabdomyosarcoma, or hypernephroma), when ^{51}Cr release of greater than 35 percent was used as a criterion of T cell-mediated cytotoxicity (one parameter of cellular immunity). Less than 1 percent of normal subjects or of household contacts of patients with the other types of tumors studied had significant cytotoxicity (normal subjects had cytotoxicity indices of less than 17 percent) with osteosarcoma (29). Similar results were obtained in a much smaller series of patients with hypernephroma and their contacts (15), and in normal controls, using hypernephroma cells as target cells in the cytotoxicity assay.

Transfer Factor Therapy

Patients with osteosarcoma were classified clinically into four groups (Fig. 14-2). Immunologic profiles on patients post-amputation were also categorized into four stages, depending on the results of their cytotoxicity and "active" and total rosette-forming cells (T-E_a and T-E_t, respectively). Stage 1 had normal values by all three laboratory parameters, Stage 2 had decreased CI but normal TE_a and T-E_t, Stage 3 showed a decrease in CI and T-E_a but not T-E_t, and Stage 4 was deficient by all three parameters.

In patients receiving no TF, the CI dropped several months after removal of the primary tumor, and it remained low. The number of T-E_a dropped approximately 60 days later, and, radiographically, metastases appeared 45 to 90 days after the drop in T-E_a. In contrast, the normal household contacts

Figure 14-2. Classification of patients in terms of the cytotoxicity of their lymphocytes for osteosarcoma cells.

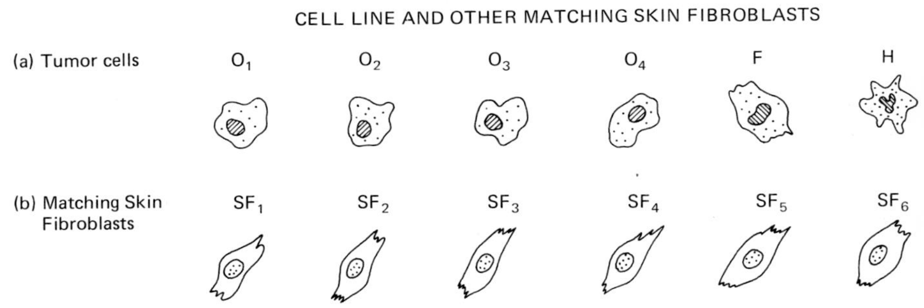

CELL LINE AND OTHER MATCHING SKIN FIBROBLASTS

		O_1	O_2	O_3	O_4	F	H
(a) Tumor cells							
(b) Matching Skin Fibroblasts		SF_1	SF_2	SF_3	SF_4	SF_5	SF_6

Lymphocytes

Donor 1	(a)	X	X	X	X	O	O
	(b)	O	O	O	O	O	O
Donor 2	(a)	O	O	O	O	O	O
	(b)	O	O	O	O	O	O

X, Marked destruction (release of ^{51}Cr)

O, Osteosarcoma

F, Fibrosarcoma or other closely related tumors

H, Hypernephroma or other nonrelated tumors

SF, Skin fibroblasts

tested maintained cell-mediated cytotoxicity for intervals ranging up to 2 years thus far, unless vigorously leukophoresed, in which case transient losses of cytotoxicity occurred (29).

These results imply a difference in immunologic memory, and perhaps in initial response (the patients rarely had the same height of ctyotoxicity index as their immune contacts, despite their presumably more intimate contact with antigen and greater antigenic mass), in individuals who develop OS upon exposure to the presumed virus and those who do not (29).

Administration of nonspecific TF_d failed to raise the cytotoxicity index or to prevent metastases. In contrast, administration of OS-TF_d raised the specific cytotoxicity index in the recipients, and, when the level decreased, re-administration of OS-TF_d again raised the level of cytotoxicity. Also, when evaluated against the natural history of this disease, specific transfer factor appeared to prevent metastases. Patients receiving nonspecific (NS)-TF_d had no rise in cytotoxicity index, but subsequent administration of OS-TF_d produced a rise. Cross-over studies between OS-TF_d and NS-TF_d showed a rise in cytotoxicity index with OS-TF_d, but a fall after NS-TF_d. In patients initially placed on OS-TF_d, each rise in index was concomitant with clinical stabilization (as mentioned, subsequent administration of NS-TF_d caused a fall in cytotoxicity). In one patient initially receiving OS-TF_d, a prolonged interval of administration of inactive TF was followed by a fall first in the index, then in T-E_a, and, finally, by the appearance of a pulmonary metastasis. We therefore feel that such prolonged control studies may be unethical.

Discussion

Based on previous inferential evidence that, in certain human tumors, a genetically determined T cell deficiency is a necessary, but not sufficient cause for development of viral neoplasia (reviewed in 10,16), we attempted to find evidence of cellular immunity to OS-associated antigens not only in first-degree relatives of OS patients but also in other close contacts (guardians, servants); such cell-mediated immunity, as measured by T cell-mediated cytotoxicity, was present in 20 percent of the contacts. We utilized a standardized ^{51}Cr release assay, because of our serious doubts regarding the interpretation of the results of the colony inhibition assay of the Hellström's (22), the standard microcytotoxicity tests employed by many investigators, and the Takasugi and Klein cytotoxicity assay (33). In individuals without tumors, such immunity persisted for long intervals; in contrast, it was usually lower in the patients, and decreased to nonimmune levels shortly after removal of the tumor. Further drops in cytotoxicity index (and, subsequently, in T-E_a) preceded evidence of new metastases. Tumor-specific transfer factor increased T cell-mediated cyto-

Phillipsburg, N. J.). The mixture was stirred at 4°C for 3 hr and pelleted at 8,000 rpm for 20 min in a Sorvall type SS-34 rotor. The pellets were resuspended in 10 ml of TNE buffer, and 20 mg of pronase (Sigma Chemical Co., St. Louis, Mo.) was added. After incubation at 37°C for 30 min, the suspension was cooled and layered over a discontinuous 20 percent and 55 percent sucrose gradient (w/v) in TNE, which was centrifuged at 27,000 rpm for 2 hr in the Beckman type SW 27 rotor. Material banding at the interphase of the gradient was collected by puncturing the bottom of the centrifuge tube and then diluted to less than 20 percent sucrose with TNE. The preparation was again incubated at 37°C for 30 min with 20 mg of pronase, cooled, and layered over a continuous 20 to 55 percent sucrose (w/v) in TNE gradient. After centrifugation at 27,000 rpm for 8 to 10 hr in a Beckman type SW 27 rotor, 1.0 ml fractions were collected from the bottom of the centrifuge tube with the aid of a Buchler piercing unit (Buchler Instruments Division, Fort Lee, N. J.). Fractions were assayed for density (calculated from refractive index) and for RT activity.

To determine the endogenous reverse transcriptase (RT) activity of the CF fractions, we used a 200-μl reaction mixture that contained, in final concentrations, 40 mM Tris HCl (pH 8.3), 60 mM NaCl, 1 mM manganese acetate, 0.2 mM each of unlabeled dATP, dCTP, dGTP, 1.9 mM dithiothreitol, 0.02 percent Triton X-100, and 3.5×10^{-7} M [^{3}H]dTTP (specific activity 57c/mmole; 53,100 cpm/pmole). The reaction mixture was incubated for 2 hr at 38°C and then precipitated with 500 μl of a solution containing equal parts of 100 percent trichloracetic acid (TCA), saturated sodium orthophosphate, and pyrophosphate (10). During this precipitation, 50 μl of yeast RNA (1 mg/ml) was used as a carrier. The acid-insoluble radioactive counts were collected onto washed 2.4 cm Whatman GF/A filters (W & R Balston, Ltd., England) and placed into vials containing 10 ml of a BBOT-toluene fluor and counted in a model LS250 Beckman scintillation counter.

The simultaneous detection assay (SDA) was done as described previously (19) with the following modifications: The endogenous RT assay was done on PEG-pronase purified fractions using 250 μl of virus preparation and 250 μl of reaction cocktail. After a 20-min incubation period at 38°C, the reaction mixture was layered over a linear 10 to 30 percent (w/v) glycerol in TNE gradient. Also, 25 μl of a 28 S ^{14}C-labeled RNA standard* was placed atop the gradient. The gradient was centrifuged at 38,000 rpm for 2 hr at 5°C in a Beckman type SW40 rotor, and 0.5 ml fractions were collected by piercing the bottom of the centrifuge tubes. The fractions were precipitated in acid, collected onto 2.4 cm Whatman GF/A glass fiber filters, which were washed

---

* The 28 S ribosomal RNA marker was prepared from ribosomes of rat embryo cells.

three times with 5 percent TCA containing 0.08 M sodium pyrophosphate and once with 80 percent (v/v) ethanol. Dried filters were counted as previously described. The sedimentation coefficient of the radioactive peaks in the gradient were calculated by the method of Martin and Ames (16).

Transformation Studies

The culture fluids from TCC cells (253J, 187G, 440P, 149J) were harvested, clarified in an International Model CS centrifuge (2,500 rpm, 5 min), and then passed through a 0.45-μm Millipore filter. To ensure that acellular fluids were used in the transformation experiments, aliquots of fluid directly from the tissue cultures, supernatants after clarification, and fluids passed through the 0.45-μm filter were placed in 25-cm^2 tissue culture flasks containing RPMI-1640 supplemented with calf serum and antibiotics. There was no cell growth in the tissue culture flasks inoculated with these fluids. Approximately 0.5 to 1.0 ml of acellular fluids that had been passed through the 0.45-μm filter was layered onto near-monolayer assay cells. The assay cells were adult human testicle, human embryonic skin, and embryonic calf urothelium. The assay cells had been maintained in tissue culture in a manner similar to that described for TCC cells.

Studies on Transformed Cells

The cells transformed by acellular fluids from human TCC in tissue culture have been characterized as to morphology by light and electron microscopy, doubling time, chromosome composition, tumor production in immunosuppressed animals, and growth in agar by methods detailed previously (6).

Transformed and control cells were also studied by indirect immunofluorescence using the sera of TCC patients, sera of patients with other genitourinary tumors, and sera from age-matched healthy controls. Transformed and control cells were grown in Leighton tubes with growth media and under the culture conditions described for TCC cells. The cells were fixed in culture, and the indirect immunofluorescence test was as described by Priori (18).

The reactivity of lymphocytes from patients with TCC against transformed and non-transformed cells was tested using the lymphocyte-mediated cytotoxicity assay described previously (13).

Results

Tissue Culture

Cells often grew out slowly from the tumor minces. In most instances, the cells were epithelial, averaged 10 μ in diameter, and multilayering was seen.

The cells grew at varying rates but most had a doubling time of approximately 48 hr. No mycoplasma was detected in these cells.

Cell Line Characterization

Seven long-term cell lines have been established from TCC; two of these, 292W and 253J, have been characterized in detail. The results of characterization studies on 253J have been submitted for publication (5), and similar unreported investigations have been carried out on 292W cells. In brief, cells from these tumors have (a) an abnormal human karyotype, (b) a doubling time from 48 to 72 hours, (3) the capacity to grow under agar, (4) the ability to produce epithelial tumors in the cheek pouches of immunosuppressed hamsters, and (e) a fine structure of epithelial cells.

Electron Microscopy

Ultrastructure studies on 33 surgical specimens of transitional cell carcinomas of the bladder, ureter, and renal pelvis revealed that 28 specimens contained virus-like particles (VLP). These VLP could be divided into two morphologic types, one of which consisted of particles with a homogenous nucleoid region, which was moderately electron dense throughout and tightly surrounded by a trilaminar envelope or unit membrane. In contrast to type-B and type-C particles, where the nucleoid is separated from the envelope by an electron translucent zone, the envelope of these particles was so closely positioned around the nucleoid that the inner leaflet of the envelope could only be seen with difficulty. The particles varied in size from 30 to 130 nm in diameter; more than 90 percent of the particles, however, were in the 30 to 80 nm range (Fig. 15-1,A). These particles resembled closely the VLP described by Feller and Chopra in human breast cancer (7). But, for convenience, we have designated these structures in TCC as type-U particles. The second type of paritcle (about 1 to 2 percent of the total VLP population) had the nucleoid set apart from the envelope by a slightly less electron dense region, 5 to 10 nm in width. The nucleoid boundaries of these particles were poorly defined and, hence, resembled the atypical type-C particles of the Mason–Pfizer virus (15). The atypical type-C particles usually were larger (70 to 130 nm) than the type-U particles. The morphology of the atypical type-C particles is illustrated in Figure 15-1,B.

Studies on grossly normal portions of transitional epithelium of the bladder and ureter near the site of the tumor revealed the presence of both type-U and type-C particles in three of four specimens. Also, both types of particles were seen in fibroblasts of the lamina propria from two of the specimens.

Ultrastructure studies on 16 transitional cell carcinomas in both primary and long-term tissue culture also demonstrated both the type-U and atypical

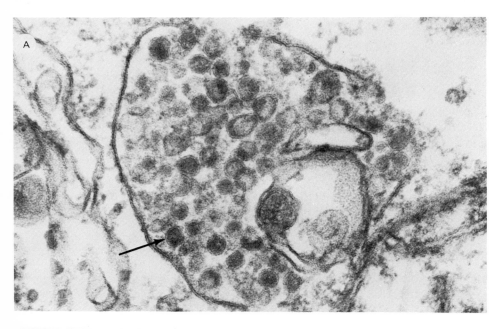

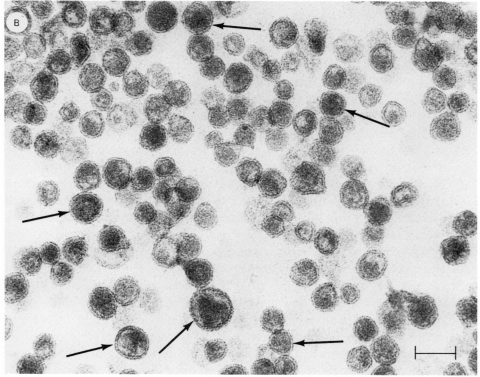

Figure 15-1. (opposite) **(A)** Thin section of a papillary tumor of the renal pelvis (patient 634S), showing many type-U particles (arrow) in a cytoplasmic vesicle of a degenerating cell. X120,000. **(B)** These particles were prepared by CF centrifugation, PEG-pronase treatment, and banding in sucrose of 253J tissue culture fluids as described in the text. Sucrose gradient fractions with bouyant densities of 1.15 to 1.18 g/ml were pooled, pelleted, and examined by thin sectioning. The pelleted material is essentially free of cellular debris and contains many type-U particles (small arrows) and several atypical type-C particles (large arrows). ×110,400. Bar represents 100 nm.

---

type-C particles in 15 cultures. The diameter of the particles in tissue culture was the same as that observed in the surgical specimens.

Both the type-U and atypical type-C particles were found in 1 to 5 percent of the cells from surgical specimens and in 1 to 10 percent of cells in tissue culture. The particles usually were found in cytoplasmic vesicles; but, they were also found free in the cytoplasm of normal and degenerating cells as well as in extracellular spaces. No virus-like particles were seen in the nucleus. How the particles mature is not clear, since budding through the cytoplasmic membrane or through other membranous systems within the cells was not seen.

No VLP were found by electron microscopy in transitional epithelium specimens from four patients with no history of carcinoma of the urinary tract. Also, 16 tumor specimens and the corresponding nontumor kidney from patients with adenocarcinoma had no VLP.

Virus Purification and Characterization

The results of a typical CF run employing clarified acellular tissue culture fluids from 292W is presented in Figure 15-2. The maximal RT activity was located in the fraction with a buoyant density of 1.17 g/ml. This sample was further purified by PEG-pronase treatment, and then it was assayed for the presence of the radioactive, high molecular weight hybrid of RNA and DNA characteristic of the oncornaviruses, using the SDA technique. The result of one such assay is shown in Figure 15-3. Two peaks of radioactivity were detected: One peak occurred between 75S and 85S and the other between 35S and 40S. Similar results have been obtained using the tissue culture fluids of 253J processed in a similar manner (1).

A preliminary characterization of the RT associated with virus particles isolated from the tissue culture fluids of cells derived from two different TCC

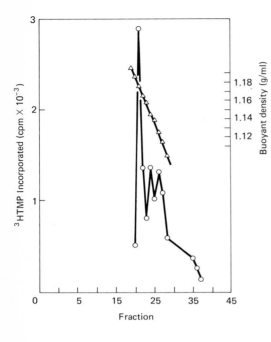

Figure 15-2. Results of continuous flow centrifugation of 5.25 liters obtained from 292W clarified fluids (see text). Each point represents 20 ml of gradient, which was processed and assayed for endogenous reverse transcriptase as described in the text. Gradient fractions were collected right to left.

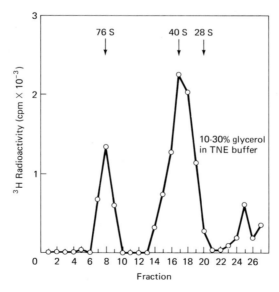

Figure 15-3. Rate-zonal centrifugation of the product of the 292W RNA-directed DNA polymerase reaction from CF 32 fraction with a density of 1.17 g/ml. Each point represents 0.5 ml of glycerol gradient, which was processed as described in text. Gradients were collected left to right.

(253J, 292W) has been done. Briefly summarized, the results indicate that the RT reaction requires Triton X-100, decreases in the absence of deoxyadenosine triphosphate, and is sensitive to treatment with 20 μg/ml of ribonuclease; manganese preferred over magnesium as the divalent cation (1).

Both type-U and atypical type-C particles were found in clarified tissue culture fluids prepared by CF centrifugation and in gradient fractions from PEG-pronase treated fractions from CF (Fig. 15-1B). The PEG-pronase treated preparations from CF fractions also were free of cellular debris (Fig. 15-1B). The particles were present in gradient fractions with buoyant densities of 1.13 to 1.19 g/ml.

Gradient fractions containing both types of particles had RT activity and high molecular weight RNA (Figs. 15-2 and 15-3). Since the type-U and the atypical type-C particle are purified together, it was not possible to determine whether one or the other, or both, had RT and high molecular weight RNA. Thus, for the purpose of this presentation, we have designated both particles as transitional cell cancer-associated virus (TCCAV).

Transformation Studies

Within 2 to 6 weeks after acellular fluids were added to assay cells, multiple discrete foci of abnormal cells were seen. The cells forming these foci exhibited malignant morphology, and multilayering was seen. The transformed cells quickly overgrew the assay cells and were subcultured by trypsinization (as described previously for TCC cells in culture). In tissue culture, the transformed cells grew rapidly, had abnormal morphology, exhibited multilayering, and grew under agar; most cells had hyperdiploid karyotypes. The transformed cells also produced epithelial-like tumors in the cheek pouches and in the subcutaneous tissues of immunosuppressed hamsters. No attempt was made to transplant tumors over a long term in animals.

The sera from twelve patients with TCC, eight patients with other tumors of the genitourinary tract and twelve healthy, age-matched controls were reacted against two of the transformed cell lines (100A-149, 100A-253J) and against untransformed control cells using the indirect immunofluorescence technique (Table 15-1). Approximately 80 percent of the sera of TCC patients reacted against the transformed cells, whereas less than 20 percent of the sera reacted against untransformed cells. By contrast, the sera of patients with other genitourinary tumors and sera from healthy controls showed little reactivity against either the transformed or the untransformed cells (Table 15-1).

Preliminary results of the lymphocyte-medicated cytotoxicity assay showed that the lymphocytes of TCC patients exhibited significant cytotoxicity against transformed cells but not against untransformed cells.

Table 15-1   Reactivity of Sera against TCC Fluid-Transformed Cells: Indirect Immunofluorescence

All tumor sera positive at 0.25 dilution or greater.

		TCC pts	Other GU tumors	Healthy, age-matched controls
Transformed cells	100a-149 Testicle	9/12[a]	1/8	1/12
	100a-253J Skin	10/12	1/8	2/12
Control cells	100a Testicle	1/12	0/8	1/12
	100a Skin	0/12	0/8	1/12

[a] Number positive/total number tested.

Discussion

TCC of the urinary tract in man has been associated with cigarette smoking, chronic phenacetin ingestion, nonnutritive artificial sweeteners, and exposure to benzidine and beta-naphthalamine. In addition, there is an increased incidence of TCC of the renal pelvis and ureter in patients with "Balkan nephropathy," and *Schistosoma haematobium* infection of the urinary bladder seems to predispose that organ to squamous cell cancer.

Other than the studies by our laboratory, published previously (1-6,9,10), there has been little evidence that a virus may play a role in the pathogenesis of urothelial tumors in any species. Olson et al. (17), however, did report the isolation of a virus from bovine papillary transitional cell tumors of the urinary bladder. The virus isolated by Olson probably was the bovine pailloma virus, a DNA virus, and its etiologic relation to the tumor is obscure.

The morphology of the atypical type-C particle associated with human transitional cell cancers of the urinary tract (TCC-UT) resembles that of Mason–Pfizer virus (15), Woolly monkey sarcoma virus (21), and particles recently described in HeLa cells (11) and in spontaneously transformed human brain cells (14). The distinguishing morphologic feature of these viruses is that they often have an irregular, poorly defined nucleoid. Gelderbloom et al. (11) recently postulated that these agents may represent a new class of "primate" oncornaviruses. But, all of these viruses, except for the virus associated with human TCC, have been demonstrated to mature by budding from the cell membrane.

The availability of virus-producing cell lines derived from human TCC has made it possible to characterize TCCAV without passage in alien cells. Thus, there is virus in the tissue culture fluids of TCC that resembles known oncornaviruses in that it has the following characteristics: (a) Its ultrastructure resembles atypical type-C virus; (b) RNA is the predominant nucleic acid; (c) its buoyant density is 1.13 to 1.19 g/ml; and (d) the virus has an RNA-directed DNA polymerase and a high molecular weight hybrid of RNA and DNA (75S to 85S), as demonstrated by the simultaneous detection technique.

The virus associated with human TCC has been linked directly to the original tumors in several ways. First, ultrastructure studies consistently demonstrated virus-like particles in the surgical specimens and in TCC cells in primary or early passage tissue culture (2,3,10). Second, acellular fluids from TCC growing in culture caused malignant *in vitro* neoplastic transformation of mammalian cells. These culture fluids were known to contain TCCAV, and furthermore, the transformed cells had VLP similar to both the type-U and atypical type-C particles (6), and the transformed cells had antigen that was recognized by sera and lymphocytes of TCC patients. Third, in data reported previously, it was demonstrated that an *in vitro* tumor-specific cytotoxicity against autochthonous transitional cell cancer in a TCC patient's serum was removed by absorption with a virus-containing pellet isolated by ultracentrifugation of supernatant fluids from cultured autochthonous TCC cells (12).

Although it now seems reasonably certain that there is an RNA virus associated with human TCC-UT, the significance of this finding is not clear. Thus, it is possible that this virus plays no role in the pathogenesis of these neoplasms but, rather, the virus may be simply a "passenger" in TCC cells. But the following observations do not support such a role. First, virus infections of the proximal urinary tract are rare in adults and usually occur only in patients who are receiving immunosuppressive therapy. Second, virus has not been detected by us in either normal adult urothelium or in normal kidney, and there is no evidence of virus in adenocarcinomas of the kidney (hypernephromas). Finally, our morphologic and characterization studies suggest that TCCAV is not a common infectious virus of man. It seems unlikely that the same commensal agent would be associated coincidentally with a series of human cancers.

As was mentioned at the outset of this discussion, TCC-UT in man have been associated with exposure to certain chemicals and drugs. It is possible to induce malignant TCC of the urinary bladder in animals with a variety of chemicals. Neither the human nor the animal tumors induced by chemical carcinogens have been studied for associated viruses. Since there is increasing evidence that viruses may play some role in what previously was thought to be purely chemically induced tumors in animals, it is possible that the chemicals may "turn on" or "activate" a virus. Therefore, it is important that the virology of chemically induced urothelial tumors of both animals and man be studied.

To prove that TCC-associated virus causes TCC in man, that is to fulfill Koch's final postulate, one would have to produce a similar tumor in humans using virus isolated directly from the human tumors. Obviously this experiment is not possible and, thus, less direct approaches to the problem are being pursued, based on concepts that have evolved from the study of virus-induced tumors in animals. These investigations should provide data (a) the identity and possibly also the origin of this virus, (b) to what degree there is biochemical or immunologic hemology between TCCAV and the recently described primate oncornaviruses or to other "candidate" human viruses, and (c) whether there is macromolecular evidence that the virus "transformed" the tumor cell. If TCCAV is an etiologic agent, virus-produced DNA transcripts should hybridize with tumor cell DNA, and this reaction could be detected by standard nucleic acid hybridization techniques.

There are at least three practical implications of the virus association with human TCC-UT. First, it should be possible to develop a highly specific screening or cancer detection test for the tumors. Such a test may be useful irrespective of whether the virus actually causes TCC-UT, since the virus is found consistently in the tumors, and because the sera of most tumor patients contain antibodies that recognize virus or virus-directed antigens. Second, since TCC cells and cells transformed by TCC tissue culture fluids appear to share common, tumor-specific antigen, it might be possible to develop antisera to this antigen that could be used in the indirect immunofluorescence technique to detect malignant exfoliated cells in the urine. The use of immunocytology should improve the accuracy and sensitivity of diagnostic urinary cytology. Third, chemoprophylaxis may control early tumors. This last postulate is based, in part, on the studies showing that a variety of drugs interfere with virus replication and the transforming capacity of the oncornaviruses (22). If antiviral chemotherapy were administered on a continuing basis to patients early in the course of their disease, tumor recurrences and the progression of benign to more malignant tumors might be obviated. But, before such a chemotherapeutic approach is tried, the many nuances of this virus-tumor system require greater understanding and better methods for assessing the status of TCCAV infection in patients must be developed.

ACKNOWLEDGMENTS

This work was supported in part by a training grant in urology from the USPHS AM 05514-08, National Cancer Grant CA 13095-03, and National Bladder Cancer Project Grant CA 15551-01.

REFERENCES

1. Castro, A. E., Bronson, D. L., Elliott, A. Y., Cleveland, P., and Fraley, E. E. Detection of RNA-directed DNA polymerase and high molecular weight RNA in particles isolated from human transitional cell cancers of the urinary tract. Nature. (Manuscript submitted.)

2. Elliott, A. Y., Fraley, E. E., Castro, A. E., Cleveland, P., Hakala, T. R., and Stein, N. Isolation of an RNA virus from transitional cell tumors of the human urinary bladder. Surgery, 74:46, 1973.

3. Elliott, A. Y., Stein, N., Fraley, E. E., and Cleveland, P. H. Replication of herpes virus of turkeys in hamster urogenital cell cultures. Am. J. Vet. Res., 34:427, 1973.

4. Elliott, A, Y., Fraley, E. E., Cleveland, P., Castro, A. E., and Stein, N. Isolation of RNA virus from papillary tumors of the human renal pelvis. Science, 179:393, 1974.

5. Elliott, A. Y., Cleveland, P., Cervenka, J., Castro, A. E., Stein, N., Hakala, T. R., and Fraley, E. E. Characterization of a cell line from human transitional cell cancer of the urinary tract. J. Nat. Cancer Inst., 53:1341, 1974.

6. Elliott, A. Y., Fraley, E. E., Cervenka, J., Cleveland, P., and Stein, N. *In vitro* neoplastic transformation of mammalian cells produced by acellular fluids of cultured human transitional cell cancers of the urinary tract. (Manuscript in preparation.)

7. Feller, W. F. and Chopra, H. C. A small virus-like particle observed in human breast cancer by means of electron microscopy. J. Natl. Cancer Inst., 40:1359, 1968.

8. Firth, J. A. and Hicks, R. M. Interspecies variation in the fine structure and enzyme cytochemistry of mammalian transitional epithelium. J. Anat., 116:31, 1973.

9. Fraley, E. E., Elliott, A. Y., and Hakala, T. R. RNA virus isolation from papillary tumors of the renal pelvis. Surg. Forum, XIII:529, 1972.

10. Fraley, E. E., Elliott, A. Y., Castro, A. E., Cleveland, P., Hakala, T. R., and Stein, N. Ribonucleic acid virus associated with human urothelial tumors: Significance for diagnosis and treatment. J. Urol., 111:378, 1974.

11. Gelderblom, H., Bauer, H., Ogura, H., Wigand, R., and Fischer, A. B. Detection of oncornavirus-like particles in HeLa cells. I. Fine structure and comparative morphological classification. Int. J. Cancer, 13:246, 1974.

12. Hakala, T. R., Castro, A. E., Elliott, A. Y., and Fraley, E. E. Humoral cytoxicity in human transitional cell carcinoma. J. Urol., 111:382, 1974.

13. Hakala, T. R., Lange, P., Castro, A. E., Elliott, A. Y., and Fraley, E. E. Cell-mediated cytotoxicity against human transitional cell carcinomas of the genitourinary tract. Cancer, 34:1929, 1974.

14. Hooks, J., Gibbs, C. J., Chopra, H. C., Lewis, M., and Gajdusek, D. C. Spontaneous transformation of human brain cells grown *in vitro* and description of associated virus particles. Science, 176,1420, 1972.

15. Kramarsky, B., Sarkar, N. H., and Moore, D. H. Ultrastructural comparison of a virus from a rhesus monkey mammary carcinoma with four oncogenic RNA viruses. Proc. Natl. Acad. Sci. USA, 68:1603, 1971.

16. Martin, R. G. and Ames, B. N. A method for determining the sedimentation behavior of enzymes: Application to protein mixtures. J. Biol. Chem. 236:1372, 1961.

17. Olson, C., Pamukcu, A. M., Brobst, D. F., et al. A urinary bladder tumor induced by a bovine cutaneous papilloma agent. Cancer Res., 19:779, 1959.

18. Priori, E. S., Wilbur, J. R., and Dmochowski, L. Immunofluorescence tests on sera of patients with osteogenic sarcoma. J. Natl. Cancer Inst., 46:129, 1971.

19. Schlom, J. and Spiegelman, S. Simultaneous detection of reverse transcriptase and high molecular weight RNA unique to oncogenic RNA viruses. Science, 174:840, 1971.

20. Spiegelman, S., Burny, A., Das, M. R., Keydar, J., Schlom, J., Travnicek, M., and Watson, K. Characterization of the products of RNA-directed DNA polymerase in oncogenic viruses. Nature, 227:563, 1970.

21. Theilen, G. H., Gould, D., Fowler, M., and Dungworth, D. L. C-Type virus in tumor tissue of a woolly monkey (*Lagothrix spp.*) with fibrosarcoma. J. Natl. Cancer Inst., 47:881, 1971.

22. Zubrod, C. G. Chemical control of cancer. Proc. Natl. Acad. Sci. USA, 69,1042, 1972.

Trials with Poly A:Poly U as Adjuvant Therapy Complementing Surgery in Randomized Patients with Breast Cancer

J. Lacour

Introduction

The experimental basis for this trial was discussed by Fanny Lacour, in this volume (Chapter 9). Poly A:poly U, when given after surgery, was found to have a definite inhibitory effect on tumor growth, at least in the case of spontaneous mammary adenocarcinoma in mice and transplantable melanoma in hamsters. As used, this complex had neither toxic nor enhancing effects. Moreover, when poly A:poly U was administered to newborn C_3H/He mice, it had a prophylactic effect, and the tumor incidence was significantly lower in the treated group than among the controls.

It was also found that rabbit pyrogenicity tests were negative at doses of 2 mg/kg, and mouse toxicity tests were negative at 250 mg/kg (the therapeutic dose being 15 mg/kg).

In view of these results, we thought it reasonable to use this complex for treatment of human cancer without clinical risk or ethical objection.

In the first trial, we gave poly A:poly U to four patients with advanced melanomas in order to assure ourselves that it would have no toxic effects in man. Intravenous injections of first 3 mg and subsequently 15 mg were given without any side effects. There was no toxicity and no pyrogenicity, nor was any modification in the blood cell count observed.

Treatment Protocol

Then, after discussions with the entire group charged with the treatment of breast cancer in our institute, we decided to start a randomized trial in patients bearing operable breast carcinomas. We followed the experimental animal model, in which poly A:poly U was given after surgical removal of the tumor, when the number of remaining cancer cells was presumed to be minimal.

Fundamental Aspects of Neoplasia,
edited by A. Arthur Gottlieb, Otto J. Plescia, and David H. L. Bishop.
© 1975 by Springer-Verlag New York Inc.

Selection of Patients

Below are the details we consider significant in the protocol used. Patients were selected if they met all of the following criteria:

1. Their tumor was an infiltrating carcinoma of medium size, 2 cm to 7 cm at its greatest diameter, without skin involvement and without complete fixation to the pectoralis major.
2. They had no palpable nodes or palpable but movable nodes.
3. There was no detectable metastasis.

According to the U.I.C.C. classification using the T.N.M. system, these patients correspond to category T_2 and part of T_3, N_0 or N_1, and M_0.

Patients with tumors of small size, namely, T_1, N_0 or N_1, M_0, were excluded from this trial since they have a sufficiently favorable prognosis to make detection of poly A:poly U effects unlikely. Such tumors, however, are being included in another trial designed to compare conservative procedures and radical surgery.

Patients with larger size tumors were also excluded; they are treated in our institute by preoperative radiotherapy followed by modified radical mastectomy. The selected patients were randomized into two groups, as follows.

Group A. Patients were treated by surgery, without any additional treatment if the nodes were free of cancer. Postoperative radiotherapy and radiotherapeutic castration were employed, if the nodes were metastatic and if the woman still menstruated or had entered the menopause within 2 years.

Group B. These patients were treated exactly as those in group A, but they also received poly A:poly U.

Analysis of Poly A: Poly U

A sample of each preparation of poly A:poly U, which was synthesized by Dr. Michelson, Directeur de Recherches au C.N.R.S., Institut de Biologie Physico-Chimique, Paris, was submitted to Dr. Plescia for an immunostimulatory assay. He determined the increase in number of murine spleen cells forming antibodies to sheep red blood cells, when stimulated by the test preparation, as a measure of its immunostimulating activity.

Injection Schedule

Fifteen milligrams of the complex were injected intravenously, twice a week for 3 weeks, into patients in Group B. The first injection was given 5 to 7 days after surgery. At the same time, and following the same schedule, patients in group A received injections of saline. Patients of both groups visited the hospital for examinations every 3 months during the first 3 years, and every 6 months thereafter.

Evaluation Criteria

The criteria of judgment were in three categories: clinical, biological, and immunological.

Clinical. The incidence of recurrences and metastases at the 3rd and 5th year; 3- and 5-year survival rates.

Biological. The red blood cell sedimentation rate and the blood cell count were determined at each examination visit.

Immunological. (a) DNCB cellular immunity tests were performed before surgery and occasionally repeated after treatment; (b) leukocyte migration inhibition test with autologous tumor extract (2) performed at the time of operation, after treatment with poly A:poly U following surgery, after 3 months, and again if the quantity of tumor antigen were sufficient; (c) rosette formation tests performed before and after treatment with poly A:poly U; and they were repeated every 3 months. Quantitative immunoglobin analyses for IgM, IgG, and IgA were also obtained each time tests of humoral immunity were performed.

Results

As of the 7th of May, 1974, 101 breast cancer patients were included in the trial that started September 1972.

Group A. Fifty-four patients represent the control group who were not given poly A:poly U but otherwise treated as the patients in Group B.

Group B. Forty-seven patients received poly A:poly U, most of them receiving 15 mg/injection with the exception of the first few who received 3 mg/injection. Total poly A:poly U injected was therefore 90 mg/patient.

We observed a slight pyrogenic effect with poly A:poly U at the 15-mg dose. About 40 percent of the patients showed a temperature elevation ranging from 0.3° to 1.7°C, usually following the first two injections generally beginning 2 to 3 hr after the injection, and lasting for 6 to 24 hr.

Immunologic Data

The MLT test in the presence of autologous tumor extract was positive in 30 percent of the patients before treatment. Among those patients who were negative, some changes were observed after treatment. Of 21 negative patients in the poly A:poly U group, 9 became positive (43 percent). Of 17 negative patients in the control group, 6 became positive after surgery (35 percent). This difference between the two groups is not statistically significant and, therefore, does not permit us to distinguish any effects of poly A:poly U from the effects due to surgery alone.

The DNCB test was positive for 70 percent of the patients before treatment. It was repeated after treatment on five negative patients, and it became positive in only one case (in the control group).

Clinical Data

Two patients, one in the control group (A) and one in the poly A:poly U group (B) died of cancer. Two patients, one in group A and one in group B, experienced recurrences or metastases. All four of these patients had had a poor prognosis, based on the presence of node metastases and histologic grade II or III, according to Bloom and Richardson (1).

These clinical observations obviously have no statistical significance for two reasons: (a) There were too few patients in each group, and (b) the follow-up time is not yet sufficiently long. Early mortality, within the first year, is not expected to be affected by immunologic stimulation, since it is most likely that patients who died already had metastases at the time of operation, even though they had not been detected clinically or radiologically.

Thus, it is too early to draw conclusions regarding possible benefits derived from postsurgical poly A:poly U treatment. But, one fact may be emphasized, that tumor enhancing or toxic effects of poly A:poly U were not observed in this trial series.

REFERENCES

1. Bloom, H. J. G. and Richardson, W. W. Histological grading and prognoses in breast cancer. British J. Cancer, 11:359, 1957.
2. Segal, A., Weiler, D., Genin, J., Lacour, J., and Lacour, F. *In vitro* study of cellular immunity against autochtonous human cancer. Int. J. Cancer, 2:417, 1972.

IV

DNA Polymerases of Malignant Cells and Associated Viruses

Endogenous RNA Synthesis Is Required for Endogenous DNA Synthesis by Reticuloendotheliosis Virus Virions

S. Mizutani and H. M. Temin

Introduction

The reticuloendotheliosis viruses are a newly described group of avian RNA viruses with a virion DNA polymerase (12,15). The reticuloendotheliosis viruses cause acute disease and reticuloendotheliosis in young fowl. The virions of reticuloendotheliosis viruses are similar to those of avian leukosis-sarcoma viruses, and their replication is also similar. Both groups of viruses have C-type virions containing a 60 to 70S RNA and a DNA polymerase. Both replicate through a DNA intermediate. The DNA intermediate of the reticuloendotheliosis viruses has been demonstrated by nucleic acid hybridization and by the isolation of infectious DNA (6,2).

The reticuloendotheliosis viruses differ from the avian leukosis-sarcoma viruses in the antigenicity of the virion proteins and in the nucleic acid sequences of the virion 60 to 70 S RNA (4,5,10). [But, there are slight serologic cross-reactions between the purified DNA polymerases from virions of these two groups (11).]

Another difference between the virions of the two groups of viruses is the lack of endogenous DNA polymerase activity in virions of reticuloendotheliosis viruses. Although virions of reticuloendotheliosis viruses contain a DNA polymerase, which is active with added templates, there is little DNA polymerase activity when templates are not added. In contrast, avian leukosis-sarcoma virions have a 20-fold greater endogenous DNA polymerase activity.

RNA Synthesis by Reticuloendotheliosis Virus Virions

A paradox therefore exists. Reticuloendotheliosis virus is replicated through a DNA intermediate, but the virion appears incapable of carrying out endogenous DNA synthesis. Many experiments have been performed using different extracts and additives to activate endogenous DNA polymerase activity (unpublished studies). All have been unsuccessful. As a working hypothesis

Fundamental Aspects of Neoplasia,
edited by A. Arthur Gottlieb, Otto J. Plescia, and David H. L. Bishop.
© 1975 by Springer-Verlag New York Inc.

to explain this paradox, the model shown in Figure 17-1 was then proposed; there is no endogenous DNA polymerase activity in reticuloendotheliosis virus virions because of the absence of an active primer. The primer had first to be formed by endogenous RNA synthesis before the virion DNA polymerase could synthesize DNA using the 3'-OH of the newly synthesized RNA as a primer. This mode of replication differed from that of avian leukosis-sarcoma viruses where the virions contain a primer (1,3).

To test this hypothesis, we first looked for RNA synthesis in disrupted virions of reticuloendotheliosis viruses. When disrupted virions of reticuloendotheliosis viruses were incubated in a system containing detergent, a divalent cation, and all four ribonucleoside triphosphates, incorporation of ribonucleoside monophosphates occurred. But, all four ribonucleoside monophosphates were not incorporated to the same extent. The nucleoside monophosphate incorporated most frequently was UMP. There was less incorporation of AMP and CMP and very little incorporation of GMP. RNA synthesis was found with disrupted virions of all four members of the reticuloendotheliosis virus group.

In Table 17-1 are listed the requirements for this RNA synthesis. There is an absolute requirement for (a) disruption of the virion by detergent, indicating that the activity is internal to the lipid-containing envelope, (b) a divalent cation, and (c) more than one ribonucleoside triphosphate. More will be said about the ribonucleoside triphosphate requirement later; it also must be realized that there are nucleoside triphosphates in virions of ribodeoxyviruses (8). The RNA synthesis was not inhibited by actinomycin D (an inhibitor of DNA-directed RNA synthesis), by α-amanitin (an inhibitor of RNA polymerase II), or by antibody to the SNV virion DNA polymerase. This antibody did inhibit the DNA polymerase activity of the same virions.

These experiments established that there was in virions of reticuloendotheliosis viruses an internal virion enzyme activity incorporating ribonucleoside monophosphates into trichloroacetic acid (TCA)-insoluble material and that this activity was different from the virion DNA polymerase activity.

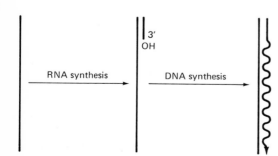

Figure 17-1. A model for DNA synthesis by reticuloendotheliosis virus virions. Only the second step appears required for *in vitro* DNA synthesis by avian leukosis-sarcoma virus virions: (−) RNA, (∼) DNA.

Table 17-1   Requirements for RNA Synthesis by
Reticuloendotheliosis Virus Virions

	[³H]UMP incorpora-tion (pmoles/mg protein/10 min)
Complete[a]	8.1
–NP-40	0.2
–MgCl₂	1.3
–MgCl₂, + MnCl₂[b]	3.8
–ATP	6.4
–ATP, CTP, GTP	2.7
+ Actinomycin D, 80 μg/ml	8.1
+ α-Amanitin, 80 μg/ml	9.6
+ Antibody[c] to TDSNV DNA polymerase	8.9

[a] Nonidet P-40–disrupted virions (40μg) of spleen necrosis virus (SNV), a member of the reticuloendotheliosis virus group, were incubated at 37°C in a total volume of 125 μl with 1 nmole each of ATP, CTP, and GTP, 0.5 nmole of [³H]UTP (22 Ci/mmole), and 1 μmole of MgCl₂ in 0.02 M Tris HCl (pH 8.0) containing 0.005 M dithiothreitol.

[b] 0.5 μmoles.

[c] The RNA synthesis was carried out after disrupted virions of SNV were preincubated at room temperature for 20 min with 50 μg of antibody, which inhibited over 95 percent of activated calf thymus DNA-directed DNA polymerase activity of disrupted virions of SNV (11).

The product was then characterized (Table 17-2). It was shown to be RNA by its resistance to deoxyribonuclease and its sensitivity to digestion by alkali and ribonuclease. The size of one-half of the native product was 4S and of the other half about 70S. After denaturation, all of the product was about 4S (data not shown).

Requirement for RNA Synthesis for Endogenous DNA Synthesis

The experiments described above established that RNA synthesis could occur in disrupted virions of reticuloendotheliosis viruses. To determine whether this RNA synthesis was required for endogenous DNA synthesis, a DNA synthesis reaction was carried out in the presence of all four ribonucleoside triphosphates. As seen in Figure 17-2, there was a five-fold stimulation of the rate of endogenous DNA synthesis in the presence of all four ribonucleoside triphosphates (or in the presence of only ATP and UTP). In the presence of ATP (or UTP) alone, there was a three-fold stimulation of the rate of DNA synthesis. It should be realized that the conditions used in this experi-

Table 17-2 Characterization of [³H]UMP-Labeled product

A reaction was carried out using the complete system described in Table 17-1. The product was purified with phenol and treated at 37°C for 1 hr as indicated. The concentrations of RNase A and DNase I were 50 μg/ml.

Treatment	Trichloroacetic acid insoluble dpm
None	2800
0.5 N NaOH	360
RNase A	340
DNase I	2200

ment were not optimal for both RNA synthesis and DNA synthesis. Therefore, these are minimal estimates of the amount of stimulation of DNA synthesis.

If the DNA was synthesized with RNA as a primer, it should be possible to isolate the covalently linked RNA–DNA intermediate and to demonstrate RNA–DNA linkage by studying the physical properties of the product and by analyzing the transfer of α-³²P from deoxyribonucleoside monophosphates to

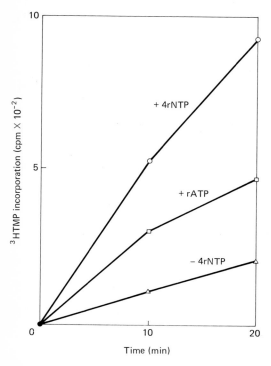

Figure 17-2. Stimulation of reticuloendotheliosis virus virion DNA synthesis by RNA synthesis. Nonidet P-40–disrupted virions of SNV (40 μg) were incubated at 37°C in a total volume of 125 μl with 1 μmole of MgCl₂, 0.5 nmoles of [³H]dTTP (18 C/mmole), and 5 nmoles each of dATP, dCTP, dGTP, (△) without any ribonucleoside triphosphates (−4 rNTP), (□) with 5 nmoles of ATP (+rATP), or (○) with 5 nmoles each of ATP, CTP, GTP, and UTP (+ rNTP) in 0.02 M Tris HCl (pH 8.0) containing 0.005 M dithiothreitol.

ribonucleoside monophosphates. To study the physical properties of the reaction product, a reaction was carried out in the presence of labeled ribonucleoside and deoxyribonucleoside triphosphates, and the product was isolated. The RNA and DNA products co-sedimented at 4S in a DMSO–sucrose density gradient. After alkali digestion, both labels sedimented more slowly than 4S, whereas, after deoxyribonuclease treatment, the DNA became TCA-soluble and the RNA still sedimented at 4S (data not shown). These results established that the DNA product was small and was linked to a 4S RNA.

RNA and DNA syntheses were then carried out in the presence of α-^{32}P-labeled deoxyribonucleoside triphosphates, and the products were digested with alkali. The results, shown in Table 17-3, indicate that some dAMP was attached to RNA, that it was almost the only deoxyribonucleoside monophosphate attached to RNA, and that 75 percent of the 3' terminal ribonucleoside monophosphates were UMP and 15 percent were AMP.

These experiments established that the reticuloendotheliosis virus virion endogenous DNA synthesis took place on an RNA primer that was about 4S and ended primarily in UMP and to lesser extent in AMP. To determine the 3' terminus of the newly synthesized RNA, a reaction was run with all four ribonucleoside triphosphates labeled, and the product was digested with alkali. The 3' terminal ribonucleoside monophosphates will become nucleosides, while the internally incorporated ribonucleoside monophosphates will become nucleotides. The results, shown in Table 17-4, indicate that 75 percent of the

Table 17-3 [^{32}P]Transfer at the RNA–DNA Linkage of the Reticuloendotheliosis Virus Virion RNA–DNA Product

RNA and DNA synthetic reactions were carried out with Nonidet P-40-disrupted virions of SNV in the presence of all four ribonucleoside triphosphates and all four deoxyribonucleoside triphosphates. One of the deoxyribonucleoside triphosphates was labeled with α-^{32}P. The product was isolated and degraded with alkali. The ribonucleoside monophosphates were separated by thin layer chromatography (14) and counted.

Labeled deoxyribonucleoside triphosphates	Percent total [^{32}P] transfer			
	Ap	CP	Gp	Vp
α-[^{32}P]dATP	15	0	0	75
α-[^{32}P]dCTP	0	0	0	0
α-[^{32}P]dGTP	0	0	0	0.5
α-[^{32}P]dTTP	1.5	0	6	2

Table 17.4   Incorporation of AMP,
UMP, CMP, and GMP by
Reticuloendotheliosis
Virus Virions

Disrupted virions of SNV were incubated in
the complete reaction mixture described in Table
17-1 with four ^{3}H-labeled ribonucleoside
triphosphates. The product was isolated and
degraded with alkali. The nucleosides and
nucleoside monophosphates were isolated by thin
layer chromatography (13,14) and counted.

	Percent pmoles	
AR	10 ⎱	
UR	30 ⎰	40
AMP	20 ⎱	
UMP	25 ⎰	45
CR, CMP, GR, GMP		15

ends were U and 25 percent were A. This distribution agrees well with the
data in Table 17-3.

In addition, the data in Table 17-4 indicate that about 40 percent of the
labeling occurred at the 3'-OH end of the RNA product. Since the product was
4S, this distribution indicates that much of the label was added to preformed
RNA molecules. In addition to this end addition, nearest neighbor analysis
and fingerprinting indicate that further RNA synthesis also occurs (data not
shown; J. Dahlberg, personal communication).

Summary and Conclusions

These data indicate that endogenous DNA synthesis by reticuloendotheliosis virus virions first requires endogenous RNA synthesis, apparently to form
the primer for the endogenous DNA synthesis. Further work is being carried
out to characterize the enzyme for the RNA synthesis, that is, whether it
is an RNA polymerase or a nucleotidyl terminal transferase. We are also
attempting to determine the nature of the template for the synthesis of the
primer and to determine whether the DNA product is synthesized using the
viral RNA as template.

The experiments reported here indicate that the mechanism of DNA synthesis by reticuloendotheliosis viruses is different from that by avian leukosis-

10. Hurwitz, J. and Leis, J. P. RNA-Dependent DNA polymerase activity of RNA tumor viruses. J. Virol., 9:116, 1972. .

11. Kawai, S. and Hanafusa, H. The effects of reciprocal changes in temperature on the transformed state of cells infected with a Rous sarcoma virus mutant. Virology, 46:470, 1971.

12. Loeb, L. A. Eucaryotic DNA polymerases. *In* Boyer, P. D., ed. The Enzymes. New York, Academic Press, Vol. X (in press).

13. Loeb, L. A., Tartof, K. D., and Travaglini, E. C. Copying natural RNAs with *E.coli* DNA polymerase I. Nature [New Biol.], 242:166, 1974.

14. McCaffrey, R., Smoler, D. F., and Baltimore, D. Terminal deoxynucleotidyl transferase in a case of childhood acute lymphoblastic leukemic. Proc. Natl. Acad. Sci. USA, 79:521, 1973.

15. Poiesz, B. J., Battula, N., and Loeb, L. A. Zinc in reserve transcriptase. Biochem. Biophys. Res. Commun., 56:959, 1974.

16. Slater, J. P., Mildvan, A. S., and Loeb, L. A. Zinc in DNA polymerase. Biochem. Biophys, Res. Commun., 44:37, 1971.

17. Slater, J. P., Tamir, I., Loeb, L. A., and Mildvan, A. S. The mechanism of *E. coli* DNA polymerase I: Magnetic resonance and kinetic studies of the role of metals. J. Biol. Chem., 247:6784, 1972.

18. Smith, G. R. and Gallo, R. C. DNA-Dependent DNA polymerase I and II from normal human blood lymphocytes. Proc. Natl. Acad. Sci. USA, 69:2879, 1972.

19. Springgate, C. F., Battula, N., and Loeb, L. A. Infidelity of DNA synthesis by reverse transcriptase. Biochem. Biophys. Res. Commun., 52:400, 1973.

20. Springgate, C. and Loeb, L. A. On mutagenic DNA polymerases in human leukemic cells. Proc. Natl. Acad. Sci. USA, 70:245, 1973.

21. Springgate, C. F., Mildvan, A. S., Abramson, R., Engle, J. L., and Loeb, L. A. *E. coli* DNA polymerase I, a zinc metalloenzyme. J. Biol. Chem., 247:6784, 1973.

22. Springgate, C. F., Seal, G., and Loeb, L. A. Infidelity of DNA replication in malignant cells. Res. Commun. Chem. Pathol. Pharmacol., 4:651, 1973.

Properties and Origin of the Subunits of Reverse Transcriptase Isolated from Avian RNA Tumor Viruses

A. Panet, I. M. Verma, and D. Baltimore

Introduction

One of the best indicators for the RNA tumor viruses group is the presence of reverse transcriptase activity in the virion (1,11). This polymerase activity can efficiently copy different RNA templates to give DNA products. Reverse transcriptases were purified from several different viruses, and their structure and activity with various templates primers were studied (6,7,12). All the isolated viral enzymes show high activity when poly(C):oligo(dG) was used as a template-primer. Subsequently, this assay became a crucial test in the search for new reverse transcriptases in various viruses or cell extracts (2). The enzymes most thoroughly studied were isolated from avian RNA tumor viruses (AMV or RSV), murine leukemia viruses (MuLV), and hamster leukemia virus (HaLV). Reverse transcriptases isolated from the different viruses have different molecular structure. Enzymes purified from AMV and RSV were shown to be composed of two polypeptides: a small subunit with molecular weights of 55,000 to 65,000 and a large subunit with molecular weights of 90,000 to 100,000 (7). The enzyme isolated from HaLV was also shown to be a two-subunit enzyme with subunit molecular weights of 53,000 and 68,000 (14). The MuLV reverse transcriptase is a single polypeptide with a molecular weight of 70,000 (10). Only reverse transcriptase isolated from avian RNA tumor viruses is capable of efficiently copying 70 S RNA isolated from the virion. The polymerases purified from MuLV and HaLV cannot efficiently transcribe isolated 70 S RNA *in vitro* (14,15).

The reverse transcriptase from avian RNA tumor viruses was shown to have ribonuclease H activity as well as polymerase activity (3,9). No ribonuclease H could be detected in the polymerases isolated from MuLV and HaLV (14,15). Grandgenett et al. (5) showed that, during purification of reverse transcriptase from AMV virions, the enzyme elutes from phosphocellulose column at two positions. The first activity was found, by glycerol gradient centrifugation, to be the small subunit (MW 65,000) that contains DNA poly-

Fundamental Aspects of Neoplasia,
edited by A. Arthur Gottlieb, Otto J. Plescia, and David H. L. Bishop.
© 1975 by Springer-Verlag New York Inc.

merase and ribonuclease H activities. The second peak of activity was found to contain two subunits (MW 65,000 and 105,000) with polymerase activity as well as ribonuclease H activity. In this chapter we describe experiments designed to study in detail the properties of the smaller subunit isolated from AMV and RSV reverse transcriptase. The two forms of the enzyme have similar enzymatic activities, but they differ in their binding affinity to the template-primer complex. In reverse transcriptase from temperature-sensitive mutant virus, the smaller subunit of the enzyme is responsible for the thermolability.

Separation of the Smaller Subunit from AMV Reverse Transcriptase

AMV reverse transcriptase was purified by sequential chromatography on DEAE-Sephadex and phosphocellulose (12). The main peak of activity from the phosphocellulose column was dialyzed against low salt buffer and rechromatographed on a second phosphocellulose column. Two peaks of reverse transcriptase activity were obtained from the second phosphocellulose column, the first peak usually constituted 3 to 7 percent of the total activity (Fig. 19-1). These two peaks of enzyme were concentrated and studied further. The difference in size between these two activities was estimated by chromatography on Sephadex G-100 column (Fig. 19-2). Whereas the main activity (peak II from phosphocellulose) appeared in the void volume of the Sephadex G-100, peak I was included in the Sephadex column and eluted only after *Escherichia coli* Pol. I (MW 109,000). Peak I was also isolated from RSV reverse transcriptase, and it comigrated on Sephadex G-100 column with peak I isolated from the AMV enzyme (Fig. 19-2).

Similarities and Differences between the Holoenzyme and the Smaller Subunit

The smaller subunit, like the honoenzyme, was found to catalyze DNA synthesis using various DNA and RNA templates, such as poly(C):oligo(dG), poly(dA-dT), and AMV 70 S RNA. Similar results were reported by Grandgenett *et al.* (5).

The common origin of peak I and peak II was tested by using antibodies, raised against the holoenzyme, to inhibit the activity of peak I. As can be seen from Figure 19-3, the polymerase activity of the holoenzyme and of the smaller subunit can be inhibited to the same extent by increasing the amounts of serum against AMV reverse transcriptase.

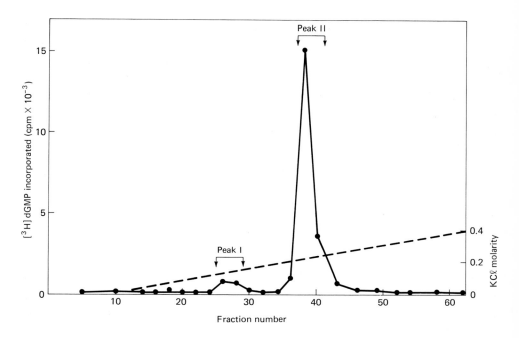

Figure 19-1. Separation of the smaller subunit on a phosphocellulose column. AMV reverse transcriptase was purified as described (12) and 370,000 enzyme units were further analyzed on a 6-ml phosphocellulose column. (A unit of enzyme is the amount of enzyme required to incorporate 1 pmole dGMP in 1 min at 37°C.) The column was washed with buffer A (50mM Tris HCl, pH8.0, 20 percent glycerol, 10 mM mercaptoethanol, 0.1 percent nonidet P40, 0.1 mM EDTA). The enzyme was eluted by washing the column with a 200 ml linear KCl gradient in buffer A from 0 to 0.4 M KCl. The fractions were assayed for polymerase activity using poly(C): oligo(dG) (12). The active fractions were pooled and concentrated on a small phosphocellulose column.

In many enzymatic systems, specific substrates are able to protect enzymes from inactivation by various factors. The extent of protection depends on the binding affinity of the enzyme for the substrate. Purified AMV reverse transcriptase can be protected from heat inactivation if the template-primer complex is added (Fig. 19-4). The effect of template-primer on the inactivation rate of the enzyme was determined by incubating the enzyme at 42°C, with or without template-primer, and assaying residual polymerase activity under standard conditions at 37°C. When poly(C):oligo(dG) were present during the preincubation of the holoenzyme, only 17 percent of the enzymatic activity was lost as compared to an 87 percent loss of enzymatic activity in a mixture that did not contain template-primer. We found that AMV 70 S RNA can

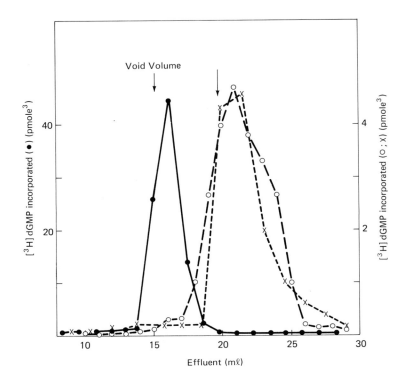

Figure 19-2. Size determination of peak I and peak II activities obtained from phosphocellulose column. The two activities from a phosphocellulose column (Fig. 19-1), peak I and peak II, were chromatographed separately on a Sephadex G-100 column (1×70 cm) with elution buffer (50 mM Tris HCl, pH 8.0; 20 percent glycerol, 0.2 M KCl, 0.1 mM EDTA, 10 mM mercaptoethanol, 0.1 percent noniodet P-40). The different fractions were assayed for polymerase activity with poly(C):oligo(dG). (×---×). *Escherichia coli* DNA Pol. I was used as an internal standard in the columns and was assayed by using poly(dA):oligo(dT)$_{12-18}$ as template-primer and [^{3}H]dTTP as substrate, (○---○) peak I of AMV, (○––○) peak I of RSV, (●—●) peak II of AMV.

protect the enzyme from inactivation better than poly(C):oligo(dG); after 30 min of preincubation at 42°C with AMV 70 S RNA, there was no apparent loss of enzymatic activity. When AMV 70 S RNA was first denatured, it lost some of its capacity to protect the enzyme as compared to native 70 S RNA; after 30 min preincubation with denatured RNA, 23 percent of the activity was lost.

The two forms of AMV reverse transcriptase (the holoenzyme and the smaller subunit) were compared for their ability to interact with the template-

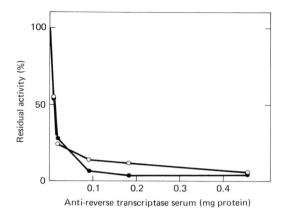

Figure 19-3. Inhibition of reverse transcriptase activity by specific antibodies. The reactions were conducted in two steps: (a) neutralization of reverse transcriptase by antibodies and (b) assay for residual reverse transcriptase activity (12). The initial reaction mixtures (50 μl) contained 10 mM Tris HCl (pH 8.3), 150 mM KCl, 20 percent glycerol, 50 μg bovine serum albumin, plus (○) 12 units peak I AMV reverse transcriptase or (●) 90 units of peak II, and rat anti-AMV reverse transcriptase serum (a gift from Dr. R. Nowinski). Incubation for 20 min at 37°C was followed by assay of the residual polymerase activity.

primer poly(C):oligo(dG) (Fig. 19-5). The thermal stability of the two forms is the same when no primer-template were present during the heating step. Where poly(C):oligo(dG) was included, the holoenzyme was protected from inactivation, and, after 30 min, only 36 percent of the activity was lost as compared to 78 percent lost in the absence of template-primer. On the other hand, the activity of the smaller subunit was not affected by poly(C): oligo(dG), and the rate of inactivation was the same with or without template-primer (Fig. 19-5).

Another line of evidence that the affinity of the smaller subunit for the template-primer is lower than that of the holoenzyme came from a study of the binding of reverse transcriptase to a DNA-cellulose column. DNA-cellulose columns are being widely used for purification of different proteins that participate in DNA metabolism and, therefore, bind very tightly to DNA-cellulose.

AMV reverse transcriptase was chromatographed on a DNA-cellulose column, and two peaks of activity were eluted by a salt gradient at 0.14M and 0.25 M KCl (Fig. 19-6). These two peaks were shown to be equivalent to respectively, peak I and peak II from phosphocellulose by a separate analysis of the DNA-cellulose fractions by exclusion chromatography on Sephadex G-100. The elution of the smaller subunit at lower salt from DNA cellulose

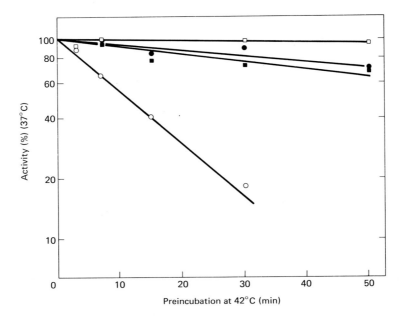

Figure 19-4. Protection of AMV reverse transcriptase from thermal inactivation by template-primer complex. Assays for heat lability were performed by preincubating the enzyme in a reaction mixture (200 μl) containing 50 mM Tris HCl (pH-8.3), 60 mM NaCl, 6 mM MgCl$_2$, 5 mM DDT, 20 μg bovine serum albumin and AMV reverse transcriptase, 1500 units: (○) without template-primer during preincubation, (●) with 10 μg poly (C) and 5 μg oligo (dG), (□) with 6 μg AMV 70 S RNA, ■ with heat-denatured AMV 70 S RNA (heated 3 min at 95°C). The mixtures were incubated at 42°C, at the times indicated, 20-μl aliquots were withdrawn, and residual enzymatic activity was measured at 37°C, using poly (C):oligo (dG) (12).

suggests that the smaller subunit has a lower affinity for DNA as compared to the holoenzyme. With this preparation of enzyme, some 25 percent of the enzymatic activity eluted from DNA-cellulose or Sephadex G-100 column as the smaller subunit. The high yield of the smaller subunit in this preparation was a result of its storage conditions. The holoenzyme was kept for 2 months in 50 percent glycerol at −20°C. Under these conditions, the dissociation of the enzyme into subunits appears to be faster than when the enzyme is kept frozen at −70°C.

The MuLV transcriptase is a single polypeptide with a molecular weight (70,000) similar to that of the smaller subunit of the AMV enzyme. It was of interest to study the effect of template-primer on the stability of MuLV reverse transcriptase as compared to the AMV enzyme. As can be seen from

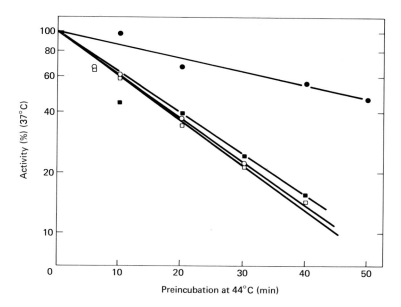

Figure 19-5. Thermal inactivation of peak I and peak II activities from phosphocellulose column chromatography. Assays for heat lability were conducted in two steps as described in Figure 19-4: (○) peak II (3,000 enzyme units) without template-primer during preincubation, (●) peak II (3,000 enzyme units) with 10 μg poly(C), 5 μg oligo(dG), (□) peak I (670 enzyme units) without template-primer, (■) peak I (670 enzyme units) with 10 μg poly(C), 5 μg oligo(dG). Preincubation was at 44°C, and residual polymerase activity was assayed at 37°C, as described (12).

Figure 19-7, MuLV reverse transcriptase is a heat-labile enzyme, and, after 30 min at 43°C, it loses more than 90 percent of its activity. Addition of poly(C):oligo(dG) or AMV 70 S RNA protects the enzyme from inactivation. After 30 min incubation in the presence of poly(C):oligo(dG), only 12 percent of the initial enzymatic activity was lost, and, when AMV 70 S RNA was present, 35 percent of the activity was lost. This result implies that the enzyme from MuLV is similar in its mode of interaction with template-primer to the holoenzyme isolated from AMV.

Characteristics of the Smaller Subunit from Temperature-Sensitive RSV Reverse Transcriptase

Verma et al. (13) have shown that reverse transcriptases purified from two temperature-sensitive mutants of RSV (*ts* 335 and *ts* 337) were thermolabile and that their heat inactivation rate was four to five times higher than the

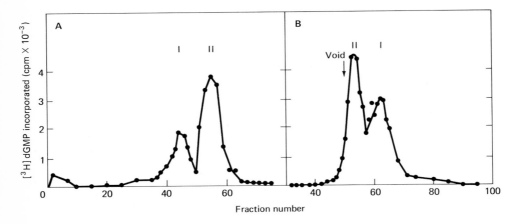

Figure 19-6. (A) Affinity chromatography of reverse transcriptase on DNA-cellulose. A DNA-cellulose column (3 ml) was washed with 50 mM Tris HCl (pH 8.0), 2 M KCl, and then equilibrated with buffer A (50 mM Tris HCl, pH 8.0, 20 percent glycerol, 10 mM mercaptoethanol, 0.1 mM EDTA, 0.1 percent Nonidet P40). Purified AMV reverse transcriptase (6,200 units) was applied to the column, and the column was washed with buffer A. The enzyme was eluted with a linear KCl gradient in buffer A (2×50 ml) 0 to 0.4 M KCl. Fractions were assayed for polymerase activity with poly(C):oligo(dG). **(B)** Chromatography of AMV reverse transcriptase on a Sephadex G-100 column. Purified reverse transcriptase (2,500 units) was chromatographed on Sephadex G-100 (1×70 cm). The column was washed with buffer A and assayed for polymerase activity as described in (A).

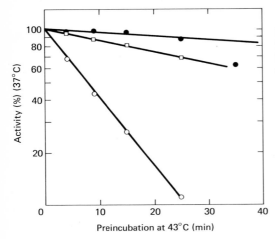

Figure 19-7. Protection of MuLV reverse transcriptase from thermal inactivation by template-primer complex. Reactions were conducted in two steps as described in Figure 19-1. Rauscher murine leukemia virus reverse transcriptase (80 enzyme units) was purified as described (5). Preincubation was at 43°C and residual polymerase activity was assayed as described (12): (○) without template-primer during preincubation, (●) with 10 μg poly(C), 5 μg oligo(dG), (□) with 6 μg AMV 70 S RNA.

rate for the wild type enzyme. Since the enzyme consists of two polypeptides, it is important to locate the mutation site responsible for this thermolability. The smaller subunit was isolated from the temperature-sensitive mutant *ts* 337 and from wild type RSV by chromatography on a phosphocellulose column, as shown in Figure 19-1. The thermolability of the smaller subunit was compared to that of the holoenzyme by preincubation of the enzymes at high temperature and measurement of the residual enzymatic activity.

The three activities of reverse transcriptase were compared using poly(C): oligo(dG) to measure RNA-dependent DNA synthesis, poly(dC):oligo(dG) to measure DNA-dependent DNA synthesis, and [^{3}H]poly(A):poly(dT) for ribonuclease H activity (Fig. 19-8). The smaller subunit isolated from *ts* 337 virions was found to be five to seven times more thermolabile than the smaller subunit of wild type origin. The DNA polymerase activity in the smaller subunit (peak I) isolated either from wild type or from *ts* 337 virions was inactivated at a rate very similar to that of the corresponding holoenzyme (peak II). For wild type enzyme and for enzyme from the mutant *ts* 337 virions, the ribonuclease H activity in the holoenzyme was found to be more temperature stable than the same activity in the smaller subunit of the same origin.

Conclusion

Very little is known about the mode of action of reverse transcriptase in the host cells. The possibility of separating the two subunits of the enzyme isolated from avian RNA tumor viruses offers a tool to study the function of each subunit. It has been shown that the isolated smaller subunit can catalyze all the three known enzymatic activities of the AMV reverse transcriptase: (a) copying RNA into DNA, (b) copying DNA into double-stranded DNA, (c) ribonuclease H. No activity could be attributed to the larger subunit. By purifying the separate smaller subunit of the DNA polymerase from a temperature-sensitive mutant of RSV (*ts* 337), it was possible to show that this subunit is encoded by the viral RNA because it retains the temperature sensitivity of the holoenzyme. The origin of the larger subunit is now under investigation. In analogy to the phage Qβ replicase, which consists of one phage-encoded subunit and three host polypeptides (4,8), one possibility is that the larger subunit is of host origin. Although no enzymatic activity could be connected with the larger subunit, its absence reduced the binding affinity of the smaller subunit to the template-primer complex.

We have isolated reverse transcriptase from chick fibroblasts transformed by RSV. Reverse transcriptase from this cell extract elutes from a phosphocellulose column as a single peak of activity at a KCl concentration of 0.25 M. This is the same salt concentration required to elute the holoenzyme purified from

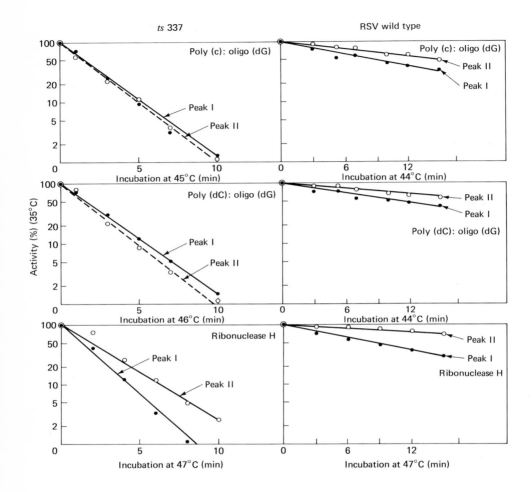

Figure 19-8. Thermal inactivation of DNA polymerase and ribonuclease H activities of smaller subunit and holoenzyme from RSV *ts* 337. Reverse transcriptase (the holoenzyme and the smaller subunit) from Rous sarcoma virus wild type or *ts* 337 were isolated as described in Figure 19-1. Assays of heat lability were performed by preincubating the enzyme in reaction mixture I, which contained 100 mM Tris HCl (pH 8.3), 20 mM dithiothreitol, 12 mM MgAc₂, and 120 mM NaCl; incubation was at high temperature. At various intervals, 0.05-ml aliquots were withdrawn and added to 0.05 ml of reaction mixture II, which contained template, primer, and substrates. mixture was kept on ice for a maximum of 10 to 15 min and then further incubated at 34°C for 15 min. Acid-precipitable radioactivity was measured as described (12). The rate of the enzyme reaction at 34°C was linear for at least 15 min. Template-primer was 1 μg poly(C) or poly(dC) with 0.5 μg oligo(dG); 20 nmoles [³H]dGTP (100 cpm/pmole) was used as substrate for DNA polymerase. Ribonuclease H was assayed by using[³H]poly(A): poly(dt) as substrate and monitoring the degradation of [³H]poly(A) to an acid-soluble substance (12).

RSV virions from phosphocellulose, which suggests that the reverse transcriptase in infected cells exists only in the form of holoenzyme. All of the reverse transcriptase activity in these transformed cells was found in the cellular membrane fraction, and no enzymatic activity could be detected in the cytoplasmic fraction (to be published).

ACKNOWLEDGMENTS

This work was supported by a contract from the Virus Cancer Program of the National Cancer Institute. One of us (D. B.) was supported by a research professorship from the American Cancer Society.
We thank Dr. Haseltine for useful discussions.

REFERENCES

1. Baltimore, D. RNA-Dependent DNA polymerase in virions of RNA tumor viruses. Nature, 226:1209, 1970.

2. Baltimore, D., McCaffrey, R., and Smoler, D. F. Properties of reverse transcriptases. *In* Fox, C. F. and Robinson, W. S., eds. New York, Academic Press, 1973, Vol. 13, p. 51.

3. Baltimore, D. and Smoler, D. Association of an endoribonuclease with the avian myeloblastosis virus DNA polymerase. J. Biol. Chem., 247:7282, 1972.

4. Blumenthal, T., Landers, T. A., and Weber, K. Bacteriophage Qβ replicase contains the protein biosynthesis elongation factors EF Tu and EF Ts. Proc. Nat. Acad. Sci. USA, 96:1313, 1972.

5. Grandgenett, D. P., Gerard, G. F., and Green, M. A single subunit from avian myeloblastosis virus with both RNA-directed DNA polymerase and ribonuclease H activity. Proc. Natl. Acad. Sci. USA, 70:230, 1973.

6. Hurwitz, J. and Leis, J. P. RNA-Dependent DNA polymerase activity of RNA tumor viruses. I. Directing influence of DNA in the reaction. J. Virol., 9:116, 1972.

7. Kacian, D. L., Watson, K. F., Burny, A., and Spiegelman, S. Purification of the DNA polymerase of avian myeloblastosis virus. Biochim. Biophys. Acta, 246:365, 1971.

8. Kamen, R. Characterization of the subunits of Qβ replicase. Nature, 228:527, 1970.

9. Molling, K., Bolognesi, D. P., Baur, H., Busen, W., Plassman, H., and Hausen, P. Association of viral reverse transcriptase with an enzyme degrading the RNA moiety of RNA–DNA hybrids. Nature [New Biol.], 234:240, 1971.

10. Ross, J., Scolnick, E. M., Todaro, G. J., and Aaronson, S. A. Separation of murine cellular and murine leukemia virus DNA polymerases. Nature [New Biol.], 231:163, 1971.

11. Temin, H. and Mizutani, S. RNA-Dependent DNA polymerase in virions of Rous sarcoma virus. Nature, 226:1211, 1970.

12. Verma, I. and Baltimore, D. Purification of the RNA-directed DNA polymerase from avian myeloblastosis virus and its assay with polynucleotide templates. *In* Moldave, K.

and Grossman, L., eds. Methods in Enzymology. New York, Academic Press, 1973, Vol. 29, p. 125.

13. Verma, I. M., Mason, W. S., Drost, S. D., and Baltimore, D. DNA polymerase activity from two temperature-sensitive mutants of Rous sarcoma virus is thermolabile. Nature, 251:27, 1974.

14. Verma, I. M., Meuth, N. L., Fan, H., and Baltimore, D. Hamster leukemia virus DNA polymerase: Unique structure and lack of demonstrable endogenous activity. J. Virol., 13:1075, 1974.

15. Wang, L. H. and Duesberg, P. H. DNA polymerase of murine sarcoma-leukemia virus: RNase H and low activity with viral RNA and natural DNA templates. J. Virol., 12: 1512, 1973.

An Inhibitor of DNA Polymerase Produced by Tumor Cells

A. A. Gottlieb, A. H. Smith, O. J. Plescia,
D. E. Nicholson, S. Bowers,
E. Pankuch, and D. Berkoben

We have previously described the isolation and partial characterization of several DNA polymerases from the murine myeloma, MOPC 21 (1,2). In particular, we have called attention to a distinct enzyme from this line of cells (R-1 polymerase), which has the ability to utilize the synthetic polynucleotide duplex poly rA:oligo(dT)$_{12-18}$ very efficiently. In this regard, R-1 polymerase resembles reverse transcriptase from the Rauscher murine leukemia virus, but it can be readily distinguished from the latter by its sedimentation coefficient and isolectric point. A summary of the comparative properties of the R-1 polymerase and the reverse transcriptase from the Rauscher murine leukemia virus are listed in Table 20-1.

In the course of our attempts to produce antibody against the Rauscher viral polymerase, we had occasion to inject Balb/c mice with the syngeneic tumor lines, MOPC-21 as well as the ascitic leukemia MCDV-12. It was observed that the sera of syngeneic tumor-bearing mice contained a factor that inhibited the R-1 polymerase. Moreover, only small amounts of inhibition were displayed by sera from allogeneic mice that had received these tumors (3). A study of the time-course of appearance of inhibitor in sera from syngeneic and allogeneic mice inoculated with the MCDV-12 leukemia line is displayed in Figure 20-1. It is clear that the level of inhibitor rises continually in the syngeneic line, but only small amounts of inhibitor appear in the serum of allogeneic mice. This observation suggests but does not prove that the inhibitory factor is produced by the tumor itself, and that the low levels observed in the allogeneic mice reflect initial growth of the tumor followed by rejection and resorption.

If allogeneic mice are immunosuppressed by radiation and then inoculated with tumor, the tumor will grow in these hosts and the level of R-1 polymerase inhibitor observed in the sera of these immunosuppressed mice is comparable to that observed when the same tumor is given to syngeneic mice (Table 20-2). Again, this suggests that the tumor cell itself is the source of the R-1 poly-

Fundamental Aspects of Neoplasia,
edited by A. Arthur Gottlieb, Otto J. Plescia, and David H. L. Bishop.
© 1975 by Springer-Verlag New York Inc.

Table 20-1   Comparative Properties of Ribopolymer-Transcribing
Polymerases

The properties described for murine myeloma R-1 polymerase and the RMLV polymerase
are those obtained in our laboratory. Sedimentation was carried out on 10 to 30 percent
gradients of glycerol containing 50 mM Tris MCl (pH 7.8); 500 mM KCl, 0.1 mM EDTA,
1 mM DDT, 0.2 percent Tween-80. The S values were computed by the formula of Martin
and Ames (7), using bovine serum albumin or bovine gamma globulin as standards.
Isoelectric focusing was carried out in 7 percent polyacrylamide gels containing 2.0 percent
of pH 3 to 10 ampholytes (LKB). After focusing was complete, the gels were sliced into
1 mm fractions and eluted into a standard assay mixture (1,2).

The data for the R-DNA polymerase were obtained from Arthur Weissbach (personal
communication), and the information on the peak A polymerase is from ref. 5. The pIs
of the R-DNA polymerase and the peak A polymerase were determined in our laboratory.

	Murine myeloma R-1 polymerase	RMLV polymerase	R-DNA polymerase (DNA Pol. III)	Peak A polymerase
Sedimentation coefficient	9.1	4.0	5.9	4.0
MW (approx.)	228,000	70,000	110,000	69,000
p*I*	5.4	4.9	5.7	5.2

merase inhibitor. This can be directly proved by culturing such tumor cells as
the MC-16 fibrosarcoma *in vitro*. The culture fluid obtained when such cells
are incubated at 37°C displays inhibitory activity against the R-1 polymerase,
whereas similar cells grown at 4°C produce very little of the inhibitor (Fig.
20-2). This result is direct evidence that the tumor cell produces the inhibitor
itself, and that the production of inhibitor is not dependent upon or influenced
by the response of the host to the tumor. Moreover, this study indicates that
only metabolically active tumor cells produce the inhibitor.

As indicated above, syngeneic mice inoculated with the MOPC-21 myeloma
cells, the MCDV-12 ascites leukemia, or the MC-16 or MCA-A fibrosarcomas
have R-1 polymerase inhibitor in their sera, whereas similar mice not challenged
with tumor have low levels of inhibitor in their sera. The levels of inhibitor
seen in the sera of normal mice are, however, significant. It is not known
whether inhibitor in normal sera is a manifestation of the rapid growth of
normal cells or a reflection of small numbers of tumor cells, which may be
present in normal mice. That question can only be resolved by further research.
In any case, the striking difference in inhibitory activity of sera from syngeneic
mice bearing tumors as compared with mice not bearing tumors suggests that

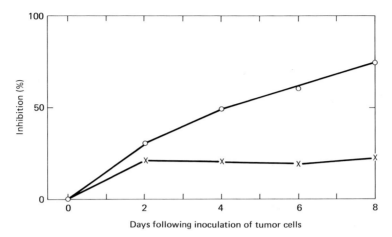

Figure 20-1. Time course of development of polymerase inhibitor in serum. On day 0 (○) syngeneic Balb/c and (X) allogeneic CFW mice were inoculated with 10^5 MCDV-12 cells. Aliquots of serum were drawn on the days indicated and 1/8 dilutions prepared in 0.02 M Tris HCl (pH 7.8), 4 mM BME, 1 mg/ml BSA, and 20 percent glycerol. A 75-μl sample of the respective dilutions was added to 8.1 μg of the R-1 polymerase in a total volume of 150 μl. After incubation at room temperature for 30 min, 50 μl of each of the mixtures was transferred to duplicate assay tubes, and incubation was continued for another 60 min at 37°. The specific activity of the [^{3}H]TTP used in these assay mixtures was 4570 cpm/pmole, and, under these conditions, this amount of enzyme catalyzed incorporation of 11.4 pmole of [^{3}H]TMP/hour. (From Gottlieb et al., ref. 3. Reprinted with permission.)

this difference in concentration of inhibitor may be used to detect the presence of small numbers of tumor cells.

At this point, it was necessary to ascertain certain of the properties of the serum inhibitor. Of interest in this regard, was the observation that this material remained soluble in 70 percent saturated ammonium sulfate solution and, as a result, could be shown to be free of gamma globulin and therefore not to be an antibody directed against the R-1 polymerase. Moreover, the inhibitor was *not* a nuclease. This could be shown by three lines of evidence:

1. The factor was capable of inactivating only the R-1 polymerase from the MOPC-21 line and the R-DNA polymerase from HeLa cells (4) or a subclone (KA 31) of Balb/3T3 A31 cells, which had been transformed by the Kirsten murine sarcoma virus (5).* It displayed no activity

* The R-DNA polymerase from HeLa cells was provided by Dr. Arthur Weissbach; the enzyme from the KA 31 cells was the gift of Dr. David Livingston.

Table 20-2   Effect of X-Irradiation of C57Bl/6 Recipient Mice on the Appearance of R-1 Polymerase Inhibitor in Serum

A group of C57Bl/6 mice (allogeneic to the MCDV-12 tumor) were X-irradiated (700 R) before receiving 10^5 MCDV-12 tumor cells or 10^8 sheep red blood cells (sRBC). Another group of C57Bl/6 mice was not irradiated but was challenged with MCDV-12 tumor cells or sRBC. Sera were collected 7 days after challenge and pooled separately from both sets of mice. 75 μl aliquots of a (1/8) dilution if these sera were mixed with 10.7 μg of the R-1 polymerase and held at room temperature for 30 min. Aliquots of 50 μl of these reaction mixtures were assayed in our standard R-1 polymerase assay as described previously (3). Samples of sera drawn before X-irradiation were tested in parallel. Results are expressed in terms of the uninhibited R-1 polymerase control.

Serum from C57Bl/6 mice	[³H]TMP incorporated (cpm)	Control (%)
Irradiated and given MCDV-12 cells	15603	47.9
Given MCDV-12 cells (no radiation)	23747	72.8
Irradiated and given sRBC	28257	86.6
Given sRBC (no radiation)	27322	83.8
Pre-irradiation	31036	95.2
R-1 enzyme control (no serum)	32601	100.0

against the polymerases from either the Rauscher murine leukemia virus (RMLV) or the avian myeloblastosis virus when the polymerases were assayed under conditions employing the same template (poly(rA):(dT)$_{12-18}$) and producing the same poly dT product (Fig. 20-3). If the inhibitor were a nuclease, one would expect it to suppress the action of these viral polymerases by degrading the template and/or the product of the reaction.

2. If sufficient inhibitor is added to the R-1 polymerase, so as to suppress the activity of the R-1 polymerase to 60 percent of the non-inhibited control reaction, the inhibition can be reversed by adding more of the R-1 polymerase (Fig. 20-4). Hence, in this study, the inhibitor did not display nucleolytic action against the polynucleotide template.

3. Direct examination of the partially purified inhibitor against a mixture of ³H-labeled synthetic ribopolynucleotides or ³H-labeled DNA from *Bacillus subtilis* indicates that the inhibitor does not possess nucleolytic properties.

Other biochemical properties of the R-1 polymerase inhibitor include: (a) approximate banding densities of 1.40 g/ml and 1.64 g/ml in equilibrium density gradients of cesium sulfate and cesium chloride, respectively and (b)

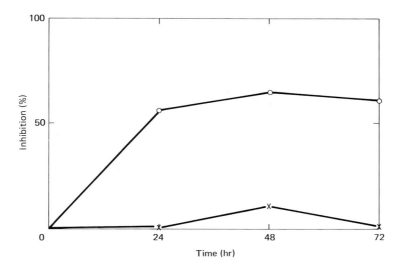

Figure 20-2. *In vitro* production by MC-16 fibrosarcoma cells of R-1 inhibitor. Aliquots of MC-16 fibrosarcoma cells were cultured at (○) 37° and (X) 4°C in minimum essential medium supplemented with 10 percent fetal calf serum. The medium from each set of cultures was collected as indicated. Ammonium sulfate was added to 70 percent saturation, and, after dialysis and reconstitution of the 70 percent supernatant to equal volume, a 0.1 dilution was tested as described in the legend to Figure 20-1. The results are expressed as a percentage of an R-1 polymerase reaction to which culture medium from an acellular culture had been added.

sensitivity of the inhibitor to a mixture of nuclease-free chymotrypsin and trypsin and to deoxyribonuclease (Table 20-3) but not to ribonuclease A. A reasonable interpretation of these results is that the inhibitor is a nucleoprotein. It is apparent from our studies that DNA in the serum of these tumor-bearing mice cannot by itself account for the observed inhibitory activity of these sera, since the concentrations of DNA present in the preparations of inhibitor as determined by the method of Kissane and Robbins (6) are not sufficient to account for the degree of inhibition observed. Moreover, the inhibitor does not inactivate DNA polymerases, which are strongly active on DNA templates, including *E. coli* DNA Pol. I. It is likely that the inhibitor is a complex of DNA and proteins of an as yet undetermined nature. A similar inhibitor has been found in the plasma of a patient with multiple myeloma. Fig. 20-5 demonstrates the comparative effects of plasma from this patient and plasma from a normal healthy individual on the R-1 and RMLV polymerases. It is clearly seen that the plasma from the patient with multiple myeloma contains an inhibitory factor directed against the R-1 polymerase but not

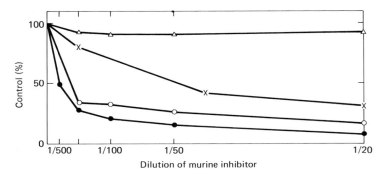

Figure 20-3. Selective action of the murine R-1 polymerase inhibitor. A preparation of the partially purified murine inhibitor containing 585 μg protein/ml prepared by ammonium sulfate fractionation was diluted as indicated, and 75 μl of these respective dilutions was added to 75 μl of enzyme dilution buffer containing 6.0 μg (●) R-1 polymerase, (○) HeLa R-DNA polymerase, (X) KA 31 R-DNA polymerase; or 9.0 μg (△) Rauscher MLV polymerase. Incubation and assay were carried out as previously described (2). Under these conditions, in which the specific activity of the [³H]TTP employed was 4,570 cpm/pmole, these amounts of R-1, HeLa R-DNA, KA 31 R-DNA, and RMLV polymerase catalyzed the incorporation of 4.5, 4.1, 2.4, and 4.7 pmole of [³H]TMP, respectively. The results are expressed as a percentage of the uninhibited controls.

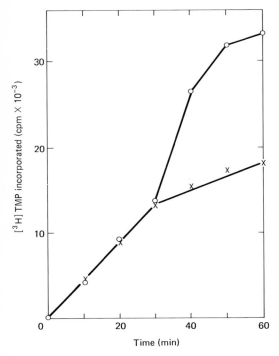

Figure 20-4. Reversal of inhibition by addition of more R-1 polymerase. Serum from MCDV-12 tumor-bearing mice was brought to 70 percent saturation in ammonium sulfate, and 100 μl of the resulting supernatant fraction was added at time 0 to two separate but identical 2.0-ml reaction mixtures, each of which represented an eightfold expansion of our standard (0.25 ml) assay mixture for R-1 polymerase activity. Each reaction mixture contained 29.5 μg of the R-1 polymerase, and [³H]TTP was supplied at a specific activity of 4,113 cpm/pmole. Incubation of each mixture was carried out at 37°C, and 0.25-ml aliquots were withdrawn at 10-min intervals for the determination of the level of incorporation of [³H]TMP into acid-precipitable form. At 30 minutes, (○) additional R-1 polymerase was added to one reaction mixture, while (X) dilution buffer only was added to the other.

Table 20-3 Effect of Pancreatic DNAse and Trypsin–Chymotrypsin on the R-1 Polymerase Inhibitor

A standard preparation of murine R-1 inhibitor, produced by ammonium sulfate fractionation, was incubated with 100 μg of deoxyribonuclease or a mixture of 100 μg trypsin + 100 μg chymotrypsin in a total volume of 3.0 ml of enzyme dilution buffer for 6 hours at 25°C. At the end of this period, the mixture was heated to 65°C for 5 minutes and washed through a CF-50A Centriflo membrane filter (Amicon), using 100 ml of 0.01 M Tris (pH 7.8)–0.01 M NaCl to remove the DNase, trypsin, and chymotrypsin, which are small enough to pass through the filter. The inhibitor remained as a concentrated solution in the filter cone and was diluted to a final volume of 1.0 ml in Tris saline, which represents a 0.1 dilution of the original inhibitor preparation. To ensure that the treated inhibitor was free of DNase, trypsin, or chymotrypsin, aliquots of enzyme dilution buffer were carried through identical treatment procedures with these enzymes, and the residue, recovered in the Centriflo cones after washing, were tested for their effects on the R-1 polymerase reaction. These control preparations are referred to as DNase control and chymotrypsin–trypsin controls. Both of these controls exhibited no inhibition of the R-1 polymerase reaction, indicating that the Centriflo procedure effectively removes these enzymes.

	[³H]TMP incorporated (cpm)	Control (%)
Pancreatic DNase		
R-1 polymerase control	23,140	100.0
R-1 polymerase + inhibitor	12,078	52.2
R-1 polymerase + inhibitor treated with DNase[a]	27,501	118.8
R-1 polymerase + inhibitor treated with DNase[a]	25,768	111.3
Trypsin-chymotrypsin		
R-1 polymerase control	23,140	100.0
R-1 polymerase + inhibitor	12,078	52.2
R-1 polymerase + inhibitor treated with trypsin-chymotrypsin[b]	21,801	94.2
R-1 polymerase + Dilution buffer treated with trypsin-chymotrypsin[b]	24,987	108.0

[a] The DNase was removed from the inhibitor by filtration through a CF-50A Centriflo membrane. The DNase passes through the membrane, while the inhibitor is retained.

[b] The trypsin and chymotrypsin were removed from the inhibitor by filtration through a Centriflo CF-50A membrane. The trypsin and chymotrypsin pass through the membrane, while the inhibitor is retained.

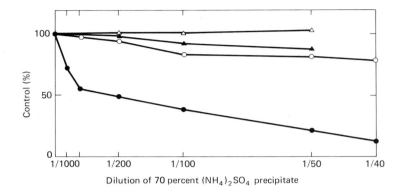

Figure 20-5. Inhibition of the R-1 polymerase by plasma from a patient with multiple myeloma. Plasma was obtained from a patient with multiple myeloma confirmed by bone marrow aspiration and 100 ml of this plasma was adjusted to 50 percent saturation in ammonium sulfate. The supernatant was recovered and additional ammonium sulfate to 70 percent saturation was added. The precipitate and supernatant fractions were recovered and dialyzed against 0.01 M Tris (pH 7.8)–0.15 M NaCl. In this case, inhibitory activity against the R-1 polymerase was detected in the precipitate but not in the supernatant fraction. [In the experiments presented herein, the greatest inhibition of the R-1 polymerase was displayed by the fraction of human myeloma plasma which was soluble in 50% saturated but precipitable at 70% saturated ammonium sulfate, and is so indicated in the material presented in this report. Investigation of other plasma and serum preparations from patients with various types of lymphoid-derived malignancies has demonstrated the presence of similar inhibitors in these sera, but, in all other cases, the bulk of the inhibitor appears in the fraction of serum which is soluble in 70% saturated ammonium sulfate. The reason for this difference in solubility between the plasma sample described herein and other plasma and serum preparations is unknown and is currently under study.] The 70 percent precipitate was diluted, as indicated, in enzyme dilution buffer, and 75 μl of three diluted fractions were added to 75 μl of enzyme dilution buffer containing 6.0 μg of the R-1 polymerase or 9.0 μg of the Rauscher MLV polymerase. Incubation and assay were carried out as described in the legend to Table 20-1. Under these conditions, in which the specific activity of the [^{3}H]TTP used was 4,715 cpm/pmole, the (●) R-1 and (▲) RMLV polymerases catalyzed the incorporation of 4.6 and 4.9 pmole of [^{3}H]TMP, respectively. Plasma from a normal individual (100 ml) was treated in a manner identical to the myeloma plasma—the fraction of normal plasma that precipitated between 50 and 70 percent ammonium sulfate was recovered, dialyzed, and assayed as above: (○) R-1 and (△) RMLV polymerases. The results are displayed as a percentage of the uninhibited control. In a separate study, the fraction of normal plasma soluble in 70-percent saturated ammonium sulfate gave no inhibition.

276

against the RMLV polymerase, while normal human plasma displays little inhibition against either polymerase.

Thus, we believe that we have clearly demonstrated that several types of mouse tumor cells produce a nucleoprotein factor that inactivates the R-1 polymerase. We have suggested that detection of such a material could be used as a basis for a test to demonstrate the presence of small numbers of tumor cells, *in vivo*. Further studies are clearly required to evaluate this suggestion, and to determine the biochemical characteristics and functions of this unusual inhibitory moiety.

ACKNOWLEDGMENTS

This work was principally supported by a grant-in-aid from the Damon Runyon–Walter Winchell Fund (DRG-1213) and additional support in the form of grants from the Metzger–Price Fund of New York (to A. A. G.) and the Ruth Estin Goldberg Memorial Fund (to O. J. P.); D. E. N. is a fellow of the Cancer Research Institute Inc.

We are gratefully indebted to Dr. Simon Sutcliffe for providing us with plasma from a patient with multiple myeloma.

REFERENCES

1. Persico, F. J. and Gottlieb, A. A. DNA polymerase of myeloma: Template and primer specificities of two enzymes. Nature [New Biol.], 239:173, 1972.

2. Persico, F. J., Nicholson, D. E., and Gottlieb, A. A. Isolation and partial characterization of multiple DNA polymerases of the murine myeloma. MOPC-21. Cancer Res. 33:1210, 1973.

3. Gottlieb, A. A., Smith, A. H., Plescia, O. J., Persico, F. J., and Nicholson, D. E. Inhibitor of DNA polymerase in sera of tumor-bearing mice. Nature, 246:480, 1973.

4. Bolden, A., Fry, M., Muller, R., Citarella, R., and Weissbach, A. The presence of a polyriboadenylic acid dependent DNA polymerase in eukaryotic cells. Arch. Biochem. Biophys., 153:26, 1972.

5. Livingston, D. M., Serxner, L. E., Hawk, D. J., Hudson, T., and Todaro, G. J. Characterization of a new murine cellular DNA polymerase. Proc. Natl. Acad. Sci. USA, 71:57, 1974.

6. Kissane, J. M. and Robins, E. The fluorometric measurement of deoxyribonucleic acid in animal tissues with special reference to the central nervous system. J. Biol. Chem., 233:184, 1958.

7. Martin, R. G. and Ames, B. A. A method for determining the sedimentation behavior of enzymes: Application to protein mixtures. J. Biol. Chem., 236:1372, 1961.

V

Viral Expression and Cell Transformation

21

In Vitro Transcription Studies with RNA Tumor Viruses

M. Jacquet, Y. Groner, G. Monroy, and J. Hurwitz

Introduction

RNA tumor viruses replicate via a pathway involving both DNA synthesis and DNA-dependent RNA synthesis (6,7,14). The first step in the pathway probably involves the action of viral RNA-dependent DNA polymerase to yield covalent RNA:DNA hybrid structures. By a mechanism, presently unknown, this intermediate is converted to DNA, which is found integrated in the host chromosome. It may be that, once integrated, viral and host genes are treated identically, and subsequent steps depend upon the nuclear transcription machinery.

In vitro analysis of viral RNA transcription of the genetic material from infected cells not only is important in elucidating the mechanism of viral expression but could also provide information on transcription in eukaryotic cells. Such studies are possible with RNA tumor viruses, since DNA complementary to viral RNA, which can be used to detect viral RNA sequences by molecular hybridization, can be readily obtained.

In this chapter, the *in vitro* transcription of viral RNA was examined using myeloblasts from chicks infected with avian myeloblastosis virus (AMV). Two types of *in vitro* transcript products were analyzed, one from isolated nuclei and the other formed from myeloblast chromatin by eukaryotic RNA polymerase. In both cases, labeled RNA formed *in vitro* yielded RNA sequences which hybridized to viral DNA probes. Similar results with nuclei isolated from Rous sarcoma, virus-infected cells have been obtained by Rymo et al. (13).

Characterization of AMV cDNA

DNA complementary to AMV RNA (cDNA) was synthesized by permeabilized AMV in the presence of high concentrations of actinomycin D (10); the latter prevents synthesis of duplex DNA, which interferes with the annealing of RNA to DNA (11). The cDNA was examined for its ability to

Fundamental Aspects of Neoplasia,
edited by A. Arthur Gottlieb, Otto J. Plescia, and David H. L. Bishop.
© 1975 by Springer-Verlag New York Inc.

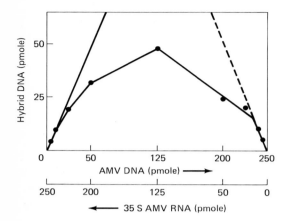

Figure 21-1. Complementarity of AMV cDNA and AMV 35 S RNA. The indicated amounts of 35 S AMV RNA and [³H]DNA (1,250 cpm/pmole of nucleotide) were incubated in the presence of 20 mM Tris Cl (pH 8.0) and 0.3 M NaCl in a total volume of 0.025 ml at 68° for 24 hr. After aliquots of the reaction mixture were treated with *Neurospora* nuclease (1.2 U/Ml) for 40 min at 37°C, the amount of acid-insoluble radioactivity remaining was determined.

hybridize to viral RNA sequences. Since virus could contain cellular RNA (9), cDNA was annealed to 35 S RNA isolated from heat-denatured AMV 70 S RNA. The hybrid structures formed were resistant to *Neurospora* nuclease, and nuclease S₁, and were sensitive to *Escherichia coli* RNase H. The hybrid material banded at a density of 1.550 g/cm³ in cesium sulfate, and melted sharply with a T_m of 88°.5C in 0.3 M NaCl. The experiment outlined in Figure 21-1 shows the stoichiometric relationship between 35 S RNA and cDNA at varying RNA:DNA ratios. The shape of the curve suggests that the RNA sequences are not equally distributed in the DNA transcript. When excess cDNA was added, the amount of DNA in hybrid was equivalent to the input RNA, indicating that all the 35 S RNA sequences were present in the cDNA. In the presence of excess RNA, more than 95 percent of the cDNA was hybridized, demonstrating that almost all the cDNA sequences correspond to 35 S RNA sequences. Thus, the cDNA is a valid probe for viral RNA sequences.

Transcription in Isolated Nuclei

RNA products synthesized *in vitro* by isolated myeloblast nuclei were examined for viral specific sequences. Myeloblast nuclei were purified by repetitive centrifugation at low speed after disruption of cellular membranes with Triton X-100. RNA synthesis was monitored by incorporation of labeled UTP into acid-insoluble material. Maximal incorporation depended upon the addition of the four nucleoside triphosphates, divalent cations, and relatively high ionic strength. The product was RNA as determined by its susceptibility to alkali and RNase A (>99 percent sensitive). α-Amanitin, a specific inhibitor of the nucleoplasmic RNA polymerase (form B) (3), reduced RNA synthesis by 80 percent. Viral sequences in nuclear transcript products were detected by hybridization with cDNA. In the experiment presented in Table 21-1, [^{32}P]RNA synthesized by isolated nuclei was incubated with an excess of cDNA at 68°C. The [^{32}P]RNA annealed with cDNA was measured by its susceptibility to RNAse H after single-stranded material had been digested with RNase A and RNase T$_1$. Approximately 2 percent of the nuclear transcript product was found in the hybrid structure. This result depended upon the addition of cDNA during annealing; RNA incubated without cDNA did not yield duplex structures. RNA synthesized in the presence of α-amanitin did not contain detectable viral RNA, indicating that the nucleoplasmic RNA polymerase B is probably responsible for the synthesis of AMV RNA sequences. Control experiments, in which RNA was synthesized in nuclei isolated from livers of uninfected chicks, yielded no detectable RNA:DNA hybrid structures with AMV cDNA.

To determine whether the amount of viral RNA synthesized *in vitro* reflected that synthesized *in vivo*, preformed nuclear RNA was examined for viral-specific sequences. The kinetics of hybridization of the nuclear RNA and

Table 21-1 AMV RNA Sequence in Nuclear Transcripts

RNA was synthesized in a reaction mixture (0.1 ml) containing 40 mM Tris Cl (pH 8.0), 100 mM (NH$_4$)$_2$SO$_4$, 4 mM ditheothreitol, 10 mM MgCl$_2$, 4 mM phosphoenol pyruvate, 0.15 unit pyruvate kinase, 2 mM sodium phosphate, 1 mM each of ATP, GTP, CTP, 20 mM α[^{32}P]UTP (10^4 cpm/pmole), and 0.09 mg myeloblast nuclei protein. When present, α-amanitin was added at a concentration of 2 μg/ml. After 20 min at 25°C, the mixture was treated with DNase (50 μg/ml) and twice extracted with phenol. Small molecular weight material was removed by gel filtration through Sephadex G-50. Annealing with cDNA was performed at 68°C in a total volume of 0.1 ml for 18 hr. Incubation without cDNA was run in parallel as a control. Duplicate aliquots of hybridization mixtures were treated with either RNases A and T$_1$ (100 μg/ml and 100 units/ml, respectively) or RNase A, T$_1$, and RNase H (40 units/ml).

Annealing conditions	Nuclei		Nuclei + α-Amanitin	
	+ cDNA	− cDNA	+ cDNA	− cDNA
RNA synthesis (cpm)				
UMP incorporated	200,000	200,000	40,000	40,000
Hybrid determination (cpm)				
RNA input	27,000	27,000	6,800	6,800
(a) RNase A+T$_1$	660	50	70	65
(b) RNase A+T$_1$+H	120	55	60	55
Hybrid (a-b)	540	<10	<10	<10

cDNA and 35 S AMV RNA and cDNA are shown in Figure 21-2. Based upon the $C_r t_{1/2}$ values, viral RNA sequences represent 0.5 percent of the total RNA in the nuclei. Because the relative amount of viral-specific RNA synthesized *in vitro* was about the same as that found in the nuclei, it is suggested that some specificity in transcription is maintained.

Transcription from Chromatin

The detection of significant amounts of viral RNA sequences in nuclear transcript products led us to examine transcription in a more purified system. The template used was chromatin isolated from myeloblast nuclei by a modification (10) of the procedure described by Huang and Huang (8). Since viral RNA sequences were apparently synthesized by the α-amanitin–sensitive RNA polymerase in nuclei, RNA polymerase form B, purified from calf thymus by a procedure adapted from Chambon et al. (3), was used to catalyze RNA synthesis. The requirements for ribonucleotide incorporation were similar to those found for isolated nuclei, except that Mn^{2+} stimulated incorporation 10- to 20-fold more than Mg^{2+}. Annealing of isolated RNA with AMV cDNA was

Figure 21-2. Kinetics of hybridization of cDNA with AMV 35 S RNA and myeloblast nuclear RNA. Incubation of 1.5 pmoles [³H]cDNA and either (○) 125 pmoles of AMV 35 S RNA or (●) 1.25 pmoles nuclear RNA from myeloblast were carried out at 68°C at the indicated $C_r t$ values. Determination of cDNA in hybrid structure was as the amount of radioactivity still acid insoluble after digestion by nuclease S_1 (1 unit/ml) for 30 min at 37°C in 0.1 M acetate buffer (pH 4.6). The results are presented as a function of the product of nucleotide concentration and time ($C_r t$).

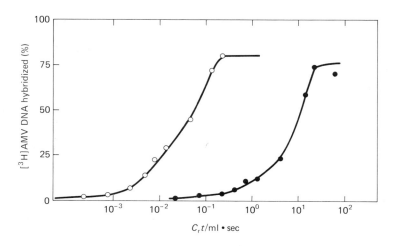

carried out under conditions that allowed hybridization of all the viral RNA sequences present in the chromatin transcript product to cDNA. After removal of single-stranded RNA with RNase A and RNase T₁, the RNA in RNA:DNA hybrid structures was determined by its susceptibility to RNase H. Approximately 1 percent of the total RNA synthesized from chromatin by the eukaryotic enzyme formed RNA:DNA hybrids with cDNA. Table 21-2 shows that a similar value was found when highly purified *E. coli* RNA polymerase (holoenzyme) was substituted for the α-amanitin–sensitive enzyme. A control run with calf thymus chromatin, a nonviral related template, yielded no hybrid with cDNA, eliminating the possibility of nonspecific hybridization. When purified DNA isolated from myeloblasts, either in a native or denatured state, was used as template, RNA:DNA hybrid structures were not detected in the transcription product, indicating that hybridizable RNA was specifically in the chromatin-directed transcript. The identity of the sequences transcribed *in vitro* from chromatin that hybridized with cDNA as viral was confirmed by competition experiments with AMV 35 S RNA (Table 21-3). Different amounts of unlabeled 35 S RNA were added during annealing, and both the DNA and RNA converted to hybrid structures were assayed. In the absence of 35 S RNA, approximately equal amounts of RNA transcript and DNA were present in the hybrid. With increasing levels of 35 S RNA, the amount of DNA in hybrid structure increased, while that of labeled transcript RNA de-

Table 21-2   Hybridization of RNA Transcribed *In Vitro* to cDNA

The products were formed in reaction mixtures (1 ml) containing 20 mM Tris HCl (pH 8.0), 100 mM (NH₄)₂SO₄, 2 mM MnCl₂, 10 mM dithiothreitol, 0.6 mM each of ATP, GTP, CTP, and 25 μM α[³²P]UTP (10⁴ cpm/pmole). Where indicated, 1.5 A₂₆₀ units of chromatin, 0.5 A₂₆₀ unit of DNA, 45 μg of protein of RNA polymerase B, and 1 μg of *E. coli* RNA polymerase were present. Reaction mixtures were incubated for 30 min at 37°C. Conditions for annealing RNA and cDNA are as described in Table 21-1. RNA in RNA–cDNA hybrid structure is defined as [³²P]RNA resistant to RNase A+T₁ but sensitive to RNase H.

Template	Enzyme	RNA (nM)	RNA in RNA: cDNA in hybrid (%)
Chromatin			
Myeloblast	Calf thymus Pol. B	1.33	0.85
Myeloblast	*Escherichia coli*	2.20	0.80
Calf thymus	Calf thymus Pol. B	1.10	<0.05
DNA			
Myeloblast (native)	Calf thymus Pol. B	0.82	<0.05
Myeloblast (denatured)	Calf thymus Pol. B	8.10	<0.03

Table 21-3 Competition between 35 S RNA and Chromatin Transcript RNA during Annealing with the AMV DNA Probe

The synthesis and isolation of [^{32}P]RNA from reaction mixtures containing calf thymus RNA polymerase B, myeloblast, chromatin, and α[^{32}P]UTP (10^4 cpm/pmole) are described in Table 21-2. Hybridization mixtures (0.2 ml) containing 150 pmole of [^{3}H]AMV DNA probe (1.2×10^3 cpm/pmole of nucleotides), 200 pmole [^{32}P]RNA, and the indicated amounts of 35 S AMV RNA were incubated 45 hr at 68°. DNA in hybrid structures was measured as DNA rendered sensitive to *Neurospora* nuclease (1.2 units/ml) by the presence of RNase H (40 units/ml). The background level of DNA resistant to *Nuerospora* nuclease in the presence of RNase H was 1.2 percent. The [^{32}P]RNA in hybrid structure was measured as the amount of ^{32}P resistant to a sequential degradation by *Neurospora* nuclease (1.2 units/ml) in 30 mM NaCl followed by RNase A and T$_1$ (50 μg/ml and 50 units/ml, respectively) in 100 mM NaCl but made acid soluble by RNase H (40 units/ml). No hybrid RNA was found in the control RNA annealed alone. The material resistant to RNase H after this treatment varies between 0.5 and 1 percent of the total RNA.

Amount of 35 S RNA present during hybridization (pmole)	DNA in hybrid (%)	[^{32}P]RNA in hybrid (%)
0	2.1	1.70
100	28.4	0.90
1500	78.0	0.03
3000	98.5	0.03

creased, showing that 35 S AMV RNA was an effective competitor.

Independent studies have shown that only 10 to 20 AMV genome equivalents are present in the DNA of infected cells (2,12). If transcription occurred randomly, *in vitro,* then the viral sequences should represent less than 0.01 percent of the total transcript. We found that the 1 percent of the RNA transcribed from chromatin that contained viral RNA sequences is similar to the amount of viral RNA synthesized by isolated nuclei. These results suggest that only selective regions of the DNA present in chromatin are available for transcription. Similar observations on globin *mRNA* transcription were reported by Axel et al. (1).

Characterization of the Chromatin Transcript Products

Since *in vivo* transcription products are mainly large molecular weight molecules (15), it was of interest to characterize the size of the *in vitro* product formed from chromatin primers and to determine the requirements for obtaining long RNA chains.

The size of RNA transcripts was determined by sedimentation velocity in SDS-sucrose gradients after heating in formaldehyde at 65°C. The results in Figure 21-3 show that RNA chains formed are heterogeneous in size, ranging from 5 to 50 S, with a broad peak in the upper part of the gradient. When heparin was added after the start of RNA synthesis, the synthesis of small RNA products was significantly reduced (Fig. 21-3,B). Multiple effects could

Figure 21-3. Size distribution of RNA products transcribed from chromatin. RNA synthesis (in 0.1 ml/nmoles) was carried out as described in Table 21-3, except in (B), where heparin (2 mg/ml) was added with [³H]UTP following a 5-min preincubation. After 20 min at 37°C, 50 mM EDTA and 0.2 percent sodium sulfate were added to stop the reaction. Samples were incubated at 65°C for 10 min in the presence of 6 percent formaldehyde and 0.1 M sodium phosphate (pH 7.0) and then layered on 10 to 30 percent sucrose gradients containing 50 mM Tris HCl (pH 8.0), 100 mM NaCl, 3 percent formaldehyde, and 0.1 percent SDS. The gradients were centrifuged for 3 hr at 49,000 rpm in an SW 50.1 rotor. Fractions (20 drops) were collected, and acid-insoluble radioactivity was determined. [¹⁴C]RNA *E. coli* ribosomal markers were in parallel gradients.

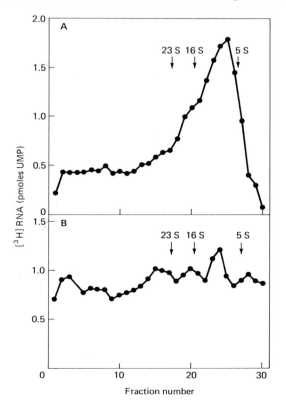

explain the change in size distribution observed in the presence of heparin. It is known, for example, that heparin inhibits nucleases, prevents reinitiation of transcription, and causes the release of certain chromatin-bound proteins (4). It is interesting to note that, in the presence of heparin, the RNA products formed have a size distribution resembling that of Hn RNA. Since the presence of large RNA molecules could result from an elongation of existing chains, it was important to determine whether new RNA chains could be initiated. Evidence for initiation was obtained from studies which showed that γ-[^{32}P]ATP and GTP were incorporated at the 5' termini end of the RNA. Alkaline degradation of γ-[^{32}P]GTP-labeled RNA yielded [^{32}P]guanosine tetraphosphate. Analysis of the γ-[^{32}P]-labeled RNA in sucrose gradient revealed that the radioactivity was distributed in products of all sizes, indicating that large RNA molecules can be synthesized *de novo* when chromatin is transcribed by RNA polymerase B.

To determine whether the nature of the DNA template affects the size of RNA product formed by the eukaryotic enzyme, well-defined DNAs isolated from phage were used as template. The results of the size distribution analyzed in sucrose gradient are summarized in Table 21-4. In contrast to *E. coli* RNA polymerase, which synthesizes large products from native DNA, calf thymus RNA polymerase B synthesized large products from single-stranded DNA and small products from native DNA. The synthesis of large RNA transcripts from the chromatin suggests that regions of the DNA, which is single stranded in

Table 21-4   Size of RNA Transcripts from Single-Stranded and Double-Stranded Phage DNA

Reaction mixtures for RNA synthesis (0.05 ml) were as described in Table 21-3, except that the following phage DNA were included as indicated: θX174 (3.5 μg), θX174-RF$_1$ (1.2 μg), native or denatured T$_2$ (1.2 μg). Either 20 μg of protein of RNA polymerase B or 1 μg of protein of *E. coli* holoenzyme was used. Formaldehyde treatment of the products and sedimentation in sucrose gradients containing formaldehyde were performed as described in Figure 21-3. The S values were calculated with reference to *E. coli* [^{14}C]RNA ribosomal markers.

DNA Template	RNA polymerase B	*Escherichia coli* RNA polymerase
Single-stranded		
θX 174	20 S	7 S
T$_2$ denatured	30 S	6 S
Double-stranded		
RF$_1$ θX 174	7 S	30 S
T$_2$ native	5 S	30 S

nature, are used as template. Further evidence supporting this interpretation was obtained from an analysis of the structure formed between RNA and its template after transcription. It is known that during RNA synthesis, the newly synthesized RNA strand is hydrogen-bonded with the DNA template. This RNA is readily displaced by the complementary strand when DNA is in duplex structure but remains in hybrid structure with single-stranded DNA templates. An analysis of the chromatin transcript synthesized by RNA polymerase B is shown in Figure 21-4. More than 70 percent of the phenol-extracted RNA

Figure 21-4. Analysis of products transcribed from chromatin. Here RNA was synthesized in 0.25-ml reaction mixture (see Table 21-3) containing chromatin (1.0 A$_{260}$ unit) and RNA polymerase B (20 μg protein). The product was extracted with phenol and filtered through Sephadex G-50. Aliquots were incubated for 30 min at 37°C with the following enzymes: (B) DNase (50 μg/ml); (C) *Neurospora* nuclease (1.2 units/ml), (D) RNase H (40 units/ml). A non-treated fraction (A) and fractions (B), (C), and (D) were diluted with 0.15 M NaCl, 10 mM sodium phosphate (pH 7.0), 5 mM EDTA, 0 025 percent sarkosyl, and Cs$_2$SO$_4$ was added to ($\triangle$) a final density of 1.550 g/ml. After the samples were centrifuged 60 hr at 30,000 rpm at 25°C in a SW 50.1 rotor, 20-drop fractions were collected from a hole pierced in the bottom of the tube. The density of each fraction was determined by measuring the refractive index, and the acid-precipitable radioactivity in each fraction was measured.

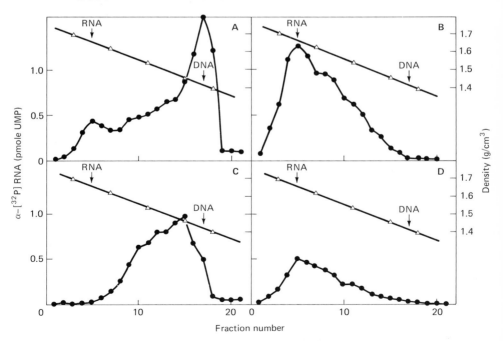

product, subjected to isopycnic centrifugation in cesium sulfate, bonded in the RNA:DNA or DNA region. Treatment of the product with DNase prior to centrifugation caused the product to band at the density of RNA, and RNase H degradation of the product lowered the amount of acid-precipitable material by 70 percent, while the remaining material banded as RNA. Treatment of the chromatin transcript product with a single-strand specific nuclease degraded 30 percent of the RNA, while the remaining material banded as RNA:DNA hybrid. These results suggest that DNA, which is effectively single stranded in nature, serves as template in chromatin. It is likely that the nucleoplasmic (as well as *E. coli*) RNA polymerase initiates synthesis at single-stranded regions, and, as RNA chains are elongated, the DNA in chromatin is converted to a single-strand state.

Summary and Conclusion

We have presented evidence that viral AMV sequences in host genetic material can be transcribed *in vitro*, either in isolated AMV-infected myeloblast nuclei or from chromatin isolated from these cells with eukaryotic RNA polymerase form B. In either system approximately 1 percent of the transcript product was found to be virus specific. This result, which is higher than expected from a random transcription of the genome, was observed with isolated chromatin as template, suggesting selection transcription of DNA. Inhibition of synthesis of viral sequences by α-amanitin, as well as the finding that RNA polymerase B catalyzes synthesis of viral sequences from chromatin, supports the hypothesis that the expression of viral information is mediated by the nucleoplasmic enzyme. Since transcription of both single-stranded DNA and chromatin by RNA polymerase B yields large RNA molecules, it is possible that gene activation in eukaryotic organisms results from the unwinding of portions of chromatin DNA (cf. ref. 5).

REFERENCES

1. Axel, R., Cedar, H., and Felsenfeld, G. The synthesis of globin RNA from duck reticulocyte chromatin *in vitro*. Proc. Natl. Acad. Sci. USA, 70:2029, 1973.

2. Baluda, M. A. and Drohan, W. N. Distribution of DNA complementary to RNA of avian myeloblastosis virus in tissues of normal and tumor-bearing chickens. J. Virol., 10:1002, 1972.

3. Chambon, P., Gissinger, F., Mandel, J. L., Kedinger, C., Gniazdowski, A., and Meihlac, M. Purification and properties of calf thymus DNA dependent RNA polymerases A and B. Cold Spring Harbor Symp. Quant. Biol., 35:693, 1970.

4. Cox, R. F. Transcription of high molecular weight RNA from hen-oviduct chromatin by bacterial and endogenous form B, RNA polymerases. Eur. J. Biochem., 39:49, 1973.

5. Crick, F. General model for the chromosome of higher organisms. Nature, 234:25, 1971.

6. Gallo, R. C. Reverse transcriptase, the DNA polymerase of oncogenic RNA viruses. Nature, 234:194, 1971.

7. Green, M. Oncogenic viruses. Ann. Rev. Biochem., 39:701, 1970.

8. Huang, R. C. and Huang, P. C. Effect of protein-bound RNA associated with chick embryo chromatin on template specificity of the chromatin. J. Mol. Biol., 39:365, 1969.

9. Ikawa, Y., Ross, J., and Leder, P. An association between globin messenger RNA and 60 S RNA derived from Friend leukemia virus. Proc. Natl. Acad. Sci. USA, 71:1154, 1974.

10. Jacquet, M., Groner, Y., Monroy, G., and Hurwitz, J. The *in vitro* synthesis of avian myeloblastosis viral RNA sequences. Proc. Natl. Acad. Sci. USA, 71:3045, 1974.

11. McDonnell, J. P., Garapin, A. C., Levinson, W. E., Quintrell, N., Fanshier, L., and Bishop, J. M. DNA polymerase of Rous sarcoma virus. Delineation of two reactions with actinomycin. Nature, 228:433, 1970.

12. Rosenthal, P. N., Robinson, H. L., Robinson, W. S., Hanafusa, T. DNA in uninfected and virus infected cells complementary to avian tumor virus RNA. Proc. Natl. Acad. Sci. USA, 68:2336, 1971.

13. Rymo, L., Parsons, J. T., Coffin, J. M., and Weissman, C. *In vitro* synthesis of Rous sarcoma virus RNA is catalyzed by a DNA-dependent RNA polymerase. Proc. Natl. Acad. Sci. USA, 71:2782, 1974.

14. Temin, H. M. and Baltimore, D. RNA-Directed DNA synthesis and RNA tumor viruses. Adv. Virus Res., 17:129, 1972.

15. Weinberg, R. A. Nuclear RNA metabolism. Ann. Rev. Biochem., 42:329, 1973.

22

Synthesis of Viral DNA and Transcription of Viral RNA during Infection and Cell Transformation by the Murine Sarcoma-Leukemia Virus

M. Green, S. Salzberg, M. S. Robin, M. C. Loni, S. Bhaduri, and G. Shanmugam

Introduction

In a study of the critical molecular events early during infection and cell transformation by tumor viruses, it is useful to analyze virus-cell systems in which most cells are rapidly infected and transformed. Although DNA tumor viruses are generally not suitable, for they transform only a small fraction of cells they infect (3), RNA tumor viruses (oncornaviruses), under suitable conditions, can efficiently infect and transform most cells in culture (4). In this process, viral RNA is reversibly transcribed to DNA, which is then integrated into the cellular genome. Integrated viral DNA is transcribed to viral mRNA molecules, some of which code for information responsible for transforming cells and maintaining the transformed state of the cell (4).

As an experimental system to study transformation of mammalian cells, we have used a clonal line of mouse 3T6 cells that is rapidly infected and transformed by the Harvey (H) strain of murine sarcoma-leukemia virus (MSV MLV). Below are described the results of studies on the synthesis of virus-specific DNA in the cytoplasm, its transport to the nucleus, its transcription to viral RNA, the formation of extra-cellular virus, and the consequent alteration of the cell surface.

Time Course of Appearance of Virus-Specific RNA, Virus Particles, and Cell-Surface Modifications in 3T6 Cells Rapidly Infected and Transformed by H-MSV MLV

The majority of cells exposed to 1 to 2 plaque-forming units/cell of MSV MLV are infected within 60 min and subsequently give rise to transformed cells (8). To measure the synthesis of viral RNA, RNA was extracted from

Fundamental Aspects of Neoplasia,
edited by A. Arthur Gottlieb, Otto J. Plescia, and David H. L. Bishop.
© 1975 by Springer-Verlag New York Inc.

cells at different times after infection and annealed with the [³H]DNA product of virion RNA-directed DNA polymerase. After 1 hr of infection, the
equivalent of 100 intracellular parental viral RNA molecules were measured.
The new synthesis of viral RNA was detected beginning at 6 to 7 hr after
infection and reached maximal levels at 25 hr. Virus particle formation was
detected at 14 to 17 hr, as assayed by the formation of extracellular particles
containing the oncornavirus-specific, RNA-directed DNA polymerase, and
reached a maximum level at 70 to 80 hr after infection (8).

Morphologic alterations of infection cells were readily detected. Uninfected
cells had a flat, stretched-out appearance. Infected cells at 24 hr consisted of
two cell types: most cells were spindle shaped but 10 to 20 percent had
acquired a rounded morphology. The number of rounded cells increased with
time of infection, to 30 to 40 percent at 48 hr and 80 to 90 percent at 74 hr.

We have previously shown that cells transformed and continuously producing MSV MLV are strongly agglutinated in the presence of the plant lectin,
concanavalin A (7). A small increase in agglutinability was observed at 22 hr
after infection of 3T6 cells by H-MSV MLV but the major increase occurred
between 22 and 63 hr. Acquisition of agglutinability by conconavalin A paralleled the increase in the fraction of 3T6 cells with a rounded morphology and
the increase in virus production.

Early Requirement for DNA Synthesis during Infection of 3T6 Cells by H-MSV MLV

The requirement for DNA synthesis early during infection and cell transformation by oncornaviruses was a major premise for the provirus hypothesis
(3,10). The discovery of the oncornavirus RNA-directed DNA polymerase
provided a mechanism for the synthesis of proviral DNA (1,11). But direct
evidence for the function of the viral DNA polymerase in the synthesis of viral
DNA *in vivo* has been difficult to obtain. Numerous studies with disrupted
virus particles and partially purified viral DNA polymerase showed that only
small fragments of single- and double-stranded DNA are formed *in vitro*; DNA
molecules the size of the viral genome were not detected (4).

In order to isolate and study the properties of intracellular virus-specific
DNA, it was first necessary to establish the time of occurrence of viral DNA
synthesis. For this purpose, we added arabinosylcytosine, a specific inhibitor of
DNA synthesis, to 3T6 cells at different times after infection and measured the
effect on subsequent virus replication and viral RNA synthesis. Our results
showed that the most critical time for viral DNA synthesis occurred between
1 and 4 hr infection (Robin, Salzberg, and Green, in preparation).

Autoradiographic Detection and Quantitation of Newly Synthesized DNA in the Cytoplasm Early After Infection of 3T6 Cells by H-MSV MLV

To establish the intracellular site of viral DNA synthesis early after infection, cell cultures were pulse-labeled for 15 min with [^{3}H]thymidine at 1-hr intervals after infection, fixed, and analyzed by autoradiography. Autoradiographic grains were readily detected in the cytoplasm at 1-hr after infection (105 grains), reaching maximal levels at 2-hr (227 grains) and 3-hr (166 grains); they decreased subsequently. Less than 1 grain/nucleus was detected in uninfected cells or when cells were treated with arabinosylcytosine. Thus, it is clear that DNA synthesis occurs in the cytoplasm of cells early after infection but not in the cytoplasm of uninfected cells.

To determine whether newly synthesized cytoplasmic DNA was transported to the nucleus, cells with irradiated with ultraviolet light to block host cell nuclear DNA synthesis, labeled with [^{3}H]thymidine for 15 min at 2 hr after infection, and chased with a 100-fold excess of unlabeled thymidine. As shown in Figure 22-1, autoradiographic grains were present in the cytoplasm of cells at 1 and 2 hr after infection, but not in the nucleus at these times. More grains appeared in the nucleus at 3, 4, and 5 hr after infection, i.e., 1, 2, and 3 hr of chase, indicating that cytoplasmic DNA was transported to the nucleus (Fig. 22-1) and suggesting that this may represent a biologic function of virus-specific DNA (Robin, Salzberg, and Green, in preparation).

The Nature of Cytoplasmic DNA Synthesized Early after Infection

Cells were labeled with [^{3}H]thymidine for 15 min at 1-hr intervals after infection and separated by differential centrifugation into cytoplasmic, postmitochondrial, and mitochondrial fractions. Although total incorporation into infected and uninfected cells was similar, larger amounts of radioactive DNA were found in the cytoplasmic fraction of infected than of uninfected cells. To determine whether newly synthesized cytoplasmic DNA was viral specific, labeled DNA was annealed with viral 60 to 70 S RNA, and the amount of DNA that formed a hybrid was determined by batch elution from hydroxyapatite (HAP) (12). A maximum of 60 percent of labeled cytoplasmic DNA at 2 and 3 hr after infection hybridized to viral RNA. The content of virus-specific DNA decreased with time of infection; at 5 hr, only 10 percent of labeled cytoplasm DNA was virus specific (Robin, Salzberg, and Green, in preparation).

The results of autoradiographic analysis and molecular hybridization de-

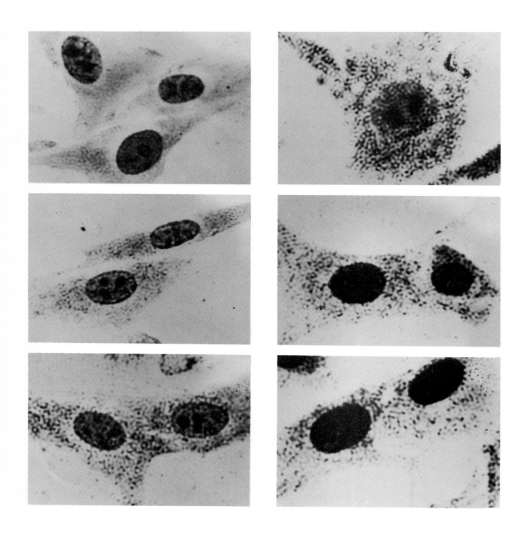

Figure 22-1. Cytologic chase of newly synthesized DNA from the cytoplasm to the nucleus of cells infected with H-MSV MLV. Immediately before infection, 3T6 cell cultures were irradiated with ultraviolet light (40 W) for 30 sec at a distance of 25 cm. Cells were labeled for 15 min with 20 μCi/ml of [^{3}H]thymidine (54 Ci/mmole) at 1 and 2 hr after infection with 1 to 2 focus-forming units/cell of H-MSV MLV. Cultures labeled at 2 hr were chased with a 100-fold excess of unlabeled thymidine for 1, 2, and 3 hr (3, 4, and 5 hr after infection, as indicated in the figure), and autoradiographs were prepared. (From Robin, Salzberg, and Green, in preparation.)

scribed above demonstrate that the synthesis of virus-specific DNA occurs in the cytoplasm early after infection. Since approximately 100 intracellular viral RNA genomes are present, in one cell, it is conceivable that cytoplasmic DNA represents mainly the abortive synthesis of nonfunctional viral DNA. But, the cytologic chase experiments, which demonstrate transport of cytoplasmic DNA to the nucleus, are consistent with a biologic function for cytoplasmic viral DNA. Our studies agree with those of Hatanaka et al. (5), who detected cytoplasmic DNA synthesis in mouse cells infected with a murine oncornavirus by autoradiography, although no evidence was presented that the DNA was viral in nature; the later times of DNA synthesis observed in the latter study may reflect less efficient infection of cells.

Association of Newly Synthesized H-MSV MLV DNA with Nuclei-In Situ Hybridization

To follow the fate of the virus-specific DNA sequences formed early during infection and transformation of 3T6 cells, we performed *in situ* hybridization with cytologic preparations. Because [³H]thymidine-labeled virus-specific DNA of high specific activity can be prepared with viral RNA-directed DNA poly-merase we have available a sensitive technique to detect small numbers of viral gene sequences in cells (2,6).

In situ hybridization was performed by annealing fixed preparations of uninfected 3T6 cells and cells at 5, 11, and 25 hr after infection with H-MSV MLV [³H]DNA fr 18 hr and exposing these preparations for 18 weeks to a photographic emulsion. An average of four grains above a background of one grain was found above interphase nuclei of uninfected cells. Infection pro-duced a profound increase in grain count. At 5 hr after infection, as shown in Figure 22-2, an average of 30 grains were found above the chromocenters of interphase nuclei, and some chromosomes were clearly labeled. The average number of grains reached 63 to 65 at 11 hr after infection and remained con-stant at 25 hr (Loni and Green, in preparation).

The specificity of these *in situ* hybridizations for viral DNA sequences was demonstrated in control experiments in which (a) autoradiographic grains were totally eliminated by pretreatment of fixed cells with DNase, (b) viral 60 to 70 S RNA and transformed cell DNA competed with the viral[³H]DNA probe during *in situ* hybridization, and (c) viral 60 to 70 S [³H]RNA gave similar results when used as a probe for *in situ* hybridization (Loni and Green, in preparation).

The autoradiographic grains detected over the nuclei of uninfected cells could represent DNA sequences of the endogenous viral genome shared with

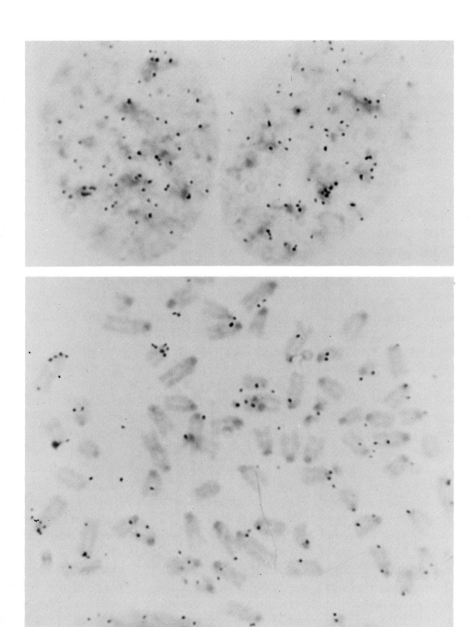

Figure 22-2. Autoradiographs of metaphase chromosomes and interphase nuclei of 3T6, clone 91 cells, 11 hr after infection. Autoradiographs show the hybridization of the viral [³H]DNA product (specific activity 6.4×10^7 dpm/μg) to some chromosomes and the dense Giemsa-stained regions of the interphase nucleus X 2038. (From Loni and Green, in preparation.)

H-MSV MLV, as implied by the oncogene hypothesis and supported by molecular hybridization experiments (4). The large increase in grain count after infection indicates that some virus-specific DNA sequences that are rapidly synthesized after infection become associated with the cell nucleus. These *in situ* hybridization data do not prove that all the newly introduced viral DNA sequences are integrated, although it is likely that a major portion of these viral sequences do become integrated late after infection.

The association between autoradiographic grains and the chromocenters of interphase nuclei of infected 3T6 cells and the centromeric heterochromatic regions of several chromosomes may be of interest (Loni and Green, unpublished data). Mouse satellite DNA has been associated with the centromeric portion of metaphase chromosomes. Perhaps the high efficiency of transformation by oncornaviruses is related to the binding of newly synthesized oncornavirus DNA to specific repetitive sequence in this region of the chromosome.

Localization and Size of Viral mRNA in MSV MLV Transformed Cells

Integrated viral DNA sequences in fully transformed, virus-producing cells are transcribed and processed to viral *m*RNA molecules and RNA precursors to the viral RNA genome. We previously detected two viral RNA species sedimenting at 35 S and 20 S RNA in cells transformed by both the Harvey and Moloney strains of MSV MLV (12). Virus-specific RNA and nascent viral polypeptides were present in free and membrane-bound polyribosomes (13). To gain insight into the function of these intracellular viral RNA species, we have analyzed the species of viral RNA in several polyribosome-containing cell fractions, using polyacrylamide gel electrophoresis and molecular hybridization (9). Electrophoresis of the RNA isolated from the postmicrosomal supernatant fraction, which contains free polyribosomes, showed a prominent viral 35 S RNA peak but no 20 S RNA (Fig. 22-3,A). Similar analysis of the microsome fraction, which contains membrane-bound polyribosomes, revealed the presence of both 35 S and 20 S RNA (Fig. 22-3,B). The RNA isolated from free and membrane-bound polyribosomes purified from these fractions by sedimentation through sucrose layers were shown to possess a similar size distribution of virus-specific RNA molecules, i.e., 35 S RNA in free polyribosomes and both 35 S and 20 S RNA in membrane-bound polyribosomes. Viral 35 S RNA probably serves both as a precursor to the viral 60 to 70 S RNA genome and as an *m*RNA in polyribosomes (4). The function of 20 S RNA is unknown; it could be a specific viral *m*RNA or a breakdown product of 35 S RNA.

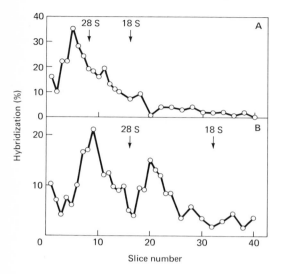

Figure 22-3. Size of virus-specific RNA in free polyribosomes (A) and membrane-bound polyribosomes (B) of MSV MLV-transformed 78A1 cells. RNA extracted from free polyribosomes (104 μg) or membrane-bound polyribosomes (30 μg) was electrophoresed on 2.5 percent polyacrylamide gels for 3 and 6 hr, respectively. The RNA in each gel slice was hybridized with the MSV MLV [³H]DNA product. [From Shanmugam, Bhaduri, and Green, 1974 (9).]

Summary and Conclusions

The early events during the efficient infection and transformation of mouse 3T6 cells by the Harvey strain of murine sarcoma-leukemia virus have been analyzed. The synthesis of DNA was detected in the cytoplasm by autoradiography of cells pulse-labeled with [³H]thymidine at 1 hr after infection, reached maximal levels at 2 hr, and decreased subsequently. Newly synthesized cytoplasmic DNA was isolated and shown to be mainly virus specific by hybridization to viral 60 to 70 S RNA.

Cytologic chase experiments, using autoradiographic analysis of ultraviolet-irradiated cells to block all cell DNA synthesis, pulse-labeled with [³H]thymidine, indicated that cytoplasmic DNA was readily transported to the nucleus. By *in situ* hybridization of fixed cell preparations with the [³H]DNA product of the viral RNA-directed DNA polymerase, newly synthesized viral DNA was shown to associate with the chromocenters of interphase nuclei by 5 hr after infection. Maximum autoradiographic grains (63 to 66 grains) of newly synthesized DNA were present in interphase nuclei by 11 hr after infection; uninfected cells contained an average of 4 grains.

The synthesis of virus-specific RNA was detected by 6 to 7 hr after infection and reached maximal levels by 24 hr. The replication of virus was detected starting between 14 and 17 hr and increased in rate until 60 to 70 hr after infection. Alterations in the cell surface as measured by cell agglutination with conconavalin A were detected starting at 24 hr after infection, paralleling the increase in virus production and acquisition of transformed cell morphology.

An established line of transformed cells replicating the murine sarcoma-leukemia virus was shown to contain two intracellular viral RNA species with $s = 20$ to 35. Free polyribosomes contain 35 S viral RNA, whereas membrane-bound polyribosomes contain the 35 S and 20 S RNA species. The 35 S RNA subunit is probably both a precursor to the viral 60 to 70 S RNA genome and an *m*RNA for the synthesis of viral proteins. Viral 20 S RNA could be a specialized viral *m*RNA or a breakdown product of 35 S RNA.

REFERENCES

1. Baltimore, D. Viral RNA-dependent DNA polymerase. Nature, 226:1209, 1970.

2. Gall, J. G. and Pardue, M. L. Formation and detection of RNA–DNA hybrid molecules in cytological preparations. Proc. Natl. Acad. Sci. USA, 63:378, 1969.

3. Green, M. Oncogenic viruses. Ann. Rev. Biochem., 39:701, 1970.

4. Green, M. and Gerard, G. RNA-Directed DNA polymerase—properties and functions in oncogenic RNA viruses and cells. *In* Davidson, J. N. and Cohn, W. E., eds. Progress in Nucleic Acid Research and Molecular Biology. New York, Academic Press, 1974, Vol. 14, p. 187.

5. Hatanaka, M., Kafefudat, T., Gilden, R. V., and Callan, E. A. O. Cytoplasmic DNA synthesis induced by RNA tumor viruses. Proc. Natl. Acad. Sci. USA, 68,1844, 1971.

6. John, H. A., Birnsteil, M. L., and Jones, K. W. RNA–DNA hybridization at the cytological level. Nature, 223:582, 1969.

7. Salzberg, S. and Green, M. Surface alterations of cells carrying RNA tumor virus genetic information. Nature [New Biol.], 240:116, 1972.

8. Salzberg, S., Robin, M. S., and Green, M. Appearance of virus-specific RNA virus particles, and cell surface changes in cells rapidly transformed by the murine sarcoma virus. Virology, 53:186,1973.

9. Shanmugam, G., Bhaduri, S., and Green, M. The virus-specific RNA species in free and membrane-bound polyribosomes of transformed cells replicating murine sarcoma leukemia viruses. Biochem. Biophys. Res. Commun., 56:697, 1974.

10. Temin, H. M. Mechanism of cell transformation by RNA tumor viruses. Ann. Rev. Microbiol., 25:609, 1971.

11. Temin, H. M. and Mizutani, S. RNA-Dependent DNA polymerase in virions of Rous sarcoma virus. Nature, 226:1211, 1970.

12. Tsuchida, N., Robin, M. S., and Green, M. Viral RNA subunits in cells transformed by RNA tumor viruses. Science, 30:1418, 1972.

13. Vecchio, G., Tsuchida, N., Shanmugam, G., and Green, M. Virus-specific messenger RNA and nascent polypeptides in polyribosomes of cells replicating murine sarcoma-leukemia virus. Proc. Natl. Acad. Sci. USA, 70:2064, 1972.

Characteristics of Cells Transformed by Rous Sarcoma Virus

J. P. Bader and D. J. Marciani

Introduction

The identification of a molecule initially responsible for the physiologic manifestation of malignancy would be a major step in resolving the general nature of the tumor cell and, eventually, in controlling cancer. Traditionally, comparisons of tumors and normal tissues, or tumors and tissues of tumor origin, have revealed biochemical differences, and when consistent differences were found among varieties of tumors and organs, theories on the nature of cancer soon followed. An extension of this approach is found in the use of cells in culture and the efficient conversion of such cells to malignant forms with viruses. Many biochemical differences have been described, and convincing arguments for the role of this or that molecule in malignancy have been presented. The inadequacy of the comparative approach in identifying a cancer-causing molecule lies in our inability to define cause–effect relationships; locating the molecular change in the sequence of changes accompanying transformation to the malignant form is impossible.

Two specific approaches offer promise in defining a molecule responsible for malignancy. One is the selection of cellular mutants with specific defects in physiologic functions known to change during transformation to malignancy. Manipulation of such cells, and especially the use of conditionally defective cells, could lead to the identification of a defective gene product, the proper function of which keeps the cell nonmalignant. This approach would almost certainly eventually reveal a molecule necessary for the maintenance of the nonmalignant phenotype, but its reliance upon hunches forebodes more frustration than gratification.

A second approach is found in the use of virus mutants that transform cells at one temperature but not at another. In some cases, particularly with RNA-containing sarcoma viruses, malignancy is probably directly brought about by the function of a viral gene product. A logical question then arises: If a viral gene product is responsible then why not simply identify the viral gene product in the infected cell? The difficulty here probably is that the viral gene

Fundamental Aspects of Neoplasia,
edited by A. Arthur Gottlieb, Otto J. Plescia, and David H. L. Bishop.
© 1975 by Springer-Verlag New York Inc.

product is identical to a cellular regulatory molecule, and the two may be distinguished only quantitatively. The potential advantage of a temperature-sensitive system is that one may hope to find a virus-coded molecule distinguishable from its cellular counterpart by its thermal sensitivity.

Temperature-Dependent Transformation by Rous Sarcoma Virus

The RNA-containing tumor viruses have a DNA replicative intermediate in their reproductive cycle (1,3,12). Meddling with this DNA by exposing newly infected cells to 5-bromodeoxyuridine resulted in the induction of mutants of Rous sarcoma virus (RSV) (2,3,4). One such mutant, RSV-BH-Ta, induced transformation in infected cells at 36°C, but, when these cells were incubated at 41°C, no transformation was seen (2). In contrast, virus reproduction occurred at both 41 and 36°C, which indicates that the gene product responsible for transformation was not important to virus production.

Cells infected with RSV-BH-Ta could be grown for several months at 41°C without becoming transformed, but, within minutes after shifting to 36°C, morphologic changes were observed. Later studies showed that 37°C was the optimum temperature for the morphologic transformation of cells infected with RSV-BH-Ta, transformation occurring more rapidly at this temperature than at 39, 38, 36, 34°C, or room temperature. The transformation was reversible, but the rapidity of the reversal depended upon the length of time the cells were kept at 37 before shifting to 41°C. This phenomenon could be explained by an accumulation of metabolic products and a generalized increase in mass of the transformed cell at 37°C, an observation described in detail in later sections.

In addition to temperature, pH was an important factor in transformation. The rapidity and degree of morphologic change was markedly dependent on pH over the range 6.6 to 7.8. Transformation of RSV-BH-Ta–infected cells increased with increasing pH, after shifting from 41 to 37°C, and was drastically inhibited at pH 6.6 and below. On the other hand, mutant-infected cells maintained at 41°C could be induced to transform by extended exposure to medium of high pH (higher than 7.6). Therefore, morphologic transformation in this system is both temperature and pH dependent.

The morphologic change in RSV-BH-Ta cells was found to occur without any requirement for new DNA, RNA, or protein synthesis. This was shown by addition of cytosine arabinoside, actinomycin D, cycloheximide, or puromycin to the medium before shifting the infected cells from 41 to 37°C. Thus, all of the requirements for informational transfer had been fulfilled at the higher temperature, and transformation in this system was dependent most probably upon a temperature-sensitive protein.

Biophysical Changes during Transformation

Several morphologic changes are observed microscopically in cells in the process of transformation, including rounding, intense vacuolization, and an apparent increase in size. In an effort to confirm this apparent size difference, cell diameters were measured, and the cells transformed by RSV-BH or RSV-BH-Ta (37°C), in fact, were found to be larger than uninfected cells or cells infected with RSV-SR or RSV-BH-Ta (41°C). Cellular volumes were determined experimentally, and the volumes of RSV-BH and RSV-BH-Ta (37°C) transformed cells also exceeded those of CE, RSV-SR, or RSV-BH-Ta (41°C) (Table 23-1).

The increase in volume was accompanied by an increase in protein, nucleic acid, and lipid, but these increases were insufficient to account fully for the size differences. The amount of protein expressed as a function of cell volume revealed that the density of protein in the nontransformed and RSV-SR cells was greater than the density of protein in RSV-BH and RSV-BH-Ta (37°C) cells (Table 23-1). These data suggested that the increases in cell mass were insufficient to explain the noted increases in cell size.

The decrease in protein density was reflected in a decrease in buoyant density, as measured in gradients of dextran T110. The RSV-BH cells (1.024 g/ml) and transformed RSV-BH-Ta cells (1.030 g/ml) were easily distinguishable from CE (1.044 g/ml) or nontransformed RSV-BH-Ta (1.042 g/ml) cells, whereas RSV-SR cells had variable intermediate densities in different experiments.

The analysis of total cellular wet and dried weights showed that the discrepancies in cell volume and cell protein were due, in fact, to differences in intracellular water (Table 23-1). The larger transformed cells contained proportionately more water than CE, RSV-BH-Ta (41°C), or RSV-SR cells.

Changes in cell diameter, volume, density of protein and buoyant density occurred without a requirement for DNA, RNA, or protein synthesis; this

Table 23-1   Volumes, Protein Densities, and Dried Weights of Transformed and Nontransformed Chick Embryo Cells

System	Volume (ml×10⁹/cell)	Protein (μg×10⁻⁴/ml cells)	Dry weight (%)
CE	2.54	11.4	16.9
CE+RSV-BH	5.94	7.7	11.6
CE+RSV-SR	3.64	10.6	16.1
CE+RSV-BH-Ta (41°C)	3.44	10.2	16.5
CE+RSV-BH-Ta (37°C)	5.10	8.6	12.7

was shown by the failure of cytosine arabinoside, actinomycin D, or cyclo-heximide to prevent the changes that occurred in RSV-BH-Ta cells after a temperature shift from 41 to 37°C.

Vacuolization

The most readily recognizable feature of cellular transformation by RSV-BH is cytoplasmic vacuolization, and vacuolization is often used as a criterion of transformation, at least by us. As indicated in our earlier discussion of transformation, shifting of RSV-BH-Ta–infected cells from 41 to 37°C results in morphologic changes observable within minutes, and vacuolization is the most prominent of these morphologic changes. This vacuolization is pH dependent and unaffected by inhibitors of DNA, RNA, or protein synthesis (2).

Cells containing vacuoles were examined by electron microscopy after being sectioned perpendicular to the plane of the substratum to which they were attached. The vacuoles were indeed in the cytoplasm, eliminating the possibility of an accumulation of a secreted substance under the cell, which could lead to fusion factor. Nothing of substance could be found in the vacuoles; histologic staining for nucleic acid, protein, lipid, glycolipid, glycoprotein, glycosoaminoglycans, or polysaccharides were invariably negative. Neutral red, however, when added to the incubation medium, was taken rapidly into the cells and vacuoles. This eliminated the possibility that the vacuoles contained gas, in a situation analogous to the gas vacuoles of certain algae (13), and demonstrated that, whatever else was in the vacuoles, water was a major constituent.

Components of the cell culture medium were examined to determine if they were essential for the vacuolization process. None of the metabolizable components, including serum, amino acids, vitamins, or glucose, were found to be essential, and no requirement for Ca^{2+}, PO_4^{3-}, or HCO_3^- could be shown (Table 23-2). But, removal of either K^+ or Mg^{2+} partially prevented vacuolization, and substitution of Li^+ for Na^+ completely prevented it. Since the uptake of water from physiologic solutions is usually accompanied by transfer of Na^+ (8), and cells accumulate water during transformation by RSV-BH-Ta, these results suggest that vacuolization may be a cellular response to an increase in cytoplasmic Na^+ and water.

Vacuolization is often considered a mark of degeneration of cells in culture. But, virtually all RSV-BH or RSV-BH-Ta (37°C) cells may be vacuolated and continue to grow and divide for many generations. Clearly, this form of vacuolization is a physiologic process, perhaps a mechanism designed to sequester excess water and Na^+. It seems unlikely, however, that the vacuoles

Table 23-2   Conditions Affecting the Development of
Vacuoles in Cells Infected by RSV-BH-Ta

Classification	Condition
Essential	Na^+
Partially essential	K^+, Mg^{2+}
Nonessential	Serum
	Amino acids
	Vitamins
	Glucose
	HCO_3^-, PO_4^{3-}, CA^{2+}
Affected by	Temperature
	pH
	Adenosine, deoxyadenosine
	Dibutyryl cAMP
	Inhibitors of cAMP phosphodiesterase

per se are responsible for the malignant properties of the transformed cell, and we are not advocating this view.

A depletion of adenosine $3':5'$-cyclic phosphate (cAMP) may be essential for the vacuolization process to occur. Addition of dibutyryl cAMP, and/or inhibitors of cAMP phosphodiesterase to RSV-BH-Ta cells before a temperature shift partially prevented vacuolization. Also, high levels of adenosine or deoxyadenosine, but no other natural ribo- or deoxyribonucleosides, inhibit vacuolization. We have not yet determined whether failure to vacuolate is due to a failure of the cell to increase its water uptake or a process that occurs subsequent to this increase in uptake of water.

Metabolic Changes Accompanying Transformation

Several metabolic differences have been observed between CE cells and RSV-BH–transformed cells, and these differences are also noted after shifting RSV-BH-Ta cells from 41 to 37°C. Glucose uptake from the medium, and the uptake of glucose analogues, is enhanced up to a fivefold increase (2,7) and the rates of uptake of galactose, leucine, uridine, and thymidine up to a twofold increase. Also, hyaluronic acid synthesis increases 5- to 10-fold within 6 hr after RSV-BH-Ta cells are shifted from 41 to 37°C (2). These increases, without exception, are prevented by actinomycin D or cycloheximide, but not by cytosine arabinoside, demonstrating that synthesis of new RNA and protein, but not DNA, is required. It is obvious, therefore, that none of these activities is responsible for the increased accumulation of intracellular water or the vacuolization occurring after a shift of mutant-infected cells from 41 to 37°C, since these changes require neither RNA nor protein synthesis.

On the other hand, deliberate manipulation of the cation content of the medium demonstrated that brief perturbations in cation exchange can affect the processes involved in glucose uptake. Deletion of K^+, or substitution of Li^+ for Na^+, results in a substantial decrease in the ability of the cells to take up glucose, whereas the addition of excess K^+ increases uptake of glucose.

Analysis of Surface Membrane Proteins

Attempts to identify, in infected cells, a specific protein responsible for transformation required a biophysical characterization of cellular proteins as a reference base. Cell membranes have been in the limelight as the residence of defects responsible for malignancy, and other studies on RSV-BH–infected cells have indicated that cell surface membrane functions might be involved in morphologic transformation. Therefore, an analysis of the protein constituents of cell surface membranes was undertaken.

Two different methods for the isolation of membranes were employed. The procedure of Brunette and Till (5) involves fixation of membranes with $ZnCl_2$ prior to cellular lysis, and yields cell "ghosts" containing membrane-associated proteins loosely attached to both internal and external surfaces. The second method, described by Perdue et al. (10), yields membranes of greater structural purity. These membranes vesicles formed during homogenization are separated from other cellular components by flotational centrifugation to density equilibrium. A preparation obtained by this latter method would contain proteins that are integral parts of cell surface membranes, whereas preparations of cell ghosts would contain, in addition, proteins that might affect the cell surface.

The protein composition of these membrane preparations was examined by electrophoresis in acrylamide gels. Gels containing sodium dodecyl sulfate and urea revealed a major change in the high molecular weight polypeptides of cell ghosts obtained from RSV-transformed cells (Fig. 23-1). Amounts of these proteins, migrating in the region of 200,000 MW, were drastically reduced in RSV-transformed cells compared to noninfected chick embryo cells, and this reduction was found also in cell ghosts from RSV-BH-Ta–infected cells grown at 37°C, as compared to those grown at 41°C. This result is similar to the results described by others (6,10,14). The decrease in high molecular weight proteins in the transformed RSV-BH-Ta cells, however, suggests that the protein is lost as a result of transformation, i.e., protein loss is a consequence rather than a cause of transformation.

A reduction in amount of a 46,000 MW polypeptide was also noted in cell

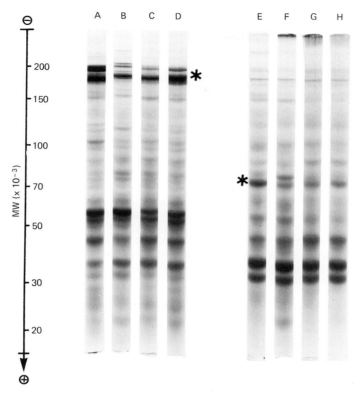

Figure 23-1. Continuous gel electrophoresis of cell ghosts and plasma membranes using sodium dodecyl sulfate and urea. Proteins (50 μg in a solution containing 1 percent SDS, 1 percent 2-mercaptoethanol, 6 percent sucrose, at pH 8.0) were layered over 5 percent acrylamide gels. Electrophoresis was carried out until the Bromophenol blue marker reached the bottom of the gel. Then the gels were fixed in propanol–acetic acid and stained with Coomassie blue. The left side of the figure shows gels of cell ghosts (5) (A) from normal chick embryo cells, (B) RSV-BH–transformed cells (C), cells transformed with the temperature-sensitive mutant, RSV-BH-Ta, growing at the transformation permissive temperature, 37°C, and (D) at the nonpermissive temperature, 41°C. The asterisk in (D) indicates the 190,000 MW region where the greatest changes were found. The right side shows gels of plasma membranes (10) isolated from (E) noninfected chick embryo cells, (F) RSV-BH–transformed cells, and cells infected with RSV-BH-Ta growing at (G) the permissive and (H) nonpermissive temperatures. The asterisk on gel (E) shows the 72,000 MW region where RSV-BH–transformed cells present a characteristic doublet.

ghosts of RSV-BH–transformed cells. A similar finding has been reported by Wickus and Robbins (14). But, this difference was not seen in RSV-BH-Ta–infected cells grown at 37 or 41°C, although it may be meaningful when the function of this protein is resolved.

These same cell ghosts were also analyzed in gels using a phenol–acetic acid–urea mixture instead of aqueous buffer (9). In this system, the charge on the protein, as well as its size, influenced mobility. As in the SDS-urea gels, transformed cells were deficient in high molecular weight polypeptides (Fig. 23-2). But, a protein identified in the 56,000 MW region in SDS–urea gels

Figure 23-2. Electrophoresis of cell ghosts and plasma membranes in the phenol–acetic acid–urea system. Protein samples were solubilized by incubation with one volume of 0.01 N NaOH–2 percent 2-mercaptoethanol for 40 min followed by the addition of four volumes of phenol–acetic acid–urea–2-mercaptoethanol (45:25:30:2, w/v/w/v) and incubation at room temperature for 15 to 20 hr. Samples were layered over 5 percent acrylamide gels, and electrophoresis was carried out using 10 percent acetic acid. The electropheretic mobilities are expressed as relative mobilities with respect to (M_c) mobility of cytochrome c. The left side of the figure shows gels of cell ghosts from (A) noninfected chick embryo cells, (B) RSV-BH–transformed cells, (C) cells infected with RSV-BH-Ta growing at 37°C and (D) at 41°C. The asterisk on (D) shows the region around 0.36 (M_c) where an alteration is detected in cells infected with RSV-BH-Ta. The right side shows gels of plasma membrane from (E) noninfected cells (F), RSV-BH–transformed cells, and RSV-BH-Ta–infected cells growing at (G) 37°C and (H) 41°C.

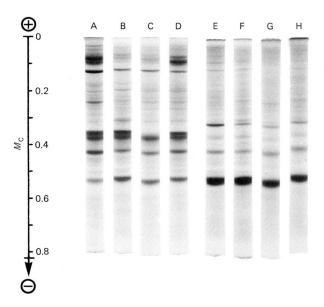

was drastically reduced in mutant-infected cells grown at the lower temperature. Isolation of proteins migrating in this region is in progress, and we intend to characterize these proteins more extensively.

Other minor differences in polypeptide patterns were found, particularly the reduction in a band of about 100,000 MW in RSV-BH cells and an increase in a band appearing at a molecular weight of 12,000. Also, an increase in the amount of a protein migrating more slowly than the heavy 50,000 to 60,000 MW protein bands was observed in phenol–acetic acid–urea gels.

When cell membrane preparations were analyzed, it was obvious that many of the polypeptides found in cell ghosts were absent or reduced, and several formerly obscure bands were enhanced. The most notable difference was in a protein of about 72,000 MW, where a major band of chick embryo cells appears as a doublet in membranes of RSV-BH–transformed cells. This was seen in both SDS–urea gels and gels containing phenol and acetic acid. This observation differs from those of Stone et al. (11), who found an increase in membrane protein in this size range in RSV-transformed cells. This difference may arise from the different procedures used in the isolation of membranes, however. No major differences in polypeptide patterns were seen in mutant-infected cells grown at the sensitive or permissive temperatures. This, of course, is expected if the hypothetical protein is a constituent in a critical concentration, which malfunctions at 41°C.

Such comparisons of proteins from RSV-BH–transformed and nontransformed cells and of RSV-BH-Ta–infected cells at transformation permissive and nonpermissive temperatures offer the hope of resolving specific proteins involved in the transformation process. We hope that the location and function of these proteins will emanate from studies on the biophysical characterization of cells transformed by Rous sarcoma virus and changes in metabolism that occur in the process of transformation.

Conclusions and Projections

Let us draw a general scheme for a sequence of physiologic changes involved in changing a cell into a malignant form (Fig. 23-3). We can suppose that a number of regulatory processes, R, are involved in maintaining cellular integrity, and that some of these may affect one or more secondary regulatory processes, R'. Alteration of the activity of R', either because of an altered R or a change in R' itself, could lead to changes in the transcription of DNA, i.e., either repression or derepression. If R' is a specific effector, then only limited regions of DNA may be affected. But, one can easily imagine an R' affecting transcription over large genetic regions, perhaps in several chromosomes, with changes resulting in a pleiotropic effect on transcription and translation. The

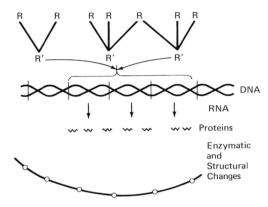

Figure 23-3. A simplified model of metabolic regulation in eucaryotic cells.

large number of new proteins resulting from this pleiotropic effect might be manifested in detectable changes in a variety of metabolic processes or structural attributes.

We have attempted in these studies to distinguish between those processes preceding and those resulting from a pleiotropic effect, using a system in which early changes can be distinguished from late changes through the use of metabolic inhibitors. Cells infected with the mutant virus, RSV-BH-Ta, behave in a normal fashion at 41°C and transform after a temperature shift to 37°C. The events preceding the pleiotropic effect include increased accumulation of water and intense vacuolization. We conclude that R is a molecule involved in the regulation of water uptake or elimination and that intracellular Na^+ and K^+ concentrations are affected (in this case, $Na^+/K^+=R'$). This perturbation of cation concentration may be sufficient to induce a pleiotropic effect on transcription and translation, resulting in increased rates of uptake of exogenous metabolites and in hyaluronic acid synthesis. Changes in cell surface proteins, as demonstrated, would not be unexpected.

This model provides an outline for projected experimentation into the nature of malignancy in the RSV-BH system: (a) the resolution of the molecule(s) primarily responsible for the early physiologic changes, (b) an analysis of intracellular ions and effects of changes in concentrations of these ions on transcription, (c) the establishment of a possible sequence of metabolic changes occurring as a result of altered transcription, (d) an analysis of the late changes to define those properties essential for the maintenance of the malignant state, and (e) a comparison of this system with others in order to determine the identity or differences in altered regulator molecules and the identity or differences in late changes of possible importance in maintaining malignancy.

REFERENCES

1. Bader, J. P. Nucleic acids of Rous sarcoma virus and infected cells. Natl. Cancer Inst. Monogr., 17:769, 1964.

2. Bader, J. P. Temperature-dependent transformation of cells infected with a mutant of Bryan Rous sarcoma virus. J. Virol., 10:267, 1972.

3. Bader, J. P. and Bader, A. V. Evidence for a DNA replicative genome for RNA-containing tumor viruses. Proc. Natl. Acad. Sci. USA, 67:843, 1970.

4. Bader, J. P. and Brown, N. R. Induction of mutations in an RNA tumor virus by an analogue of a DNA precursor. Nature [New Biol.], 234:11, 1971.

5. Brunette, D. M. and Till, J. E. A rapid method for the isolation of L-cell surface membranes using an aqueous two-phase polymer system. J. Membr. Biol., 5:215, 1971.

6. Bussell, R. H. and Robinson, W. S. Membrane proteins of uninfected and Rous sarcoma virus-transformed avian cells. J. Virol., 12:320, 1973.

7. Hatanaka, M. and Hanafusa, H. Analysis of a functional change in membrane in the process of cell transformation by Rous sarcoma virus: Alteration in the characteristics of sugar transport. Virology, 41:647, 1970.

8. Kleinzeller, A. Cellular transport of water. In Hokin, L. E., ed. Metabolic Pathways. New York, Academic Press, 1972, Vol. VI, pp. 92–132.

9. Marciani, D. J. and Kuff, E. L. Isolation and partial characterization of the internal structural proteins from murine intracisternal A-particles. Biochemistry, 12:5075, 1973.

10. Perdue, J. F., Kletzien, R., and Miller, K. The isolation and characterization of plasma membrane from cultured cells. I. The chemical composition of membrane isolated from uninfected and oncogenic RNA virus-converted chick embryo fibroblasts. Biochim. Biophys. Acta, 249:419, 1971.

11. Stone, K. R., Smith, R. E., and Joklik, W. K. Changes in membrane polypeptides that occur when check embryo fibroblasts and NRK cells are transformed with avian sarcoma viruses. Virology, 58:86, 1974.

12. Temin, H. M. Nature of the provirus of Rous sarcoma virus. Natl. Cancer Inst. Monogr., 17:557, 1967.

13. Walsby, A. E. Structure and function of gas vacuoles. Bacteriol. Rev., 36:1, 1972.

14. Wickus, G. G. and Robbins, P. W. Plasma membrane proteins of normal and Rous sarcoma virus-transformed chick-embryo fibroblasts. Nature [New Biol.], 245:65, 1973.

24

Synthesis and Integration of Rous Sarcoma Virus Proviral DNA in Duck Embryo Fibroblast Cells

R. V. Guntaka, J. M. Bishop, and H. E. Varmus

Introduction

Early studies with inhibitors of nucleic acid synthesis resulted in the proposal of a DNA intermediate called a "provirus" in the life cycle of RNA tumor viruses (14). Further studies have provided substantial evidence for the synthesis of proviral DNA (pDNA) upon infection of cells with RNA tumor viruses and a role for the provirus in virus replication and cellular transformation (3,4). The mechanics by which pDNA is synthesized and integrated into the host cell genome, however, remain to be elucidated. There are conflicting reports on the site of pDNA synthesis in an infected cell (5,9), and size and other characteristics of pDNA have not been established. In this report we summarize our results on the synthesis and characteristics of pDNA and the effect of ethidium bromide on integration of pDNA into host cell DNA.

In brief, we present evidence to show that the proviral DNA of avian sarcoma virus is synthesized in the cytoplasm early after infection and then transported into the nucleus where integration occurs. Prior to integration, proviral DNA is a duplex with a molecular weight of 6 to 7×10^6 daltons; at least some of this DNA is in a closed circular form. Integration of proviral DNA into host genome appears to be a prerequisite for virus production and cellular transformation.

Site of Proviral DNA Synthesis

We have used molecular hybridization to detect pDNA in cytoplasmic and nuclear fractions of duck cells infected with the B77 strain of Rous sarcoma virus. Proviral DNA can be detected in the cytoplasm from 3 to 6 hr following infection, but, 9 hr after infection, most of the pDNA is localized in the nucleus (Table 24-1). The appearance of pDNA in the nucleus coincides with its disappearance from the cytoplasm. We have presented evidence elsewhere that detection of pDNA in the cytoplasm is not a result of nuclear breakage or

Fundamental Aspects of Neoplasia,
edited by A. Arthur Gottlieb, Otto J. Plescia, and David H. L. Bishop.
© 1975 by Springer-Verlag New York Inc.

Table 24-1 Site of Proviral DNA Synthesis

Duck cells were infected with RSV-B77 at a multiplicity of infection (m.o.i.) of 5 to 6 (experiment I) or lower multiplicity (experiment II) in the presence of 2 μg/ml polybrene. At the indicated times, cells were collected and fractionated into cytoplasm and nuclei; DNA extracted from both sources was assayed for virus-specific DNA by reassociation kinetics (18). Copy numbers per cell for cytoplasmic DNA or per genome for nuclear DNA were computed, taking into account the number of cells employed to recover cytoplasmic DNA.

Time after infection (hr)	Number of copies/cell					
	Cytoplasm		Nucleus		Nuclear (%)	
	I	II	I	II	I	II
3.0	0.60	0.40	0.00	0.00	0	0
6.0	0.80	0.40	0.18	0.05	18	12
9.5	0.10	0.05	0.80	0.30	90	86
24.0	0.05	0.05	1.5	0.70	97	93

selective leakage of pDNA from nucleus to cytoplasm during cell fractionation (8). From these results we conclude that pDNA synthesis occurs in the cytoplasm of acutely infected cells. This conclusion is further strengthened by evidence obtained with enucleated cells. Infection of duck cells with B77 following enucleation of the cells in the presence of cytochalasin B results in the synthesis of both strands of pDNA as assayed by hybridization to 70 S RNA or to complementary DNA synthesized *in vitro* (8).

Characteristics of Proviral DNA

All RNA tumor viruses so far studied contain a 70 S RNA (MW 10×10^6), which is dissociated into 35 S (3×10^6) subunits when treated with denaturants (heat or solvent), which disrupt hydrogen bonds (6). These viruses also contain an RNA-dependent DNA polymerase, which utilizes virion RNA as a template to synthesize DNA (15). But, the *in vitro* product is generally very short (80 to 100 nucleotides, or about 1 percent of the 35 S subunit) and transcribed disproportionately from the genome (7,17). Studies with RSV mutants bearing temperature-sensitive, RNA-dependent DNA polymerase indicate that the viral enzyme carries out pDNA synthesis *in vivo* (11; Varmus et al., unpublished data).

The size of the pDNA present in the cytoplasm of infected cells was determined by centrifugation of DNA from cytoplasmic extracts in both neutral and alkaline sucrose gradients. Proviral DNA was assayed by annealing each fraction with labeled cDNA synthesized *in vitro* (this assay measures the viral DNA strand of the same polarity as genomic RNA). Two peaks at 26 and 21 S could be resolved when native DNA was analyzed on a 5 to 20 percent neutral sucrose gradient (Fig. 24-1) (the peak at 26 S is more discrete in other gradients). In addition, some pDNA at 16 S was found as a shoulder to the 21 S peak in some experiments or as a distinct peak in others. A clear peak at 9 S was also observed in some experiments. Although the relative amounts of these species vary in different experiments, at least one-third of the total pDNA sediments at 21 S. Assuming that all these size classes are linear molecules, the calculated molecular weights are 10×10^6, 6×10^6, 3.5×10^6 and 0.5×10^6 daltons for the 26, 21, 16 and 9 S species, respectively. Any conformational change due to tertiary structure, however, would yield different sedimentation coefficients for the same molecular weight species. For example, if a 21 S linear molecule also exists in a closed circular form, then it would sediment at 26 S.

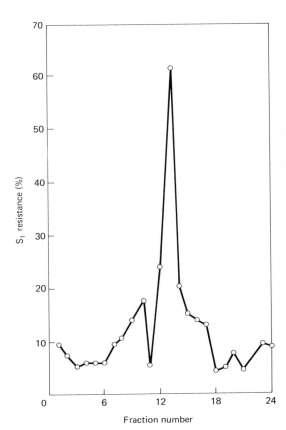

Figure 24-1. Molecular weight determination of proviral DNA in neutral sucrose gradient. Cytoplasmic DNA was isolated from duck cells infected with B77 virus for 4.5 hr and layered on top of a 5 to 20 percent sucrose gradient in 0.1 M NaCl–20 mM Tris HCl (pH 8.1)—1 mM EDTA. Centrifugation was for 5 hr in a SW 41 rotor at 40,000 rpm and 20°C. Fractions were collected, and each fraction was treated with 0.3 M NaOH for 16 hr at 37°C to eliminate any residual RNA, neutralized, and assayed for virus-specific DNA with ^{3}H-labeled complementary DNA (cDNA). The ^{3}H-labeled M13 DNA (kindly donated by Dr. M. Goulian) was centrifuged in a parallel gradient to serve as a marker.

R. V. Guntaka, J. M. Bishop, and H. E. Varmus

It has been shown previously that integration of pDNA into cell DNA begins around 10 hr after infection (18). Therefore, it was thought that by this time most of the molecules might be complete and assume their natural configuration before integration occurs. Native unintegrated pDNA can be separated from integrated DNA by Hirt fractionation (1,10). This fractionation depends on the fact that large molecular weight DNA is precipitated with SDS and NaCl and therefore can be separated by centrifugation at $17,000 \times g$. At least a large fraction of unintegrated pDNA will remain in the supernatant under these conditions. Analysis of the unintegrated DNA from 8-hr–infected cells on a neutral sucrose gradient gave a pattern similar to that of cytoplasmic pDNA (Fig. 24-1) except that relatively more pDNA sedimented at 26 S.

Analysis of the same preparation of pDNA in an alkaline sucrose gradient demonstrated a major component with a size of about 3.5×10^6 daltons (22 to 24 S). About 20 percent of the total virus-specific DNA was relatively small, with a molecular weight ranging from 0.5×10^6 to 1.0×10^6 daltons. In addition, about 30 percent sedimented at 63 to 65 S under these conditions (Fig. 24-2). This result would be expected if the 26 S material observed under neutral conditions represents a closed circular form. The experiment described below lends support to this notion.

Proviral DNA has a G+C content of about 50 percent, whereas duck DNA

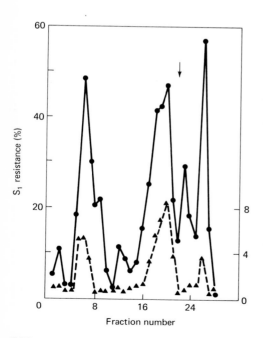

Figure 24-2. Molecular weight determination of proviral DNA in alkaline sucrose gradient. Duck cells were infected with B77 virus for 8 hr. DNA was extracted from Hirt supernatant and centrifuged in a 5 to 20 percent alkaline sucrose gradient (0.7 M NaCl—0.3 M NaOH–1 mM EDTA). Centrifugation was for 3 hr in a SW 41 rotor at 40,000 rpm and 20°C. Fractions were collected and assayed for virus-specific DNA by hybridization with (–●–) [³H]cDNA or (–▲–) 70 S [³²P]RNA.

318

has a G+C content of 42 percent. Therefore, in a cesium chloride gradient, we would expect pDNA to band at a buoyant density heavier than the duck DNA. But this would be true only with unintegrated pDNA because, once integration takes place, the pDNA would band at a density corresponding to the duck DNA. In agreement with these expectations, unintegrated pDNA banded at a density of 1.712 g/ml and integrated DNA at 1.698 g/ml (Fig. 24-3). This experiment does not distinguish circular DNA from open or linear DNA. Ethidium bromide (EB) binds to DNA and causes the molecule to unwind. Closed circular DNA binds less EB than linear DNA binds, and this results in a buoyant density difference between the closed and open circular or linear molecules (12). To explore the possibility that pDNA exists in a closed

Figure 24-3. Tertiary structure of pDNA. Duck cells were infected with B77 virus for 10 hr at m.o.i. of about four. High molecular weight DNA was precipitated by adding sodium dodecyl sulfate and NaCl as described previously (10). About 50 percent of the total pDNA remained in the supernatant. DNA was extracted from the supernatant and pellet and centrifuged in cesium chloride or casium chloride containing 300 μg/ml EB (12). Centrifugation was for 66 hr at 33,000 rpm in a type 40 rotor at 20°C. Fractions were collected and assayed for pDNA by hybridization with ^{3}H-labeled cDNA. Centrifugation of unintegrated and integrated DNA was performed in cesium chloride (A) or cesium chloride containing EB (B), (C). (–●–) unintegrated DNA, (–▲–) integrated DNA.

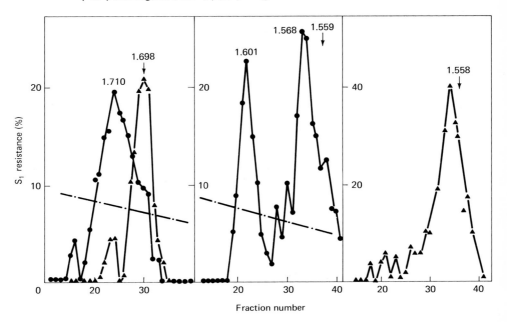

circular form, free pDNA was isolated from cells infected for 10 hr with B77 virus and subjected to equilibrium centrifugation in cesium chloride containing EB. Fractions were collected and assayed for virus-specific sequences (Guntaka et al., in preparation). About 40 percent of the unintegrated pDNA banded at 1.601 g/ml and the remainder at 1.568 g/ml (Fig. 24-3). Under similar conditions, the buoyant density difference between closed and open circles of SV40 DNA was found to be 0.035 g/ml. The buoyant density difference of 0.033 g/ml between the two main bands of pDNA is close to that observed for SV40; consequently, we have reached the provisional conclusion that pDNA exists in a circular form. In contrast, all the pDNA from a Hirt pellet (integrated DNA) had a buoyant density of 1.558, similar to that for the duck DNA (Fig. 24-3). These results suggest that pDNA circularizes before integration, but we consider these results provisional and in need of confirmation.

Integration of Proviral DNA into the Cell Genome

Proviral DNA, which is synthesized in the cytoplasm of infected duck cells, migrates to the nucleus between 6 and 9.5 hr after infection (8). Although 20 percent of the total pDNA can be detected in the nucleus by 6 hr, none of it is integrated. About 30 percent of pDNA found in the nucleus is integrated by 10 hr and, by about 20 to 30 hr, virtually all the pDNA is covalently connected to cell DNA (18). Transcription of viral RNA, on the other hand, could not be detected earlier than 10 to 15 hr post-infection (Mahy, unpublished data). This sequence of events (integration followed by virus production) suggests that integration might be a mandatory precedent to the syntheses of viral RNA. The relationship between these events can ideally be investigated by isolating viral or cell mutants defective in integration. To date, no such mutants have been isolated, and we have approached this problem by seeking specific inhibitors of integration.

Recently we found that ethidium bromide specifically blocks integration of provirus into the host cell genome (Guntaka et al., in preparation). Duck cells, pretreated for 4 hr with ethidium bromide (1.0 μg/ml), were infected with B77 virus in the presence of the dye for 40 hr. High molecular weight DNA was isolated and assayed for integration by the "network" test described previously (18). Under these conditions, there is no decrease in the amount of pDNA made, but the extent of integration was reduced by a factor of at least five. Virus production, as measured either by incorporation of [³H]uridine into particles banding at a density of 1.15 to 1.17 g/ml in a equilibrium sucrose gradient, or by focus formation, is proportionately diminished (Table 24-2). Virus-specific RNA, as monitored by hybridization to complementary DNA, is

Table 24-2 Effect of EB on Integration and Virus Production

Duck cells were pretreated with 1.0 μg/ml EB for 4 hr and infected with B77 virus for 40 hr. Control culture did not receive EB. The DNA was isolated after 40 hr and tested for integration (18). One plate from each batch was labeled for 12 hr with [³H]uridine (8 μCi/ml; 27 Ci/mmole). Virus was banded in a 15 to 55 percent sucrose gradient, and fractions were collected and precipitated with TCA. The virus particles banded at a density of 1.16 g/cc³. Samples were titered for focus formation on chicken cell monolayer 48 hr after infection (16).

	Copies/cell	Integration (%)	Incorporation of [³H]uridine into virus (cpm)	Virus production (FFU/ml)
Control	1.72	100	3095	1.5×10^5
EB (1.0 μg/ml)	1.55	17	417	8.5×10^3

Figure 24-4. Effect of varying concentrations of EB on integration and virus production. Cells were pretreated for 3 hr with varying concentrations of EB and infected for 38 hr. The DNA was isolated and tested for integration. Virus production was monitored as described above. Labeling was for 12 hr. (–○–) percent integration, (–●–) percent virus production. Percent virus production in transformed cells (□) after 24 hr or (■) 48 hr of EB (1.0 μg/ml) treatment is given in the same figure.

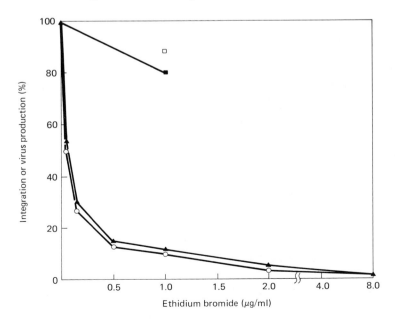

also proportionately decreased in the presence of EB. Similar results were obtained with 0.5 μg/ml EB, but the inhibition of integration and virus production was less at low concentrations of EB (Fig. 24-4). In contrast we found that virus production in infected and transformed duck cells was only minimally affected by 1.0 μg/ml EB even after 48 hr.

In concentrations greater than 1.0 μg/ml, EB not only blocks integration but also suppresses pDNA synthesis and is toxic to duck cells. Ethidium bromide also reduces cellular transformation, and this reduction is proportional to the inhibition of integration. These results suggest that virus production and cellular transformation depend upon integration of the provirus into cell DNA.

Our results contradict those of Richert and Hare (13) and Bader (2) who found that EB at 1.0 μg/ml does not affect the replication of RSV after infection of chick embryo fibroblasts. Substantial differences in the experimental design might explain the contradiction in part. It is unlikely that duck cells are more sensitive to EB than chicken cells, since we found that 1.0 μg/ml EB inhibits virus production to the same level in chicken as well as in duck cells.

The mechanism of inhibition of integration by EB is presently unknown. In view of our observation that pDNA probably exists in a circular form before integration, we speculate that EB binds to newly synthesized pDNA and interferes with the process of circularization.

ACKNOWLEDGMENTS

We thank Suzanne Heasley, Jean Jackson, and Lois Fanshier for technical assistance. This work was supported by grants from the American Cancer Society (VC-70A), USPHS (AI 08864, CA 12705, AI 06862, AI 00299), and Contract No. NO1 CP-33293 within the Virus Cancer Program of the National Cancer Institute. R.V.G. acknowledges the support by a Senior Dernham Fellowship (D-235) of the American Cancer Society, California Division; H.E.V. is a recipient of a Research Career Development Award (CA 70193) from the National Cancer Institute.

REFERENCES

1. Ali, M. and Baluda, M. A. Synthesis of avian oncornavirus DNA in infected chicken cells. J. Virol., 13:1005, 1974.

2. Bader, A. V. Role of mitochondria in the production of RNA-containing tumor viruses. J. Virol., 11:314, 1973.

3. Baluda, M. and Nayak, D. P. DNA complementary to viral RNA in leukemic cells induced by avian myeloblastosis virus. Proc. Natl. Acad. Sci. USA, 66:329, 1970.

4. Bishop, J. M. and Varmus, H. E. The molecular biology of RNA tumor viruses. *In*

Becker, F., ed. Cancer: A Comprehensive Treatise. New York, Plenum Press (in press), 1974.

5. Dales, S. and Hanafusa, H. Penetration and intracellular release of the genomes of avian RNA tumor viruses. Virology, 50:323, 1972.

6. Duesberg, P. On the structure of RNA tumor viruses. Curr. Top. Microbiol. Immunol., 51:79, 1970.

7. Garapin, A. C., Varmus, H. E., Faras, A. J., Levinson, W. E., and Bishop, J. M. RNA-Directed DNA synthesis by virions of RSV: Further characterization of the templates and the extent of their transcription. Virology, 52:264, 1973.

8. Varmus, H. E., Guntaka, R. V., Fan, W. J. W., Heasley, S., and Bishop, J. M. Synthesis of viral DNA in the cytoplasm of duck embryo fibroblasts and in enucleated cells after infection by avian sarcoma virus. Proc. Natl. Acad. Sci. USA, 71:3874, 1974.

9. Hatanaka, M., Kakefuda, T., Gilden, R. V., and Callan, E. A. O. Cytoplasmic DNA synthesis induced by RNA tumor viruses. Proc. Natl. Acad. Sci. USA, 68:1844, 1971.

10. Hirt, B. Selective extraction of polyoma DNA from infected mouse cell culture. J. Mol. Biol., 26:365, 1967.

11. Linial, M. and Mason, W. S. Characterization of two conditional early mutants of Rous sarcoma virus. Virology, 52:258, 1973.

12. Radloff, R., Bauer, W., and Vinograd, J. A dye-buoyant density method for the detection and isolation of closed circular duplex DNA: The closed circular DNA in HeLa cells. Proc. Natl. Acad. Sci. USA, 57:1514, 1967.

13. Richert, N. J. and Hare, J. D. Distinctive effects of inhibitors of mitochondrial function on Rous sarcoma virus replication and malignant transformation. Biochem. Biophys. Res. Commun., 46:5, 1972.

14. Temin, H. M. Mechanism of cell transformation by RNA tumor viruses. Ann. Rev. Microbiol., 25:609, 1971.

15. Temin, H. M. and Baltimore, D. DNA-Directed DNA synthesis and RNA tumor viruses. Adv. Virus Res., 17:219, 1972.

16. Temin, H. M. and Rubin, H. Characteristics of an assay for Rous sarcoma virus and Rous sarcoma cells in tissue culture. Virology, 6:669, 1958.

17. Varmus, H. E., Levinson, W. E., and Bishop, J. M. Extent of transcription by the RNA-dependent DNA polymerase of Rous sarcoma virus. Nature [New Biol.], 233:19, 1971.

18. Varmus, H. E., Vogt, P. K., and Bishop, J. M. Integration of DNA specific for Rous sarcoma virus after infection of permissive and nonpermissive hosts. Proc. Natl. Sci. USA, 70:3067, 1973.

Control of the Epstein–Barr Virus Genome by Mammalian Cells

R. Glaser and F. Rapp

Introduction

The Epstein–Barr virus (EBV) originally described in 1964 by Epstein and Barr (1) and EBV-specific antigens have been observed in lymphoblastoid cell lines from Burkitt tumors. Established lymphoblastoid cell lines examined to date are of two types: those that contain EBV markers, such as the early antigens (EA), virus capsid antigen (VCA), membrane antigen (MA), and virus particles, such as P3J-HR-1 (HR-1), and cells that do not produce antigens or virus particles, such as Raji cells. All cell lines, however, whether positive or negative for EB virus markers, contain EBV-specific nucleic acid associated with the genome of the cell (4,16,18). The EBV genome, however, is maintained in a repressed state, i.e., total repression in EB negative cells and partial repression in EB producer cells. What controls the repressed state and regulates the expression of the EB virus genome is central to an understanding of the relationship of the transforming virus and the transformed cell in which the virus genome resides.

We have attempted to elucidate the nature of the association of the EBV and the host cell and the role cellular regulation plays in the repression–derepression of the EBV genome described by several workers. The use of somatic-cell hybridization has proved to be a useful tool in studying the association. The approach offers a means for studying the expression of the EB virus in a variety of cell types.

Production of Somatic-Cell Hybrids of Burkitt Lymphoblastoid Cells

Under certain conditions, heterokaryons resulting from cell fusion initiated by inactivated Sendai virus have developed into replicating somatic-cell hybrid cell lines containing chromosomes of both parental cell lines and expressing the sum total of the genotypic information contained in the nuclei of the hybrid cells.

The fusion of Burkitt lymphoblastoid cells to other cell types proved to be

Fundamental Aspects of Neoplasia,
edited by A. Arthur Gottlieb, Otto J. Plescia, and David H. L. Bishop.
© 1975 by Springer-Verlag New York Inc.

Table 25-1   Chromosome Analysis of Human–Human Hybrid Cell Lines and Parental Lines (D98 and HR-1)[a]

Cell line	Chromosome number/number of cells with:																		
	44	45	46	47	48	51	52	56	57	58	61	62	63	80	82	89	92	93	94
HR-1	1	2	13	33	1														
D98	1					1	1	1	1	2	14	20	10						
D98/HR-1 Clone 2														1	1	3	1	1	1
D98/HR-1 Clone 7																1			

[a] From Glaser and O'Neill, ref. 6. Copyright 1972 by the American Association for the Advancement of Science.

difficult. But, by selecting a human cell (D98) that was deficient in hypoxanthine-guanine phosphorylbosyl transferase (HGPRT) (which will not grow in HAT selective medium) and by washing out the lymphoblastoid cells, we were able to select for hybrid cells (6). Confirmation of hybridization was accomplished using chromosome analysis (Table 25-1) and by human enzyme analysis (6,7).

Biologic Properties of Burkitt Somatic-Cell Hybrids

D98 cells are epithelial-like cells, which presumably are one of several variants of HeLa cells (Fig. 25-1) (2,7). Burkitt tumor cells are small lymphoblastoid cells which grow in suspension. Hybrid cells between D98 and HR-1 cells (designated D98/HR-1) (Fig. 25-2) and D98 and Raji cells (designated D98/Raji) are large epithelial-like cells, which grow as a monolayer similar to D98 cells. But, there are some important differences in the growth properties between the D98 parent and the D98/HR-1 hybrid. The D98 cells are contact inhibited, i.e., they do not spontaneously form multi-layered foci *in vitro*. The D98/HR-1 and D98/Raji cells grow frequently in multi-layered foci (10; unpublished data).

Since the ability to grow in soft agar is a characteristic of transformed cells, we measured the cloning efficiency of the D98 cells and D98/HR-1 hybrid cells (7). The results are shown in Table 25-2. The D98/HR-1 hybrid cells have a cloning efficiency three times greater than the D98 cells. Based on the D98 cell history, they are transformed cells. The enhancement of two properties characteristic of transformed cells in the D98/HR-1 hybrid, however, may

Chromosome number/numbered cells with:																			
95	97	98	99	100	101	102	103	104	105	106	107	108	109	110	111	112	113	134	138
1	1	2		3	5	5	6	5	6	3	5	2	1	1			2		
			1				4	1	4	6	8	19	9	1	2	1	1		1

be a result of the expression of the repressed EB virus genome. To further substantiate this, we have now obtained hybrids between mouse LM TK⁻ (CLID) cells and HR-1 cells (CLID/HR-1) that do not contain detectable amount of EBV DNA or other markers, but do contain at least 13 human chromosomes (unpublished data). When the cloning efficiencies were compared between the CLID parent and the EB-negative CLID/HR-1 hybrid, no significant difference was observed. In addition, neither the CLID nor CLID/ HR-1 cells form multi-layered foci *in vitro* (unpublished data). Whether these apparent changes in growth characteristics described depend on the EBV genome remains to be clarified.

Expression of the EB Virus in Hybrid Cells

When the D98/HR-1 and D98/Raji somatic-cell hybrids were examined for EBV-specific antigens by the immunofluorescence test, no antigens were detected (5,6,10). But, both hybrid cell types contained EBV DNA, as determined by nucleic acid hybridization (5,6,8). Attempts were made to induce the EB virus from the hybrid using the halogenated pyrimidine, 5'-iododeoxyuridine (IUdR). The hybrid cells were grown on glass cover slips in medium containing 60 μg/ml IUdR for 3 days at 37°C, the medium was replaced with normal medium (containing no drug) and examined for the presence of EBV EA, VCA, and MA, using the immunofluorescence test, and virus particles by electron microscopy. Only EA was synthesized while the cells were grown in the presence of IUdR (Fig. 25-3) (Table 25-3); VCA and MA were observed in addition to EA but only after removal of medium containing IUdR. Both VCA

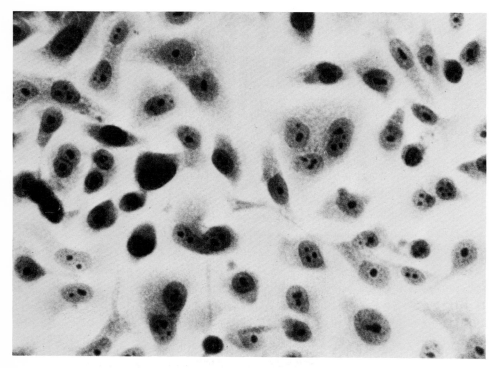

Figure 25-1. Photomicrograph of D98 cells stained with hematoxylin and eosin. X 569.

and MA appeared within 24 hr after the change of medium. EB virus DNA synthesis was absent in cells synthesizing EA (in the presence of IUdR) (Table 25-4) but increased rapidly after removal of the drug (Fig. 25-4) (8). Since it was shown that herpes simplex virus (HSV) may code for a virus-specific thymidine (TdR) kinase in virus-infected cells, we examined D98/HR-1 cells after activation of the EB virus for evidence of a new TdR kinase. When experiments were performed assaying TdR kinase in IUdR-treated and untreated D98/HR-1, HR-1, and D98 cells, an increase in TdR kinase was observed only in cells containing the EBV genome (D98/HR-1 and HR-1) and only after virus induction (9) (Table 25-5 and Fig. 25-5). This increase in TdR kinase occurs only after removal of IUdR when, as previously described, there is an increase in EBV DNA. We are currently examining the induced TdR kinase to determine if the enzyme is a new EBV-coded TdR kinase or a derepressed-cell TdR kinase resulting from the induction of the EBV.

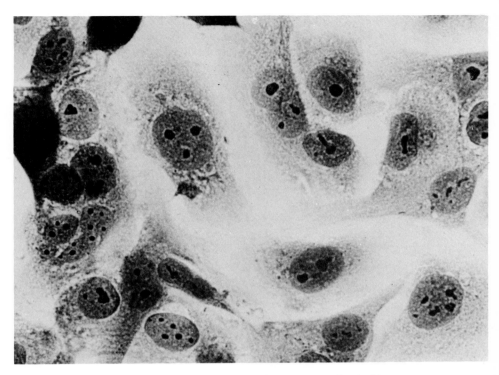

Figure 25-2. Photomicrograph of D98/HR-1 cells stained with hematoxylin and eosin. X 569.

Table 25-2   Cloning Efficiency of
D98/HR-1 Cells in
Soft Agar[a]

Cell line	Cloning efficiency (%)
D98[b]	9.4
HR-1[c]	50
D98/HR-1 cl 1[a]	28
D98/HR-1 cl 3[a]	26

[a] From Glaser et al., ref. 7.

[b] 1000 cells seeded/plate.

[c] 500 cells seeded/plate.

Table 25-3   Induction of EBV Antigens in
Hybrid Cells Treated with IUdR as
Measured by Indirect
Immunofluorescence Test[a,b]

	EBV antigens		
Day	EA	VCA	MA
1	+	−	−
2	+	−	−
3	+	−	−

[a] From Glaser et al., ref. 8.

[b] Treated with 60 μg/ml IUdR at 37°C. Cells were maintained in medium containing the drug.

Role of the Cell in the Maintenance of the EBV Genome and the Control of Virus Expression

As indicated earlier, Burkitt lymphoblastoid cell lines are of two types. Those in which the EB virus is spontaneously expressed in about 1 to 10 percent of the cell population, e.g., HR-1, as measured by the synthesis of virus-specific antigens (by the immunofluorescence test) and those in which 0 to

Figure 25-3. Immunofluorescence photomicrograph of D98/HR-1 cells containing EBV antigens after treatment with IUdR. X 437.

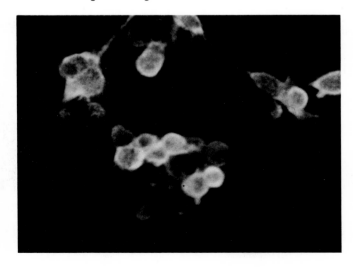

Table 25-4 DNA–RNA Hybridization of Specimens Prepared from D98/HR-1 Cells Grown in Medium Containing IUdR[a]

Time treated with IUdR (Days)	cRNA hybridized (cpm/50 μg DNA)[b]	Genome equivalent per cell (No.)
1	761	16
2	725	15
3	573	11

[a] From Glaser et al., ref. 8.

[b] The hybridized value for D98 cell DNA (159 cpm) was subtracted to estimate virus genome number equivalents.

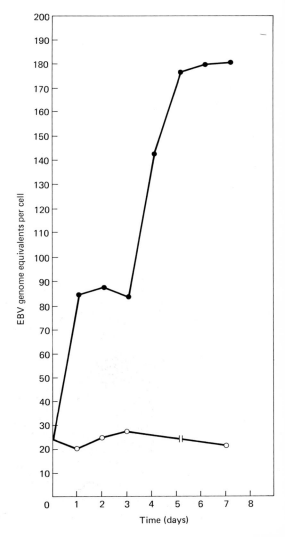

Figure 25-4. Induction of EBV DNA in D98/HR-1 cells as measured by DNA–cRNA hybridization: (●) cells treated with 60 μg/ml IUdR for 3 days and then examined for EBV genome equivalents. The hybridized value for D98 cell DNA, 159 cpm, was subtracted to estimate EBV genome equivalent (1.5×10^5 cpm of cRNA was used for each test). (○) control, cells grown in normal Eagle's medium. (From Glaser et al., ref. 8.)

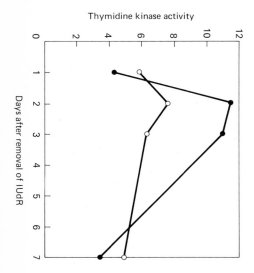

Thymidine kinase activity

Days after removal of IUdR

Figure 25-5. Activity of TdR kinase in control and IUdR-treated D98/HR-1 clone 1 hybrid cells: D98/HR-1 clone 1 cells were treated with 60 µg/ml of IUdR for 3 days. The IUdR supplemented medium was removed, fresh medium was added, and the cells were harvested at the times indicated. The TdR kinase was assayed in cell-free extracts, with TdR kinase activity represented as mµmoles of phosphorylated TdR/mg protein/15 min at 38°C. (●) IUdR-treated D98/HR-1 clone 1 hybrid cells, (○) control D98/HR-1 clone 1 hybrid cells. (From Glaser et al., ref. 9.)

<1 percent of the cells are positive, e.g., Raji cells. It has been shown by cloning experiments that all HR-1 cells are capable of allowing the spontaneous expression of EBV EA and VCA (14). One is left with the conclusion that the EBV genome is repressed totally in Raji and other "negative" lymphoblastoid cells and repressed in about 90 percent of the HR-1 cells at any given time. Furthermore, when HR-1 cells were hybridized to D98 cells, the virus genome from the HR-1 producer cell line was "turned off." This suggests that some factor(s) in D98 cells can totally repress the EBV genome. We have shown that dibutyryl cyclic AMP (Bt_2-cAMP) affects induction of EBV

Table 25-5 TdR Kinase Activity in Somatic Cell Hybrids of Burkitt Lymphoblastoid and Human Cells[a,b]

	Cell assayed		
Time of assay	D98	D98/HR-1 clone 8	HR-1
Day 1	3.2	5.7	9.7
Day 2	5.2	9.4	10.8
Day 3	3.4	10.5	12.3
Day 7	4.2	5.1	4.8

[a] From Glaser et al., ref. 9.

[b] TdR kinase activity is shown as mµmoles [^{14}C]TdR phosphorylated/mg protein/15 min at 38°C.

[c] Cells were treated with IUdR (60 µg/ml) at 37°C for 3 days, at which time medium with IUdR was replaced by medium without IUdR. "Day 1" means one day after removal of IUdR.

from D98/HR-1 cells (Table 25-6) (17), and it has also been shown that cAMP affects cellular regulation (13). This work supports the concept of cellular control of the expression of the EBV.

When lymphoblastoid cells are treated with IUdR, a number of EBV markers are synthesized. The number of both EA and VCA synthesizing HR-1 cells increases; only the EA component, however, is synthesized in Raji cells exposed to IUdR (3,5,11). We had previously suggested that this observation could be explained if the genome in EB-negative lymphoblastoid cells was defective and could not code for late virus functions (10). To test this hypothesis, we made hybrid cells by fusing D98 cells to Raji cells (D98/Raji). After cloning, the D98/Raji hybrid cells were examined for EB virus markers. Although the hybrid cells did contain EBV DNA (5), the D98/Raji cells were negative for expression of virus-specific antigens.

Both Raji and D98/Raji were treated with IUdR as previously described and examined for an increase in EBV DNA by nucleic acid hybridization, virus antigens by the immunofluorescence test, and virus particles by electron microscopy. Raji cells only synthesized EA (5), which agrees with already published data. When D98/Raji cells were exposed to IUdR, EA, VCA, and virus particles were synthesized (Table 25-7) (5). There was no increase in the number of EBV genome equivalents in Raji cells after induction, although a large increase in EBV DNA was observed in the D98/Raji cells (Table 25-8) (5).

Table 25-6   Induction of EBV Antigens in D98/HR-1 Hybrid Cells Following Treatment with IUdR and Bt$_2$-cAMP[a]

	Percent of cells positive for EBV antigens[b]				
	No IUdR		IUdR pretreatment[c]		
			No Bt$_2$-cAMP	2mM Bt$_2$-cAMP	No Bt$_2$-cAMP	2mM Bt$_2$-cAMP
Day	EA	VCA	EA	EA	VCA	VCA
2	0	0	6	18	5	10
3	0	0	10	20	8	27
4	0	0	16	37	12	26

[a] From Zimmerman et al., ref. 17.

[b] Immunofluorescence tests were performed on acetone-fixed cells at the designated times. Sera positive for either anti-EA or anti-VCA were used in the indirect immunofluorescence test along with rabbit anti-IgG conjugated to fluorescein isothiocyanate. Percentages were determined by viewing >300 cells in each of five independent experiments.

[c] IUdR (60 μg/ml) was added to the culture medium for 3 days. The medium was then replaced with fresh Eagle's medium containing 2 mM Bt$_2$-cAMP.

Table 25-7 Induction of EBV Antigens and Virus Particles
in Raji and D98/Raji Cells as Measured by the
Indirect Immunofluorescence Test[a] and
Electron Microscopy[b]

Cell line	EBV antigens[c]		Virus particles[d]
	EA	VCA	
Raji	+	−	−
D98/Raji[e]	−	−	−
D98/Raji	+	+	+

From Glaser and Nonoyama, ref. 5.

[a] As previously described (10,8).

[b] As previously described (10).

[c] Treated with 60 μg/ml IUdR for 3 days at 37°C. Cells were maintained in normal medium for an additional 3 days.

[d] Treated with 60 μgm/ml IUdR for 3 days at 37°C. Cells were maintained in normal medium for an additional 7 days.

[e] Control no IUdR.

From these studies, the following points can be made: (a) spontaneous expression of EBV antigens is repressed in D98/Burkitt somatic-cell hybrids made with both producer and non-producer lymphoblastoid cell lines, and (b) although spontaneous expression of the EBV genome is repressed in D98/Raji and Raji cells, the regulatory mechanisms controlling virus induction in D98/Raji appears to be different from the regulatory mechanism in Raji cells. The concept of the host cell interacting with the EBV genome resulting in at least some cellular control of virus expression is supported in other studies with lymphoblastoid cells. Hampar et al. (12) recently reported that the replication

Table 25-8 DNA–RNA Hybridization Tests[a]

DNA on filter		cRNA hybridized (cpm/50 μg DNA)	Estimated number of genome equivalents per cell
Raji		5,000	50
Raji[b]		5,206	54
D98/Raji	clone 4	143	3
D98/Raji[b]	clone 4	27,672	346

[a] From Glaser and Nonoyama, ref. 5.

[b] Treated with 60 μg/ml IUdR for 3 days, followed by growth in normal medium for an additional 3 days.

of the EBV genome is synchronized with the replication of cell DNA (in Raji cells) in early S phase (S_1) of the cell cycle, the same phase that data suggest is critical for induction of the virus genome with drugs (11). In addition, Miller and Lipman (15), working with EBV-transformed, simian lymphoblastoid cells, also suggested cellular control over the expression of EB virus. They found that different clones of transformed human, squirrel monkey, and marmoset lymphoblastoid cells differed in the amount of virus released and that this characteristic was stable. In addition, they found that two non-producer clones (not releasing virus) could not be superinfected with EBV.

Therefore, three lines of evidence including: (a) manipulation of the EB virus genome from one cell type to another by somatic-cell hybridization, (b) examination of the expression and replication of the EBV genome as these two functions relate to normal cell replication, and (c) study of the expression of the virus genome in clones of a variety of cells transformed by the same virus, all indicate that the host cell plays an important part in the overall expression of the latent EB virus. Whether this is true for all virus-transformed cells remains to be determined.

REFERENCES

1. Epstein, M. A. and Barr, Y. M. Cultivation *in vitro* of human lymphoblasts from Burkitt's malignant lymphoma. Lancet, 1:252, 1964.

2. Gartler, S. M. Apparent HeLa cell contamination of human heteroploid cell lines. Nature, 217:750, 1968.

3. Gerber, P. and Lucas, S. Epstein–Barr virus-associated antigens activated in human cells by 5-bromodeoxyuridine. Proc. Soc. Exp. Biol. Med., 141:431, 1972.

4. Glaser, R. and Nonoyama, M. Epstein–Barr Virus: Detection of genome in somatic cell hybrids of Burkitt lymphoblastoid cells. Science, 179:492, 1973.

5. Glaser, R. and Nonoyama, M. Host cell regulation of induction of Epstein–Barr Virus. J. Virol., 1974 (in press).

6. Glaser, R. and O'Neill, F. J. Hybridization of Burkitt lymphoblastoid cells. Science, 176:1245, 1972.

7. Glaser, R., Decker, B., Farrugia, R., Shows, T., and Rapp, F. Growth characteristics of Burkitt somatic cell hybrids *in vitro*. Cancer Res., 33:2026, 1973.

8. Glaser, R., Nonoyama, M., Decker, B., and Rapp, F. Synthesis of Epstein–Barr virus antigens and DNA in activated Burkitt somatic cell hybrids. Virology, 55:62, 1973.

9. Glaser, R., Ogino, T., Zimmerman, J., Jr., and Rapp, F. Thymidine kinase activity in Burkitt lymphoblastoid somatic cell hybrids after induction of the EB virus. Proc. Soc. Exp. Biol. Med., 142:1059, 1973.

10. Glaser, R. and Rapp, F. Rescue of Epstein–Barr virus from somatic cell hybrids of Burkitt lymphoblastoid cells. J. Virol., 10:288, 1972.

11. Hampar, B., Derge, J. G., Martos, L. M., Tagamets, M. A., Chang, S.-Y., and Chakrabarty, M. Identification of a critical period during the S phase for activation of the Epstein–Barr virus by 5-iododeoxyuridine. Nature [New Biol.], 244:214, 1973.

12. Hampar, B., Tanaka, A., Nonoyama, M., and Derge, J. G. Replication of the resident repressed Epstein–Barr virus genome during the early S phase (S-1 period) of nonproducer Raji cells. Proc. Natl. Acad. Sci. USA, 71:631, 1974.

13. Hsie, A. W., Jones, C., and Puck, T. T. Further changes in differentiation state accompanying the conversion of Chinese hamster cells to fibroblastic form by dibutyryl adenosine cyclic 3':5'-monophosphate and hormones. Proc. Natl. Acad. Sci. USA, 68: 1648, 1971.

14. Maurer, B. A., Imamura, T., and Wilbert, S. M. Incidence of EB virus-containing cells in primary and secondary clones of several Burkitt lymphoma cell lines. Cancer Res., 30:2870, 1970.

15. Miller, G. and Lipman, M. Comparison of the yield of infectious virus from clones of human and simian lymphoblastoid lines transformed by Epstein–Barr virus. J. Exp. Med., 138:1398, 1973.

16. Nonoyama, M. and Pagano, J. S. Detection of Epstein–Barr viral genome in nonproductive cells. Nature [New Biol.], 233:103, 1971.

17. Zimmerman, J. E., Jr., Glaser, R., and Rapp, F. Effects of dibutyryl cyclic AMP on the induction of Epstein–Barr virus in hybrid cells. J. Virol., 12:1442, 1973.

18. zur Hausen, H. and Schulte-Holthausen, H. Presence of EB virus nucleic acid homology in a "virus-free" line of Burkitt tumour cells. Nature, 227:245, 1970.

The Regulation of Deoxypyrimidine Kinases in Normal, Transformed, and Infected Mouse Cells in Culture

E. H. Postel and A. J. Levine

Introduction

The small DNA tumor viruses, such as SV40 and the adenoviruses, contain a limited amount of genetic information and yet can initiate a large number of changes in the cells they infect. For example, infection of resting or confluent monolayer cultures of mouse cells with SV40 results in an abortive (no virus production), nonkilling response where at least some early viral functions are expressed (10). A number of alterations in cellular functions have been detected as well. There is an increase in the specific activities of several enzymes involved in the biosynthesis of the deoxypyrimidine neucleotides and deoxyribonucleic acid (12). The rate of cellular DNA synthesis is markedly increased after viral infection, and these cells usually undergo one or several rounds of cell division (11). Infected cells frequently have an altered cell morphology and can divide even in the absence of normal cell serum factors (13). This series of complex events has been termed abortive transformation (15). Established mouse cell lines, such as 3T3 cells, grow until they reach characteristically low saturation densities, at which time the rate of cell division is drastically reduced. Viral-transformed cells have apparently overcome this regulatory control and grow to much higher saturation densities (18). It has been suggested that one or a limited number of viral gene products can alter the regulation of this type of growth control (9).

In order to study the basis of altered growth control by the DNA tumor viruses, we have investigated the regulation of several cellular gene products in normal, transformed, and abortively infected mouse cells under a variety of physiologic conditions. The deoxypyrimidine kinases (deoxycytidine, deoxyuridine, and deoxythymidine kinases) were chosen because (a) several lines of evidence suggest that each enzyme might occur in multiple forms in the cell (1,8,17), (b) they are regulated in specific ways during the cell cycle (16), and (c) these enzyme activities are among those specifically increased after nonproductive infection of mouse cells with SV40 (12). Consequently, the

Fundamental Aspects of Neoplasia,
edited by A. Arthur Gottlieb, Otto J. Plescia, and David H. L. Bishop.
© 1975 by Springer-Verlag New York Inc.

deoxypyrimidine kinases represent a group of cellular gene products whose expression may be altered in response to the physiologic state of the cell or by viral infection.

Our examination of the regulation of the deoxypyrimidine kinases in mouse cells has shown: (a) multiple forms of each of these enzymes can be demonstrated in mouse cells, (b) these multiple forms of deoxypyrimidine kinases are regulated by the physiologic state of the cell, (c) viral infections result specifically in the induction of only a limited number of these multiple enzyme forms and (d) the regulation of the deoxypyrimidine kinases in normal and transformed cells is qualitatively similar.

Multiple forms of deoxypyrimidine kinases have been demonstrated in a number of other systems. The possibility that two different forms of deoxythymidine kinase exist has been suggested by nucleotide inhibition data in rat liver extracts (5) and by subcellular fractionation in mouse liver extracts (1). By examining a number of properties, such as electrophoretic mobility, pH optima, heat stability, nucleotide inhibition, and phosphate donor specificity, it could be demonstrated that human fetal and human adult tissue also contain different molecular forms of deoxythymidine kinase (17). Chinese hamster fibroblasts in culture contain two biochemically distinct deoxycytidine kinases as shown by DEAE cellulose chromatography: a cytoplasmic activity and a mitochondrial activity (8). It will be shown in the present work that mouse cells may express, at different times, three different forms each of deoxycytidine, deoxythymidine, and deoxyuridine kinases and that some of these activities are substrate specific whereas others are multifunctional, i.e., apparently a single activity can phosphorylate two or three of the deoxyribonucleoside substrates.

It has been a general observation that, in rapidly growing tissues from a number of sources, including fetuses (17), virus-infected cells (6,12), regenerating mouse liver (1), and mammalian tumors (4,5,14), deoxythymidine kinase activity is greatly enhanced. Several hypotheses have been entertained concerning the regulation of the level of deoxythymidine kinase activity in these tissues. For example, increased activity may reflect a general responsiveness to changes in cellular function and growth requirements. Others have suggested a developmental sequence of controls, with the existence of distinct fetal and adult deoxythymidine kinases (6,17). It is also conceivable that the state of differentiation may affect the expression of kinase activities. To date, the possibility that the SV40-induced kinases in mouse cells are viral modified cellular enzymes has not been conclusively ruled out, although it is assumed that many of the induced enzymes are cellular proteins, since the viral genome is too small to code for all the induced proteins in addition to its own structural proteins.

Our evidence favors the hypothesis that the regulation of deoxypyrimidine kinases is governed by the physiologic state of the cells. It will be shown that actively growing mouse cells, whether normal tissue culture cell lines, fetal liver cells, virus-infected cells, or transformed cells, express specific kinase activities, which, by five different sets of criteria, are similar in all of these growing cells. Resting cells, on the other hand, whether normal tissue culture cells, adult liver cells, or transformed cells at very high saturation densities, have their own specific enzyme activities, which differ from the growing cell kinase activities. Hence, the regulation of deoxypyrimidine kinases in all these different mouse cell systems appears to be qualitatively similar and perhaps served by a unique regulatory mechanism.

Results

Multiple Forms of Deoxypyrimidine Kinases as a Function of the Physiological State of the Cells

In order to detect multiple forms of deoxythymidine kinase, deoxyuridine kinase, and deoxycytidine kinase in mouse cells in culture, five sets of criteria were developed to distinguish between these different enzymes. These criteria were: (a) electrophoretic mobility in polyacrylamide gels, (b) substrate specificty, (c) sensitivity to *para*-hydroxymercurobenzoate (*p*HMB), (d) the use of ribonucleotides other than riboadenosine triphosphate (r-ATP) as a phosphate donor for the deoxyribonucleoside substrate, and (e) feedback inhibition by deoxythymidine triphosphate (dTTP) of enzymatic activity. The standard experimental procedure was to prepare soluble extracts from mouse cells, which were then electrophoresed through a discontinuous 4 to 7 percent polyacrylamide gel system. The gels were sliced and the enzyme activities were eluted and tested for the above criteria by determining the conversion of labeled deoxyribonucleosides to deoxyribonucleotides using DEAE cellulose filter papers. Although the recovery of enzymatic activities eluted from the gel slices varied from experiment to experiment (35 to 95 percent) the results were qualitatively identical between experiments and quantitatively identical within any experiment. For this reason, only qualitative or very large quantitative differences between multiple enzyme activities were acceptable.

The multiple forms of deoxypyrimidine kinases were clearly observed in NIH Swiss 3T3 mouse cells in culture by analyzing these enzymatic activities in extracts prepared from actively growing or resting cells. Growing 3T3 cells contained a deoxythymidine kinase activity (Fig. 26-1, Table 26-1) that migrated in polyacrylamide gels in a heterogeneous fashion and used deoxyuridine poorly as a substrate. No detectable deoxycytidine kinase activity was

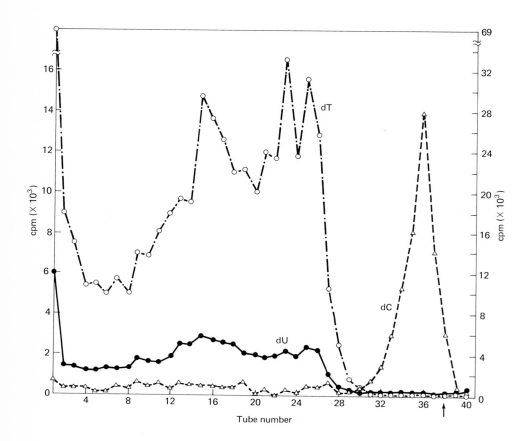

Figure 26-1. Polyacrylamide gel profile of the deoxypyrimidine kinase activities found in actively growing NIH Swiss 3T3 cells 3 days in culture: (○) deoxythymidine kinase, (●) deoxyuridine kinase, (△) deoxycytidine kinase. Soluble cell extracts (340 μg of protein) were electrophoresed on polyacrylamide gels. These gels were sliced and the enzyme activities were eluted and assayed for the phosphorylation of the three different deoxypyrimidine nucleosides as described elsewhere.

associated with this enzyme. This growing cell enzyme activity was sensitive to pHMB (0.8 mM), resistant to dTTP (0.1 mM) feedback inhibition, and employed r-CTP poorly as a phosphate donor (Table 26-1). These same growing cells also contained a deoxycytidine kinase that migrated in these gels with an R_f of 0.9 (Fig. 26-1, Table 26-2). This enzymatic activity used only deoxycytidine as a substrate, was sensitive to pHMB (0.8 mM), resistant to dTTP (10 mM) feedback inhibition, and employed r-UTP two to five times better as a phosphate donor, than did r-ATP (Table 26-2).

Table 26-1 Deoxythymidine Kinase Activities

Property	Enzyme activities		
1. Polyacrylamide gel electrophoresis R_f	Heterogeneous	0.3 (3T3, Balb/c-3T3) 0.4 (129-3T3)	0.6
2. Stage of growth where enzyme activities are observed	Growing cells	Resting cells	Mainly resting cells
3. Substrate specificity	dT dU (poor)	dT,dU,dC	dT,dU,dC
4. Sensitivity to pHMB	Sensitive	Resistant	Sensitive (3T3) Resistant (Balb/c-3T3)
5. dTTP feedback inhibition	Resistant	Resistant (3T3, Balb/c-3T3) Sensitive (129-3T3)	Sensitive (3T3) Resistant (Balb/c-3T3)
6. r-CTP as a phosphate donor (CTP/ATP)	Poor (0.2)	Very good (2 to 5) (3T3, Balb/c-3T3) same (1.0) (129-3T3)	Good (1.0)

Table 26-2 Deoxycytidine Kinase Activities

Property	Enzyme activities		
1. Polyacrylamide gel electrophoresis R_f	0.3	0.6	0.9
2. Stage of growth where enzyme activities are observed.	Resting cells	Mainly resting cells	Growing cells
3. Substrate specificity	dC,dT,dU	dC,dT,dU	dC only
4. Sensitivity to pHMB	Resistant	Resistant (Balb/c-3T3)	Sensitive
5. dTTP feedback inhibition	Resistant (3T3, Balb/c-3T3) Sensitive (129-3T3)	Stimulated (5×) (3T3, Balb/c-3T3)	Resistant (3T3, Balb/c-3T3, 129)
6. r-UTP as a donor (UTP/ATP)	very good (2 to 3x) (3T3, Balb/c-3T3)	same (1.0) (3T3, Balb/c-3T3)	Very good (2 to 3×) (3T3, Balb/c-3T3, 129)

As these 3T3 cells pass from an actively growing (Fig. 26-1) to a resting state (Figs. 26-2 and 26-3), new enzymatic activities began to appear, and the level of the growing cell kinases decrease. There were two major deoxythymidine kinase activities detected in resting cell extracts (Fig. 26-3, Table 26-1). The major activity had an R_f of about 0.3 and employed deoxythymidine, deoxyuridine, and deoxycytidine as substrates. These enzymatic activities were resistant to *p*HMB (0.8 mM) and employed r-CTP two to five times better than r-ATP as phosphate donor (Table 26-1). When several mouse cell lines of different origins and genetic backgrounds (NIH Swiss 3T3; Balb/c-3T3; 129 3T3) were compared for their phosphate donor specificity or sensitivity to dTTP feedback inhibition, there appeared to be some strain variability (Table 26-1). The 129/3T3 cell line (derived from the 129 Sv inbred strain of mouse) contained a slightly faster migrating major resting cell enzyme ($R_f \sim 0.4$) (Table 26-1) that differed from Balb/c-3T3 and NIH Swiss/3T3 activities in two of the criteria employed here (Table 26-1).

The 0.3 or 0.4 R_f enzyme activity phosphorylated deoxythymidine, deoxyuridine, and deoxycytidine. It was possible that the phosphorylation of deoxy-

Figure 26-2. Polyacrylamide gel profile of the deoxypyrimidine kinase activities observed in NIH Swiss 3T3 cells 6 days in culture approaching a confluent monolayer (resting) condition. Conditions and key are given in Figure 26-1. In this gel, 820 μg of protein were electrophoresed.

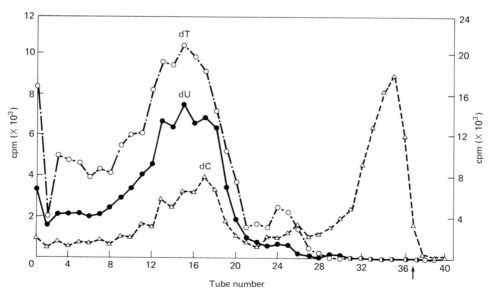

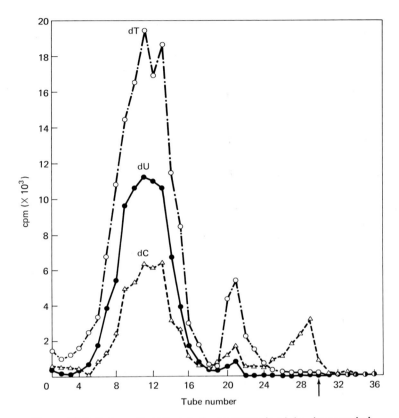

Figure 26-3. Polyacrylamide gel electrophoresis of the deoxypyrimidine kinase activities detected in NIH Swiss 3T3 cells 9 days in culture (3 days in depleted medium) and resting at a confluent monolayer. Conditions of the assay and key are given in Figure 26-1 (900 μg of protein were applied to this gel).

cytidine by this enzyme activity was due to a deoxyuridine kinase activity contaminated with deoxycytidine deaminase. This latter enzyme would convert the substrate, deoxycytidine, to deoxyuridine. The deoxyuridine could then be phosphorylated by deoxyuridine kinase, yielding a false positive for deoxycytidine kinase activity. This possibility was ruled out by thin layer chromatography of the phosphorylated product of the 0.3 R_f enzyme employing deoxycytidine and deoxyuridine as substrates, and in each case, more than 90 percent of the product of this reaction was dCMP and dUMP, respectively.

A second thymidine kinase activity, with an $R_f = 0.6$ was also present in NIH Swiss and Balb/c-3T3 cell lines. This enzyme activity has not been detected in the 129/3T3 line employed in these studies. As will be discussed in the next section, this activity is most likely due to mitochondrial enzyme and is more prevalent in extracts prepared from resting cells than from growing cells. The 0.6 R_f thymidine kinase activity coelectrophoreses with enzymatic activities that phosphorylate deoxycytidine and deoxyuridine (Fig. 26-3) and does not employ r-CTP as a phosphate donor better than r-ATP (Table 26-1). Again, strain differences between NIH Swiss/3T3 and Balb/c-3T3 cell lines have been detected when sensitivity to *p*HMB or dTTP feedback inhibition were tested (Table 26-1). The properties of the two 0.6 R_f deoxy-cytidine kinases found in resting cell extracts are reviewed in Table 26-2. The 0.9 R_f growing cell enzyme is found in lower amounts in resting cells (Fig. 26-3) and is not detectable in cultures kept in depleted medium for 5 days (Fig. 26-4).

It should be noted at this point that there has been some variability in the presence of one or both of these two multiple forms (0.3 and 0.6 R_f enzymes) of resting cell kinases. Any one of three patterns of resting cell kinases have been observed in each of several separate experiments. Either both the 0.3 and 0.6 R_f enzyme activities were present in resting cells (Fig. 26-3) or only the 0.3 R_f enzyme activity was detected (Fig. 26-4), or only the 0.6 R_f activity appeared in resting normal 3T3 cell extracts (Fig. 26-5). The variables that give rise to these apparent alternatives of resting cell gene expression are under investigation.

The above experiments demonstrate the following points: (a) There are at least three deoxythymidine, deoxyuridine and deoxycytidine kinases that can be found in mouse cells in culture. (b) These deoxypyrimidine kinase activities appear to be expressed (in normal 3T3 cell lines) as a function of the physiologic state of the cell, i.e., growing vs. resting culture conditions. (c) Although there are some mouse cell culture strain differences in the properties of these enzymes, the criteria reviewed in Tables 26-1 and 26-2 serve to distinguish between the multiple enzyme forms.

Deoxypyrimidine Kinases in 3T3 TK⁻ Cells

Variants of mouse cell lines can be obtained, by appropriate selection with antimetabolites, that contain very little deoxythymidine kinase (2) or deoxy-cytidine kinase (8) activity. Growth in the presence of bromodeoxyuridine (BUdR) selects for cells that contain only the mitochondrial form of deoxy-thymidine kinase (3T3TK⁻) (2,3). When growing and resting cell extracts prepared from 3T3TK⁻ cells were electrophoresed on polyacrylamide gels and examined according to our standard set of criteria to determine which of the multiple forms of enzymes were present or absent, the only thymidine kinase activity detected in these cells was the 0.6 R_f enzyme (Fig. 26-6). These data tentatively assign this enzyme activity as the mitochondrial form (3). Isola-

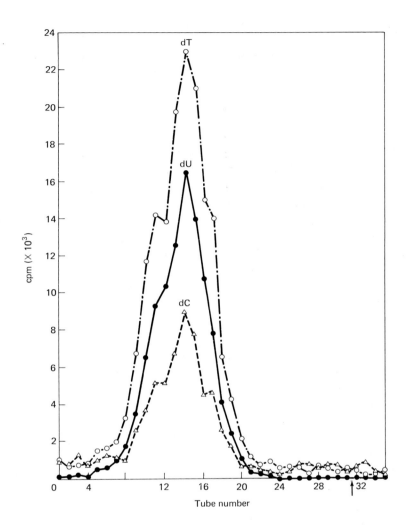

Figure 26-4. Polyacrylamide gel electrophoresis of the deoxypyrimidine kinase activities found in resting Balb/c-3T3 cells in a confluent monolayer 9 days in culture (5 days in depleted medium). Conditions for the enzyme assays and key are given in Figure 26-1 (300 μg of protein were applied to this gel).

tion of purified mitochondria and analysis of that enzyme will serve to confirm this assignment. Of some interest here is the observation (Fig. 26-6) that selection with BUdR against the 0.3 R_f resting cell enzyme also eliminated the deoxycytidine and deoxyuridine kinase activities at this R_f value. This finding suggests that the 0.3 R_f thymidine kinase is a trifunctional enzyme that also phosphorylates deoxycytidine and deoxyuridine and is, therefore, a deoxy-

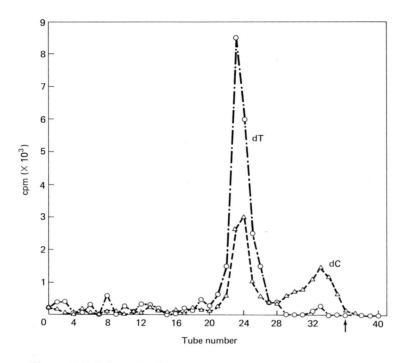

Figure 26-5. Polyacrylamide gel profile of the deoxyuridine kinase activities found in resting NIH Swiss-3T3 cells in a confluent monolayer 9 days in culture (3 days in depleted medium). Note that normal resting 3T3 cells in a confluent monolayer may yield a pattern of resting cell deoxypyrimidine kinase activity as observed in Figures 26-3, 26-4, or 26-5. The exact variable that determines these alternative forms of resting cell gene expression are not clear. The assay conditions and key are given in Figure 26-1 (200 μg of extract were applied to this gel).

pyrimidine kinase. That BUdR does not select against the substrate specific, 0.9 R_f deoxycytidine kinase activity in these same cells serves as a control against the possibility that BUdR might mitigate against the production of deoxycytidine kinase as well as deoxythymidine kinase.

Deoxypyrimidine Kinases of Transformed Cell Lines

How does viral transformation of 3T3 cells affect the regulation of these deoxypyrimidine kinases? Do the small DNA tumor viruses permanently turn on the growing cell forms of these kinases as part of the transformed cell phenotype, as has been suggested (6,17), or does the regulation of the deoxy-pyrimidine kinases continue to reflect the state of growth of transformed cells?

As a test of these alternative models, soluble extracts were prepared from

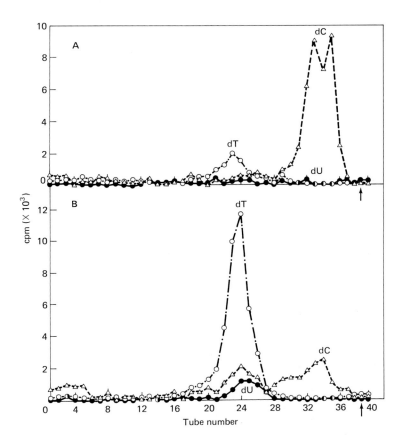

Figure 26-6. Polyacrylamide gel profile of the deoxypyrimidine kinase activities found in NIH Swiss 3T3TK⁻ cells (A) actively growing in culture (2 days) or (B) resting in a confluent monolayer (5 days). The assay conditions and key are given in Figure 26-1. (460 μg of protein in the 2-day extract and 630 μg of protein in the 5-day extract were applied to the gels).

actively growing SV40-transformed 3T3 cells and from transformed cells after they had reached very high saturation densities and effectively stopped growing. The kinase activity profiles following electrophoresis of these extracts are presented in Figure 26-7,A. By all criteria tested (Tables 26-1 and 26-2), the deoxypyrimidine kinase activities found in growing transformed cells were identical to those found in growing normal 3T3 cells. At very high saturation densities, under conditions of minimal cell division, these transformed cells contained the enzymatic activities characteristic of resting normal 3T3 cells (Fig. 26-7,B). Here again, the major resting cell kinase activity could be either

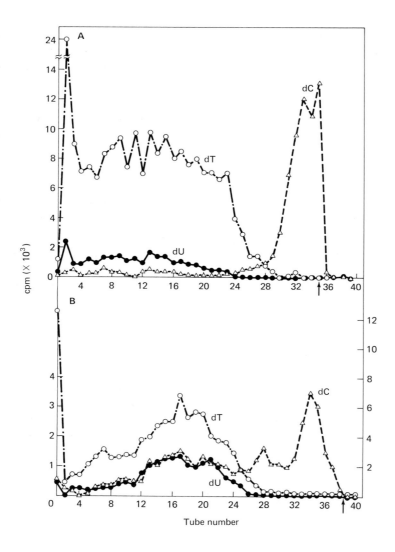

Figure 26-7. Polyacrylamide gel profile of the deoxypyrimidine kinase activities found in SV 40-transformed NIH Swiss 3T3 (SV 3T3-101) cells either (A) actively growing (1.5 days in culture) or to cells (B) at high saturation densities (3 days in culture). Assay conditions and key are given in Figure 26-1.

the 0. 3 R_f or the 0.6 R_f enzyme. It is clear, then, that the deoxypyrimidine kinases of SV40-transformed cells are regulated by the physiologic state of the cell, i.e., growing vs. resting state. The only difference between normal and SV40-transformed cells, with regard to the regulation of their deoxypyrimidine kinases, is that transformed cells grow to higher saturation densities and consequently retain the growing cell kinases for longer periods of time in culture. There appears to be no permanent block in the switch from growing to resting state kinases in these cells.

Viral Induction of Deoxypyrimidine Kinases

Infection of 129-3T3 cells with SV40 or type-5 adenovirus resulted in a dramatic increase in the specific activity of each of the deoxypyrimidine kinases (Table 26-3). Do these viruses increase the activity of a particular kinase or are all of the multiple forms of the deoxypyrimidine kinases affected by these agents? Figure 26-8 presents a profile of the kinase activities in type-5 adenovirus–infected and mock-infected resting 129-3T3 cells following electrophoresis. After either SV40 or type-5 adenovirus infection, the growing cell activities of deoxythymidine kinase and deoxycytidine kinase were increased. By all criteria tested (Tables 26-1 and 26-2) the viral-induced kinase activities appear identical to the normal 3T3 growing cell kinases. If the resting cell enzymatic forms of these kinase are affected at all in the viral-infected cell, they appear to be present in depressed levels compared to a mock-infected resting cell (Fig. 26-8).

At least in the case of the SV40-infected resting mouse cells, there is an induction of cellular DNA synthesis and a stimulation in the rate of cell division (mitotic index) 30 to 72 hr after infection (11,13). This is consistent

Table 26-3 SV40 and Type-5 Adenovirus–Induced Deoxypyrimidine Kinases in 129-3T3 Cells

| | Specific activity (S.A.) ($\mu\mu$moles of substrate phosphorylated/ μg of protein in 20 min at 34°C) | | | | | |
| | dT Kinase | | dU Kinase | | dC Kinase | |
Extracts	S.A.	Increase	S.A.	Increase	S.A.	Increase
1. Mock-infected cells	0.6	—	0.37	—	0.09	—
2. Adenovirus-infected cells	18.3	30	4.12	11	0.17	2
3. SV 40-infected cells	27.0	45	7.0	19	0.47	5

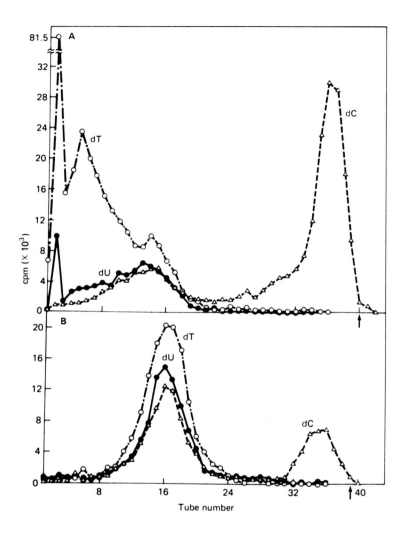

Figure 26-8. Polyacrylamide gel profiles of the deoxypyrimidine kinase activities found (B) in mock-infected 129-3T3 cells or (A) type-5 adeno-virus-infected 129-3T3 cells. Very similar results were obtained after SV 40 infection. This 129-3T3 cell line does not contain detectable 0.6 R_f enzyme activity, but 129 SV mice and a second SV129-3T3 cell line do have 0.6 R_f enzyme activities. The stimulation of the deoxypyrimidine kinases after viral infection (m.o.i.=100 PFU/cell) is best observed in 129-3T3 cells and only poorly expressed in Balb/c-3T3 cells (1040 μg of protein from mock-infected cells and 1400 μg of protein from infected cells were applied to these gels). Assay conditions and key are given in Figure 26-1.

with the specific increase in the growing cell forms of thymidine and deoxy-cytidine kinase observed in these infected cells.

Discussion

The results presented in this paper demonstrate the existence of multiple forms of deoxythymidine, deoxyuridine, and deoxycytidine kinases in mouse cells in culture. These enzymatic activities can be distinguished by the criteria reviewed in Tables 26-1 and 26-2. These multiple activities have been detected in three different mouse cell lines of different origins and different genetic background. The multiple forms of deoxypyrimidine kinases appear to be regulated by the physiologic state of the cell, i.e., growing vs. resting cells. Growing mouse cells in culture contain a substrate-specific deoxycytidine kinase. The growing cell thymidine kinase activity phosphorylates deoxyuridine poorly and has a highly heterogeneous electrophoretic mobility (Fig. 26-1, Table 26-1). Whether this activity represents a single protein species that is aggregated or associated with cellular components or several overlapping enzyme activities is not yet clear. Because this heterogeneous collection of activities behaves in an identical fashion for all other criteria tested (*p*HMB, dTTP, rCTP, substrate specificity) (Table 26-1) and all the growing cell thymidine kinase activity is lost in 3T3TK⁻ cells, (Fig. 26-6) it appears likely (but it has not been shown) that this is a single enzyme activity with a heterogeneous electrophoretic mobility, for some reason. The growing cell deoxycytidine, deoxyuridine, and deoxythymidine kinases can be found in growing 3T3 cells, growing SV40-transformed 3T3 cells, and after viral infection of resting 129-3T3 cells. We have also detected these same enzyme activities in fetal 129Sv mice (12 to 18 days of fetal life) and in young mice. These enzyme activities are absent or much reduced in resting normal and transformed cells. Several organs (liver, brain, kidney, or heart) from adult 129Sv mice (about 6 months of age) contain very little of the growing cell kinases (Yau and Postel, unpublished observations).

The two major resting cell kinases migrate in polyacrylamide gels with R_fs of approximately 0.3 and 0.6. The 0.3 R_f activity appears to be a multifunctional enzyme, which phosphorylates deoxythymidine, deoxyuridine, and deoxycytidine. The 0.6 R_f deoxythymidine kinase coelectrophoreses with a deoxyuridine and deoxycytidine kinase activity and appears to be the mitochondrial form of thymidine kinase. This enzyme activity can be observed in low levels in growing cells in culture and in fetal and young mice. Interestingly, it is the major deoxythymidine kinase activity found in adult mouse liver, kidney, and heart. In resting normal 3T3 cells or in resting viral-transformed cells in tissue culture, either the 0.3 R_f or the 0.6R_f or both enzymes, are observed to be the major resting cell kinases. The reason for this variability in tissue culture cells is not clear.

Several of the criteria employed to distinguish between the multiple forms of deoxypyrimidine kinases (Tables 26-1 and 26-2) show some variation when different cell lines are tested. These results are being repeated with extracts prepared from tissues of different inbred strains of mice. If these differences found in tissue culture truly reflect variations between different inbred mouse strains, it will be possible to map some of these enzyme activities in the mouse genetically. It will clearly be useful to know if these kinase activities are closely linked and if they segregate together or segregate independently. An analysis of the genetics of this system could be useful in understanding the level of regulation of these enzymes.

The results presented here indicate that the deoxypyrimidine kinases of the mouse are regulated by the physiologic state of the cell, i.e., growing vs. resting conditions. This level of control is independent of the origin of the cells examined, be they normal 3T3, transformed, or infected 3T3 cells. Prior interpretations of derepressed fetal gene products, to explain the differences between the deoxythymidine kinases found in fetal, normal adult, transformed, or viral-infected cells (6,17), appear to us to imply a developmental level of control that is not compatible with the available evidence. Clearly, the growing cell enzymes can be found in so-called normal 3T3 cells, and the resting cell enzymes have been observed in transformed cells.

Finally the evidence presented here is consistent with the observation that SV40 or adenovirus stimulates a cellular deoxythymidine, deoxyuridine, and deoxycytidine kinase after infection. Polyoma-infected 3T3TK⁻ cells do not contain a deoxythymidine kinase activity stimulated after infection (2). It is the growing cell kinases that are specifically stimulated by these viruses. It may well be that SV40 infection of mouse cells results in a stimulation of the growing cell kinases because this virus induces one of several rounds of cell division.

REFERENCES

1. Adelstein, S. J., Baldwin, C., and Kohn, H. I. Thymidine kinase in mouse liver: Variations in soluble and mitochondrial-associated activity that are dependent on age, regeneration and starvation and treatment with actinomycin D and puromycin. Dev. Biol., 26:537, 1971.

2. Basilico, C., Matsuya, Y., and Green, H. Origin of the thymidine kinase induced by polyoma in productivtly infected cells. J. Virol., 3:140, 1969.

3. Berk, A. J. and Clayton, D. A genetically distinct thymidine kinase in mammalian mitochondria. J. Biol. Chem., 248:2722, 1973.

4. Bresnick, E. and Karjala, R. End-product inhibition of thymidine kinase activity in normal and leukemic human leukocytes. Cancer Res., 24:841, 1974.

5. Bresnick, E., Thompson, U., Morris, H., and Liebelt, A. Inhibition of thymidine kinase activity in liver and hepatomas by TTP and dCTP. Biochem. Biophys. Res. Comm., 16:278, 1964.

6. Bull, D. L., Taylor, A. T., Austin, D. M., and Jones, O. W. Stimulation of fetal thymidine kinase in cultured human fibroblasts transformed by SV40 virus. Virology, 57:279, 1974.

7. Cohen, G. Ribonucleotide reductase activity of synchronized KB cells infected with Herpes Simplex virus. J. Virol., 9:408, 1972.

8. DeSaint Vincent, B. R. and Buttin, G. Studies on 1-β-Darabinofuranosylcytosine resistant mutants of chinese hamster fibroblasts. Eur. J. Biochem., 37: 481, 1973.

9. Dulbecco, R. and Eckhart, W. Temperature-dependent properties of cells transformed by a thermosensitive mutant of polyoma virus. Proc. Natl. Acad. Sci. USA, 67:1775, 1970.

10. Green, H. and Todaro, G. J. On the mechanism of transformation of mammalian cells by SV40. *In* Colter, J. and Paranchych, W., ed. Molecular Biology of Viruses. New York, Academic Press, 1967, p. 667.

11. Henry, P., Black, P. H., Oxman, M. M., and Weissman, S. M. Stimulation of DNA synthesis in mouse cell line 3T3 by Simian Virus 40. Proc. Natl. Acad. Sci. USA, 56: 1170, 1966.

12. Kit, S., Piekarski, L. J., and Dubbs, D. R. DNA polymerase induced by Simian Virus 40. J. Gen. Virol., 1:163, 1967.

13. Smith, H., Scher, C. D., and Todaro, C. J. Induction of cell division in medium lacking serum growth factor by SV40. Virology, 44:359, 1970.

14. Sneider, T. W., Potter, V. R., and Morris, H. P. Enzymes of thymidine triphosphate synthesis in selected Morris Hepatomas. Cancer Res., 29:40, 1969.

15. Stoker, M. Abortive transformation by polyoma virus. Nature, 218:234, 1968.

16. Stubblefield, E. and Mueller, G. C. Thymidine kinase activity in synchronized HeLa cell cultures. Biochem. Biophys. Res. Commun., 20:535, 1965.

17. Taylor, A. T., Stafford, M., and Jones, O. Properties of thymidine kinase partially purified from human fetal and adult tissue. J. Biol. Chem., 247:1930, 1972.

18. Todaro, G. J. and Green, H. An assay for cellular transformation by SV40. Virology, 23:117, 1964.

VI

Tumor Cell Growth and Regulation

27

Studies on the Cellular Mechanisms of Chemical Oncogenesis in Culture

C. Heidelberger

Introduction

It is now almost 200 years since the remarkable paper by Percivall Pott called attention to the high incidence of cancer of the scrotum among the chimney sweeps of London and correctly attributed this to their continual contact with coal tar. Thus, 1776, in addition to being the birth date of our country was also the birth date of cancer research and of chemical carcinogenesis. It has been a repeated tragedy that many chemicals have been found to induce cancer in man before carcinogenic activity has been detected in animal tests. At present, about 20 different chemicals have been unequivocally found to produce cancer in humans, usually as a result of industrial exposure. It is now generally accepted by most epidemiologists that chemicals are the cause of 80 to 90 percent of all human cancers (17).

In the course of this brief presentation, I wish to make four points: (a) chemicals are the major cause of cancer in humans, (b) those chemical carcinogens that are not themselves chemically reactive must be converted metabolically into a chemically reactive form in order to produce their noxious effects, (c) cell culture model systems are now available for quantitative studies of chemical oncogenesis that make it possible to ask and answer, for the first time, critical questions about the cellular mechanisms of chemical oncogenesis, and (d) these are exciting times in the field of chemical oncogenesis.

Activation of Chemical Carcinogens

The necessity for the metabolic activation of most carcinogenic chemicals emerged from the brilliant research of my colleagues, James and Elizabeth Miller. They showed that the aromatic amino carcinogens, N-acetylaminofluorene and p-dimethylaminoazobenzene, required metabolism by the microsomal mixed-function oxidases to electrophilic forms, and they elucidated the chem-

Fundamental Aspects of Neoplasia,
edited by A. Arthur Gottlieb, Otto J. Plescia, and David H. L. Bishop.
© 1975 by Springer-Verlag New York Inc.

ical and enzymatic properties of these conversions (25,26). In our laboratory we have long been interested in the cellular and molecular mechanisms of oncogenesis by polycyclic aromatic hydrocarbons (12,13), and our contribution to the elucidation of a mechanism of their metabolic activation will be given below.

Some time ago I decided that, in order to answer critical questions about the cellular mechanisms of chemical oncogenesis, it would be necessary to develop quantitative systems in which the phenomenon could be reproduced in cell cultures. In the course of our work, Leo Sachs beat us to it with his development of the hamster embryo cell system (2), with which he has done so many fruitful studies. This system has also been adopted and widely studied by DiPaolo and his colleagues (7,8).

Methods

My colleagues and I have developed two such systems, using fibroblastic cell lines derived from the prostate glands of adult C3H mice (4,5,6) and from C3H mouse embryos (35,36). These cell lines are highly susceptible to postconfluence inhibition of cell division, remain flat in confluent dishes, have a low saturation density, have a very low incidence of spontaneous malignant transformation, and do not produce tumors when inoculated into immuno-suppressed C3H mice. These cells can also be cloned with high efficiency. When these cells are treated in culture with oncogenic polycyclic aromatic hydrocarbons, such as methylcholanthrene (MCA), the social behavior of the cells is changed: they pile up in distinct colonies after a monolayer is reached, and they produce malignant fibrosarcomas upon inoculation into isologous mice. Thus, in these systems, morphologic and malignant transformation are equated. Moreover, there was an excellent correspondence between the number of transformed colonies a given oncogen produces in both systems and its *in vivo* oncogenic activity. Quantitative dose-response curves showed that the processes of malignant transformation and cytotoxicity are unrelated (6,35), confirming the conclusion reached by Huberman and Sachs (20) with the hamster embryo cells. I have recently reviewed various aspects of chemical oncogenesis in cultures (14,15,16).

Since these model systems can be considered as somewhat artifactual, it is continually necessary to validate them with respect to carcinogenesis *in vivo*. Thus, we were encouraged to find that the complicated situation of individual non-cross–reacting cell surface transplantation antigens that was known for chemically induced sarcomas in mice (33) was also found in our chemically transformed clones in culture (9,27,29).

Metabolic Activation

Returning now to the matter of the metabolic activation of polycyclic hydrocarbons, the extensive studies on their metabolism in liver preparations by Boyland and Sims led to the postulation, in 1950, that epoxides (arene oxides) could account for the metabolic products that were produced: phenols, *trans*-dihydrodiols, and glutathione conjugates (3). When the concept of metabolic activation was understood, it became evident that epoxides could also be a metabolically activated form. In fact, we were able to isolate an epoxide as an intermediate in the microsomal metabolism of the carcinogen, dibenz[*a,h*]anthracene (37). Moreover, Grover and Sims showed that labeled epoxides could react covalently in the test tube with DNA and proteins (10). In collaboration with Grover and Sims, we found that epoxides were much more active than the parent hydrocarbons in producing malignant transformation, and that the other metabolites were inactive (11,19,24); the epoxides were also bound covalently to DNA, RNA, and proteins of transformable cells to a greater extent than the parent hydrocarbons (21,22). Furthermore, we showed that inducers of the microsomal mixed-function oxidases increased malignant transformation produced by MCA, whereas inhibition of the enzyme system abolished transformation (23). This demonstrated that metabolic activation is required for hydrocarbons to produce transformation.

Cellular Mechanisms

I can now pose three fundamental questions about the cellular mechanisms of chemical oncogenesis: (a) Does the chemical transform nonmalignant cells into malignant cells, or, as had been postulated by Prehn (34), does the chemical somehow select for preexisting malignant cells? (b) If the chemical does produce a direct transformation, does it do it by itself, or does the chemical "switch on" a "latent" oncogenic virus, which produces the transformation? (c) If the chemical does produce transformation by itself, does it do it by a mutational mechanism (defined as the result of an alteration in the primary sequence of DNA) or by some nonmutational perpetuated effect on gene expression (cf. ref. 32)?

The proposal postulated in the first question was examined using the prostate fibroblast system, and it was possible to produce malignant transformation in high efficiency when single individual cells were treated with MCA (28). This experiment clearly eliminated the possibility of selection and shows that the chemical *does* directly transform nonmalignant cells to malignancy.

The second question was approached in collaboration with Drs. Robert Nowinski and Ulf Rapp. A number of untransformed and chemically transformed clones derived from C3H mice were examined for the gs-1 antigens of the oncornaviruses and for infectious viruses; all were negative. A series of clones, both untransformed and transformed, derived from AKR mice were similarly examined. All of these clones produced infectious viruses and expressed gs-1 antigens (Rapp, Nowinski, Reznikoff and Heidelberger, in preparation). Therefore, we can conclude that the cell genotype determines the expression of oncornavirus particles, and that the transformed phenotype does not. Since the chemical oncogen in the process of malignant transformation does not "switch on" intact virions, it is now necessary to determine whether it will "switch on" viral information. This is being investigated by appropriate DNA–RNA molecular hybridization experiments.

Oncogenic vs. Mutagenic Activity

The question of the relationship between oncogenic and mutagenic activities has been discussed frequently (cf. refs. 15 and 16). It now seems clear that whenever activated forms of chemical oncogens have been examined they are mutagenic; this also applies to epoxides of polycyclic hydrocarbons in mammalian cells in culture (18). But, analogies between the two processes studied in different organisms and cells are not sufficient to establish a mechanism, and it is necessary to attempt to perform critical experiments. One approach to this stems from our finding that, in cells synchronized by four different methods, there is a very sharp cell cycle dependency for transformation produced by the short-acting oncogen, N-methyl-N'-nitro-N-nitrosoguanidine (MNNG). The sensitive phase always occurs about 4 hr prior to the onset of DNA synthesis in synchronized 10T½ cells (1). In this specific system, we examined the production and repair of single-stranded breaks in the DNA produced by MNNG under conditions where transformation is and is not produced. Using alkaline sucrose gradient sedimentation of pre-labeled DNA, we were unable to discern any relationship between transformation and DNA repair (30,31). Obviously, additional experiments, using different techniques, will be necessary before the relationship between DNA repair and oncogenic transformation can be established. We are currently engaged in other experimental approaches toward the determination of the relationship between chemical mutagenesis and oncogenesis.

REFERENCES

1. Bertram, J. S. and Heidelberger, C. Cell cycle dependency of oncogenic transformation induced by N-methyl-N'-nitro-N-nitrosoguanidine in culture. Cancer Res., 34:526, 1974.

2. Berwald, Y. and Sachs, L. *In vitro* transformation of normal cells to tumor cells by carcinogenic hydrocarbons. J. Natl. Cancer Inst., 35:641, 1965.

3. Boyland, E. The biological significance of metabolism of polycyclic compounds. Symp. Biochem. Soc., 5:40, 1950.

4. Chen, T. T. and Heidelberger, C. Cultivation *in vitro* of cells derived from adult C3H mouse ventral prostate. J. Natl. Cancer Inst., 42: 903, 1969.

5. Chen, T. T. and Heidelberger, C. *In vitro* malignant transformation of cells derived from mouse prostate in the presence of 3-methylcholanthrene. J. Natl. Cancer Inst., 42:915, 1969.

6. Chen, T. T. and Heidelberger, C. Quantitative studies on the malignant transformation of mouse prostate cells by carcinogenic hydrocarbons *in vitro. Int. J. Cancer*, 4:166, 1969.

7. DiPaolo, J. A., Donovan, P. J., and Nelson, R. L. Quantitative studies of *in vitro* transformation by chemical carcinogens. J. Natl. Cancer Inst., 42:867, 1969.

8. DiPaolo, J. A., Nelson, R. L., and Donovan, P. J. Morphological, oncogenic, and karyological characteristics of Syrian hamster embryo cells transformed *in vitro* by polycyclic hydrocarbons. Cancer Res., 31:1118, 1971.

9. Embleton, M. J. and Heidelberger, C. Antigenicity of clones of mouse prostate cells transformed *in vitro*. Int. J. Cancer, 9:8, 1972.

10. Grover, P. L. and Sims, P. Interaction of the K-region epoxides of phenanthrene and dibenz[*a,h*]anthracene with nucleic acids and histone. Biochem. Pharmacol., 19:2251, 1970.

11. Grover, P. L., Sims, P., Huberman, E., Marquardt, H., Kuroki, T., and Heidelberger, C. *In vitro* transformation of rodent cells by K-region derivatives of polycyclic hydrocarbons. Proc. Natl. Acad. Sci. USA, 68:1098, 1971.

12. Heidelberger, C. Studies on the cellular and molecular mechanisms of hydrocarbon carcinogenesis. Eur. J. Cancer, 6:161, 1970.

13. Heidelberger, C. Chemical carcinogenesis, chemotherapy: cancer's continuing core challenges—G.H.A. Clowes Memorial Lecture. Cancer Res., 30:1549, 1970.

14. Heidelberger, C. *In vitro* studies on the role of epoxides in carcinogenic hydrocarbon activation. *In* Nakahara, W., Takayama, S., and Sugimura, T., eds. Topics in Chemical Carcinogenesis. Tokyo, University of Tokyo Press, 1972, pp. 371–386; discussion, pp. 387–388.

15. Heidelberger, C. Current trends in chemical carcinogenesis. Fed. Proc., 32:2154, 1973.

16. Heidelberger, C. Chemical oncogenesis in culture. Adv. Cancer Res., 18:317, 1973.

17. Higginson, J. *In* Environment and Cancer, 24th Symp. Fundamental Cancer Res., Baltimore, Williams & Wilkins, 1972, pp. 69–92.

18. Huberman, E., Aspiras, L., Heidelberger, C., Grover, P. L., and Sims, P. Mutagenicity to mammalian cells of epoxides and other derivatives of polycyclic hydrocarbons. Proc. Natl. Acad. Sci. USA, 68:3195, 1971.

19. Huberman, E., Kuroki, T., Marquardt, H., Selkirk, J. K., Heidelberger, C. Grover, P. L., and Sims, P. Transformation of hamster embryo cells by epoxides and other derivatives of polycyclic hydrocarbons. Cancer Res., 32:1391, 1972.

20. Huberman, E. and Sachs, L. Cell susceptibility to transformation and cytotoxicity by the carcinogenic hydrocarbon benzo[*a*]pyrene. Proc. Natl. Acad. Sci. USA, 56:1123, 1966.

21. Kuroki, T. and Heidelberger, C. Determination of the h-protein in transformable and transformed cells in culture. Biochemistry, 11:2116, 1972.

22. Kuroki, T., Huberman, E., Marquardt, H., Selkirk, J. K., Heidelberger, C., Grover, P. L., and Sims, P. Binding of K-region epoxides and other derivatives of benz[*a*]-anthracene and dibenz[*a,b*]anthracene to DNA, RNA, and proteins of transformed cells. Chem.-Biol. Interact. 4:389, 1971/72.

23. Marquardt, H. and Heidelberger, C. Influence of "feeder cells" and inducers and inhibitors of microsomal mixed-function oxidases on hydrocarbon-induced malignant transformation of cells derived from C3H mouse prostate. Cancer Res., 32:721, 1972.

24. Marquardt, H., Kuroki, T., Huberman, E., Selkirk, J. K., Heidelberger, C., Grover, P. L., and Sims, P. Malignant transformation of cells derived from mouse prostate by epoxides and other derivatives of polycyclic hydrocarbons. Cancer Res., 32:716, 1972.

25. Miller, J. A. Carcinogenesis by chemicals: An overview—G. H. A. Clowes Memorial Lecture. Cancer Res., 30:559, 1970.

26. Miller, E. C. and Miller, J. A. Mechanisms of chemical carcinogenesis: nature of proximate carcinogens and interactions with macromolecules. Pharmacol. Rev., 18:805, 1966.

27. Mondal, S., Embleton, M. J., Marquardt, H., and Heidelberger, C. Production of variants of decreased malignancy and antigenicity from clones transformed *in vitro* by methylcholanthrene. Int. J. Cancer, 8:410, 1971.

28. Mondal, S. and Heidelberger, C. *In vitro* malignant transformation by methylcholanthrene of the progeny of single cells derived from C3H mouse prostate. Proc. Natl. Acad. Sci. USA, 65:219, 1970.

29. Mondal, S., Iype, P. T., Griesbach, L. M., and Heidelberger, C. Antigenicity of cells derived from mouse prostate cells after malignant transformation *in vitro* by carcinogenic hydrocarbons. Cancer Res., 30:1593, 1970.

30. Peterson, A. R., Bertram, J. S., and Heidelberger, C. DNA damage and its repair in transformable mouse fibroblasts treated with N-methyl-N'-nitro-N-nitrosoguanidine. Cancer Res., 34:1592, 1974.

31. Peterson, A. R., Bertram, J. S., and Heidelberger, C. Cell cycle dependency of DNA damage and repair in transformable mouse fibroblasts treated with N-methyl-N'-nitro-N-nitrosoguanidine. Cancer Res., 34:1600, 1974.

32. Pitot, H. C. and Heidelberger, C. Metabolic regulatory circuits and carcinogenesis. Cancer Res., 23:1694, 1963.

33. Prehn, R. T. Tumor-specific antigens of putatively nonviral tumors. Cancer Res., 28:1326, 1968.

34. Prehn, R. T. A clonal selection theory of chemical carcinogenesis. J. Natl. Cancer Inst., 32:1, 1964.

35. Reznikoff, C. A., Bertram, J. S., Brankow, D. W., and Heidelberger, C. Quantitative and qualitative studies of chemical transformation of cloned C3H mouse embryo cells sensitive to postconfluence inhibition of cell division. Cancer Res., 33:3239, 1973.

36. Reznikoff, C. A., Brankow, D. W., and Heidelberger, C. Establishment and characterization of a cloned line of C3H mouse embryo cells sensitive to postconfluence inhibition of division. Cancer Res., 33:3231, 1973.

37. Selkirk, J. S., Huberman, E., and Heidelberger, C. An epoxide is an intermediate in the microsomal metabolism of the chemical carcinogen, dibenz[*a,b*]anthracene. Biochem. Biophys. Res. Commun., 43:1010, 1971.

28

Growth Control and the Mitotic Cell Surface

R. J. Mannino, Jr. and M. M. Burger

Introduction

It is becoming increasingly clear that the cell surface is a highly specialized organelle capable of regulating intracellular events. Changes in the configuration of the surface are detectable with a number of biochemical probes, the most notable being the lectins. Lectins are molecules that specifically agglutinate animal cells. They are available from many sources, but are most commonly isolated from plant seeds. A number of these lectins have been shown to differentially agglutinate untransformed and transformed cells. Two lectins that clearly discriminate between normal and transformed cells and have been widely studied are Concanavalin A (ConA), an agglutinin isolated from jack bean, and wheat germ agglutinin (WGA).

Saturation Density of Lectin Agglutination

In a number of the tissue culture cell lines studied, a good correlation has been demonstrated between the saturation density and agglutinability by lectins. For example, Pollack and Burger (13) have shown, using 3T3 mouse fibroblasts and a number of transformed lines derived from the 3T3 cell line, that the higher the saturation density in tissue culture, the lower the concentration of WGA necessary for half-maximal agglutination, i.e., the higher the saturation density, the higher the agglutinability, by certain lectins.

A correlation between *in vitro* saturation density and *in vivo* tumorogenicity has been demonstrated by Aaronson and Todaro (1). Using tissue culture cells derived from inbred mice, they demonstrated that the higher the saturation density in tissue culture, the greater the neoplastic potential of a cell upon introduction into a mouse. Thus, it has been suggested that, at least for the cell types that have been studied, a lectin-detectable cell surface configuration is associated both with uncontrolled cell growth and with neoplastic potential.

Fundamental Aspects of Neoplasia,
edited by A. Arthur Gottlieb, Otto J. Plescia, and David H. L. Bishop.
© 1975 by Springer-Verlag New York Inc.

Lectin Surface Configuration and Transformation

The relationship between a lectin-detectable cell surface configuration and the transformed state has also been suggested in a variety of studies using cell lines that are temperature sensitive for transformation (5,7,12). At a permissive temperature, the cells grow as transformed cells and are highly agglutinable, whereas, at a nonpermissive temperature, the cells return to normal, controlled growth, and concomitantly, are no longer agglutinable with lectins.

Studies of the binding of fluorescent-labeled WGA (and, more recently, of fluorescent-labeled ConA) to normal and transformed cells have demonstrated that untransformed cells in interphase bind very little fluorescent lectin, whereas transformed cells are highly fluorescent. Unexpectedly, however, untransformed cells in mitosis were shown to bind fluorescent-labeled lectin at levels approximately equal to those of the transformed cells (8). Subsequently it was shown that untransformed cells undergoing mitosis bind approximately as much ^{3}H-labeled ConA as transformed cells and three- to five-fold more than untransformed interphase cells (10) and that untransformed cells in mitosis are as agglutinable as transformed cells (11).

Since a lectin-detectable cell surface configuration apparently is not a peculiar property of transformed cells but is also demonstrable in untransformed, mitotic cells, it was of interest to investigate whether this cell surface configuration is only an indication of the "proliferating" state or whether it plays an active role in the mechanisms regulating cellular growth.

Mild proteolytic treatment of the surfaces of untransformed cells in a density-inhibited monolayer results in both the appearance of the agglutinable state and of one round of cell division (2,3,14). Other treatments that induce growth in density-inhibited cells, such as insulin, serum stimulation, and urea (15), also induce the agglutinable state. Thus, a treatment that induces the lectin-detectable cell surface change results in at least one round of cell division.

It has also been possible to "cover" this agglutinable cell surface through the binding of the lectin ConA (6). This lectin is toxic in its native, agglutinable form, a fact that necessitated the preparation of a "monovalent" ConA, a molecule that binds to the cell surface but does not cause agglutination. When monovalent ConA, prepared by chymotrypsinization (6), was added to polyoma virus-transformed 3T3 cells, the cells grew to densities similar to those of untransformed cells. Upon removal of the nonagglutinating ConA, the cells once again grew to high saturation densities. Therefore, the "covering-up" of the lectin sites results in untransformed growth, whereas their subsequent exposure leads to a return to uncontrolled growth.

All of these data have led to the proposal that the lectin-detecable cell sur-

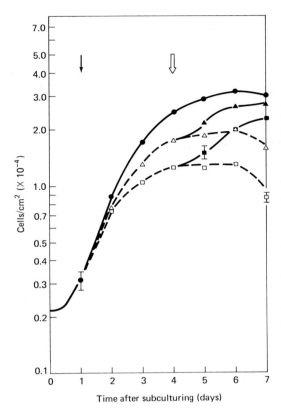

Figure 28-1. Growth inhibition of 3T3 cells induced by Suc ConA. Here 3T3 cells were subcultured in 3.5-cm Falcon plastics tissue culture dishes containing Dulbecco's modified Eagles medium (DME) containing 10 percent calf serum. The arrows indicate the times at which the medium was changed to DME + 5 percent calf serum ± Suc ConA. Cells were removed from the dishes with EDTA–trypsin solution and counted in a Coulter counter. Duplicate dishes were counted for each point: (●——●) control, no Suc ConA, (△——△) 250 μg/ml Suc ConA on days 1 and 4, (□——□) 500 μg/ml Suc ConA days 1 and 4, (▲——▲) and (■——■), fresh medium without Suc ConA on day 4.

face change accompanying mitosis of untransformed cells is involved in producing the signal that commits a cell to enter the next round of cell division (8). Since a transformed cell is constantly in the "mitotic configuration," it is constantly being induced to grow.

If the surface configuration permanently exhibited by transformed cells is related to the cell surface change accompanying mitosis of untransformed cells, and the interaction of nonagglutinating ConA with transformed cells results in decreased cell growth, it should follow that high enough concentrations of non-agglutinating ConA would also inhibit the growth of untransformed cells. The results of such an experiment are illustrated in Figure 28-1.

Non-Agglutinating ConA

When 3T3 cells are grown in the presence of a preparation of non-agglutinating ConA, they grow to a density that is below the level of the saturation density of control cells. The extent of this inhibition of growth depends upon the concentration of non-agglutinating ConA present, i.e., the higher the concentration of non-agglutinating ConA, the lower the density at which cell growth stops. This growth inhibition can be reversed by removing the medium containing the non-agglutinating ConA and replacing it with ConA-free medium.

The non-agglutinating ConA used in these studies was prepared by succinylation, according to Gunther et al. (9), rather than by enzymatic methods. Succinylated ConA (Suc ConA) sediments as a dimer in the analytic ultracentrifuge ($s_{20,w}=4.0$) in contrast to native ConA, which is a tetramer ($s_{20,w}=6.1$). Of the 13 free amino groups present per ConA monomer, approximately 10 groups are succinylated. The Suc ConA retains the ConA sugar-binding specificity, as demonstrated by its ability to bind on Sephadex and by its specific elution with glucose (0.1 M). In contrast to ConA, which precipitates glycogen at levels as low at 0.05 mg/ml, Suc ConA shows no detectable glycogen precipitation with concentrations as high as 3 mg/ml. With higher concentrations, glycogen precipitation is visible. We believe this is due to a small amount of tetrameric ConA contaminating the Suc ConA preparation. Indeed, analysis of schlieren patterns obtained from analytic ultracentrifugation shows approximately 5 percent tetramer ConA contamination. The banding patterns of native ConA and Suc ConA on SDS-polyacrylamide disc-gel electrophoresis are essentially identical.

Growth Termination by Suc ConA

An interesting characteristic of Suc ConA-induced growth inhibition is that, for a given concentration of Suc ConA, the cell density at which growth terminates is *independent of the initial cell density*. That is to say, for a given concentration of Suc ConA, the density at which growth ceases is highly dependent upon the final cell density, but is independent of the initial cell density (Fig. 28-2). Furthermore, growth inhibition by Suc ConA appears to involve specific binding, since succinylated bovine serum albumin has no inhibitory effect on cell growth and 5×10^{-3}M α-methyl-D-mannopyranoside, a specific inhibitor of ConA-mediated cell agglutination, blocks inhibition of growth by Suc ConA. It appears, therefore, that Suc ConA-induced growth inhibition involves some function of *both* Suc ConA–cell interactions and cell–cell interactions. This suggests that the effect of Suc ConA is neither toxic nor directly inhibitory to some metabolic process, such as protein synthesis.

Growth termination in the presence of Suc ConA is preceded by a decrease in the rate of [³H]thymidine incorporation per cell. Cultures that have stopped growing under the influence of Suc ConA show a rate of [³H]thymidine incorporation per cell that is identical to that of a density-inhibited monolayer.

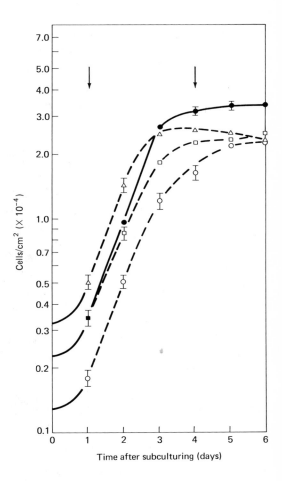

Figure 28-2. Growth inhibition induced by Suc ConA is dependent upon final cell density and independent of initial cell density. Growth conditions and cell counting were as described in Figure 28-1: (●———●) control, no Suc ConA, (○———○) cells subcultured at ~0.12× 10^4 cells/cm²+250 μg/ml Suc ConA, (□———□) cells subcultured at 0.23× 10^4 cells/cm²+250 μg/ml Suc ConA, (△———△) cells subcultured at ~0.32×10^4 cells/cm²+250 μg/ml Suc ConA. Note that at this high density, cell increase exceeds the final density, and then the culture slowly becomes less dense.

Upon removal of the Suc ConA, the observed increase in cell growth is preceded by an increase in the rate of [³H]thymidine incorporation. Measurements of the DNA content per cell through impulse cytophotometry show that Suc ConA-inhibited cells accumulate in the G_1 phase of the cell cycle, as in the case of density-inhibited cells.

The saturation density of 3T3 cells depends on the serum conditions in which the cells are grown; the saturation density can be adjusted upward or downward by either increasing the percentage of serum in the medium or changing the medium more or less frequently. Cells growing in the presence of Suc ConA show a serum dependence very similar to that of the untreated cells. It is very important to note that, for a given concentration of Suc ConA, *the ratio of the final density of cells whose growth has been inhibited by Suc ConA to the saturation density of control cells grown under*

369

identical conditions is constant. Suc ConA-inhibited cells show the same sensitivity to serum pulses in the presence of Suc ConA that untreated cells show in the absence of Suc ConA. We believe this indicates that Suc ConA does not exert its inhibitory effect by removing necessary growth factors from the serum but, rather, that it interacts directly with the cells.

It should be mentioned here that native ConA, in our hands, has never induced a reversible inhibition of growth of 3T3 cells. At low doses (25 to 50 μg/ml) it appears to slow growth of 3T3 cells, and, at higher doses, it is toxic. Native ConA, even at low doses, causes the cells to attach more firmly to the tissue culture dish substratum. This property of strong adhesion is most easily demonstrated by treatment with an EDTA–trypsin (0.05 percent) solution. Whereas control cells detach within 5 to 10 min, ConA-treated cells will remain attached up to 30 min, and pieces of cells will remain attached even after cell lysis has occurred. In our experience, Suc ConA has never caused cells to become more firmly attached to the growing surface; the adherence of Suc ConA-treated cells to the substratum is essentially indistinguishable from that of control cells, as measured by the ease of EDTA–trypsin removal from the substratum.

By all the parameters measured thus far, cells whose growth has been inhibited by Suc ConA are similar to untreated density-inhibited cells, and our working hypothesis is that Suc ConA interacts with 3T3 cells by a mechanism that mimics the phenomen of density-dependent inhibition of growth.

At this point, it was of interest to determine whether or not Suc ConA exerts its growth inhibitory effect at a particular point during the cell cycle. To test this, 3T3 cells were synchronized by plating into medium containing only 2 percent serum. Under these conditions, the cells go through approximately one round of cell division, and then stop in the G_1 phase of growth as demonstrated by impulse cytophotometry. Upon replacement of the old medium with fresh medium containing 10 percent serum, the resting cells begin to grow and go through mitosis approximately 26 to 30 hr after medium replacement. With such a synchronized population of cells at a low density it was then possible to add Suc ConA at various times during the cell cycle and to observe the effect of Suc ConA on growth. This experiment was designed so that the density of the cells at the time of the medium change would be the same as the expected final density of cells grown from day 1 in a given concentration of Suc ConA. Therefore, if Suc ConA could exert its growth inhibitory effect at the time of the medium change, no growth of the Suc ConA-treated cells would be expected.

In contrast to what was expected, in the presence of Suc ConA the cells went through one round of cell division, i.e., through the remainder of G_1 all of S, G_2 and M, before growth was inhibited (Fig. 28-3). If Suc ConA were added at the time of the first medium change, but removed just before mito-

Figure 28-3. Growth inhibition by Suc ConA can only occur by interaction with cells in mitosis. The 3T3 cells were subcultured in DME+2 percent calf serum. When growth had become stationary, the medium was replaced with DME+10 percent calf serum±Suc ConA. The medium was replaced again 23 hr later, just before mitosis. The (+ −) cells received Suc ConA at the first medium change, none at the second; (− +) cells received no Suc ConA at the first medium change, but Suc ConA at the second; and so on. Cell counting was as described in Figure 28-1. We believe that the 10 to 15 percent differences between the (+ +) and (− +) and (+ −) and (− −) curves are a result of the occurrence of some cell death, rather than of a growth inhibition effect.

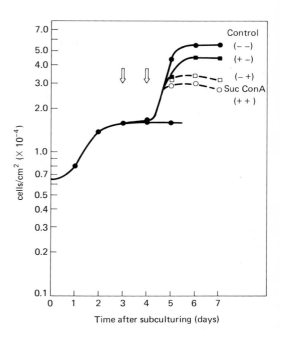

sis, growth continued past the first round of cell division. If Suc ConA were added just before the cells entered mitosis, the cells stopped growing after the completion of cell division. These data suggest to us that Suc ConA exerts its growth inhibitory effect during the mitotic phase of the cell cycle. Experiments are currently in progress to examine the effect of Suc ConA on the mitotic phase of the cell cycle in more detail in order to obtain a better understanding of Suc ConA-induced growth inhibition.

The finding that Suc ConA causes growth inhibition by specifically interacting with cells during mitosis correlates well with the earlier data that WGA and ConA bind to untransformed cells in mitosis but do not bind to interphase cells. In Figure 28-4, we present a diagrammatic representation of some of the factors regulating cellular growth in our system, as well as some theoretical explanations concerning their interrelationship.

STOP and GO Signals and Cell Growth

Untransformed 3T3 cells proceed through the cell cycle and are triggered into a new round of the cell cycle by a "GO" signal read early in the mitosis of the previous cycle. It has been demonstrated that compounds that induce cell growth in 3T3 cells cause a very rapid drop in the intracellular levels of cyclic AMP (cAMP)(4). An inhibition of this decrease in the intracellular cAMP level inhibits entrance into S phase (DNA synthesis) (4). A similar

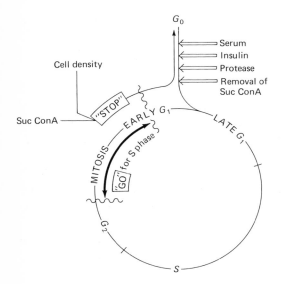

Figure 28-4. Proposed interrelationships of various factors regulating the growth of 3T3 cells and the involvement of the mitotic cell surface configuration. The GO signal occurs early in mitosis, concomitant with the change to the agglutinable state; the STOP signal must be received before the cells revert back to the non-agglutinable state, some time early in the G_1 period of the cell cycle during which the cells are agglutinable. Note that the G_0 cells are past the point at which cells can receive the STOP signal.

drop in the intracellular level of cAMP also occurs during mitosis (4), and it is possible that a decrease in the level of cAMP plays a part in this GO signal.

When the cell density of a growing culture reaches a certain level, growth stops, and the cells accumulate in G_0, a specific stage of G_1. We believe that a STOP signal exists that commits the cell to G_0 and inhibits cell growth. This STOP signal must come after the GO signal but, obviously, before G_0. Studies using density-inhibited cells synchronized using 50 percent serum, show that a decrease in the intracellular level of cAMP occurs even in the mitosis immediately before the entrance of the cell into G_0 (Bombik and Burger, unpublished observation). Thus, inhibition of the decrease in cAMP levels is probably not the natural mechanism of growth control.

Our working hypothesis is that Suc ConA mimics the mechanism of density-dependent inhibition of growth and works through the same STOP signal to route the cells into G_0. Studies are underway, however, to establish the effect (if any) of Suc ConA on changes in intracellular cAMP levels.

Cells that have stopped growing and are resting in G_0 can be induced to re-enter the growth cycle by a number of treatments, including serum stimulation, insulin treatment, mild proteolysis, and, in the case of Suc ConA-inhibited cells, removal of Suc ConA. Serum stimulation, insulin treatment and mild proteolysis all rapidly induce the agglutinable state in the surface membrane. This membrane-mediated change is accompanied by a rapid decrease in the intracellular cAMP levels (4) and eventually leads to DNA replication and to one round of cell division.

If Suc ConA is added concomitantly with a serum pulse, cell division is not inhibited, even though the agglutinable surface configuration is known to be present. This suggests to us that not only is a specific cell surface configuration required for Suc ConA to exert its inhibitory effect, but that the particular surface requirement must occur during the mitotic stage of the cycle. We suggest, therefore, that cells are capable of acting upon a STOP signal only in mitosis and early G_1, i.e., that part of the cell cycle when untransformed cells exhibit the lectin-detectable cell surface configuration. If growing cells proceed through this period in the cell cycle without receiving a STOP signal, they are committed both to a complete round of DNA replication and to cell division. Cells that do receive the STOP signal accumulate in G_0 and are also "past the point of no return." If G_0 cells are stimulated to re-enter the growth cycle, they are unable to respond to a STOP signal, either from Suc ConA or from high cell density, until they have proceeded through the entire cell cycle, entered mitosis, and assumed an agglutinable surface configuration.

Summary

Our present working hypothesis is that growing untransformed cells, upon entering mitosis, undergo a lectin-detectable surface membrane change and receive a GO signal, which initiates the next round of cell division. Sometime thereafter, but before the surface membrane returns to the non-agglutinable state, the cells receive a STOP signal that initiates the resting, G_0 state. If the cells do not receive the STOP signal, they are committed to another complete round of cell division.

ACKNOWLEDGMENTS

The authors wish to express their appreciation to Ms. Mary Beth Hatten for her comments and critical review of this manuscript.

This work was supported by the Swiss National Foundation (Grant No. 3.1330.73 SR).

REFERENCES

1. Aaronson, S. and Todaro, G. Basis for the acquisition of malignant potential by mouse cells cultivated *in vitro*. Science, 162:1024, 1968.
2. Burger, M. A difference in the architecture of the surface membrane of normal and virally transformed cells. Proc. Natl. Acad. Sci. USA, 62:994, 1969.
3. Burger, M. Proteolytic enzymes initiating cell division and escape from contact inhibition of growth. Nature, 227:170, 1970.

4. Burger, M., Bombik, B., Breckenridge, B., and Sheppard, J. Growth control and cyclic alterations of cyclic AMP in the cell cycle. Nature [New Biol.], 239:161, 1972.

5. Burger, M. and Martin, G. Agglutination of cells transformed by Rous sarcoma virus by wheat germ agglutin and concanavalin A. Nature [New Biol.], 237:9, 1972.

6. Burger, M. and Noonan, K. Restoration of normal growth by covering of agglutin sites on tumour cell surface. Nature, 228:512, 1970.

7. Eckhart, W., Dulbecco, R., and Burger, M. Temperature-dependent surface changes in cells infected or transformed by a thermosensitive mutant of polyoma virus. Proc. Natl. Acad. Sci. USA, 68:283, 1971.

8. Fox, T., Sheppard, J., and Burger, M. Cyclic membrane changes in animal cells: Transformed cells permanently display a surface architecture detected in normal cells only during mitosis. Proc. Natl. Acad. Sci. USA, 68:244, 1971.

9. Gunther, C., Wang, J., Yahara, I., Cunningham, B., and Edelman, G. Concanavalin A derivatives with altered biological activities. Proc. Natl. Acad. Sci. USA, 70:1012, 1973.

10. Noonan, K. and Burger, M. Binding of ^{3}H-Concanavalin A to normal and transformed cells. J. Biol. Chem., 248:4286, 1973.

11. Noonan, K. and Burger, M. Induction of 3T3 cell division at the monolayer stage. Exp. Cell Res., 80:405, 1973.

12. Noonan, K., Renger, H., Basilica, C., and Burger, M. Surface changes in temperature-sensitive simian virus 40 transformed cells. Proc. Natl. Acad. Sci. USA, 70:347, 1973.

13. Pollack, R. and Burger, M. Surface-specific characteristics of a contact-inhibited cell line containing the SV40 genome. Proc. Natl. Acad. Sci. USA, 62:1074, 1969.

14. Sefton, B. and Rubin, H. Release from density dependent growth inhibition by proteolytic enzymes. Nature, 227:843, 1970.

15. Weston, J. and Hendricks, K. Reversible transformation by urea of contact inhibited fibroblasts. Proc. Natl. Acad. Sci. USA, 69:3727, 1972.

Changes in Cytoplasmic Poly(A)-Rich RNA in WI-38 Cells Stimulated to Proliferate

A. M. Novi and R. Baserga

Introduction

Several lines of evidence indicate that activization of the genome is one of the early events in the pre-replicative phase of WI-38 human diploid fibroblasts stimulated to proliferate by a change of medium (5,11,30,31). An increase in chromatin template activity occurs within 1 hr after stimulation and is paralleled by an increase in incorporation of [³H]uridine into nuclear RNA (11).

Recent studies have shown that poly(A)-rich regions are a structural feature common to most eukaryotic messenger RNAs (8,10,12,13,17,19,21-23,27,29, 34,35). In fact, the presence of poly(A) segments in *m*RNA has been used to separate *m*RNA from other cytoplasmic RNAs (8,14,19,25,29,33,34).

The present investigation was undertaken to determine changes in poly(A)-rich cytoplasmic RNA occurring in WI-38 cells stimulated to proliferate by a change of medium. The results indicate that (a) some of the rapidly labeled polysomal RNA of WI-38 cells contains poly(A)-rich sequences, (b) stimulation of cell proliferation by a change of medium induces a biphasic increase in the incorporation of [³H]adenosine into poly(A)-rich cytoplasmic RNA, and (c) the early increase in [³H]adenosine incorporation into poly(A)-rich cytoplasmic RNA is related to the subsequent stimulation of DNA synthesis.

Experimental Procedures

Cell culture. The WI-38 cells, purchased from Flow Laboratories (Rockville, Md.), were grown as previously described (11), and used for experiments at passage 27, when confluent (7 days after plating). Unless otherwise stated, cells were stimulated to proliferate by replacing the old medium with fresh medium containing 10 percent fetal calf serum (30).

Fundamental Aspects of Neoplasia,
edited by A. Arthur Gottlieb, Otto J. Plescia, and David H. L. Bishop.
© 1975 by Springer-Verlag New York Inc.

Preparation of WI-38 Polysomal RNA

The WI-38 cells were harvested and lysed according to the procedure of Lazarides et al. (18). The scraped cells were collected by sedimentation at $700 \times g$ for 1 min, resuspended in 0.12 M sucrose in 0.12 M KCl, 7.5 mM $MgCl_2$, 0.5 mM $CaCl_2$, and 0.02 M Tris HCl (pH 8.5) (Buffer A) containing 2 mg/ml of bentonite, and lysed by adding 2 volumes of a solution containing 1 percent Triton X-100 and 0.4 percent sodium deoxycholate in buffer A. The lysate was centrifuged at $17,000 \times g$ in a Sorvall Model RC-2 refrigerated centrifuge for 10 min, and 2-ml portions of the supernatant were layered over a discontinuous gradient (5 ml of 0.5 M sucrose over 2 ml of 2.0 M sucrose in buffer A) and centrifuged at $136,000 \times g$ for 12 hr using a Spinco 50 rotor. The polysomal pellet was redissolved in 0.01 M Tris buffer (ph 7.4), containing 1 mM EDTA, 0.1 M NaCl, and 0.5 percent sodium dodecyl sulfate. The RNA was extracted according to the chloroform–phenol procedure of Perry et al. (28), with slight modifications. The chloroform–phenol phase and interphase were re-extracted with 0.5 volumes of chloroform and 0.5 vol of 0.1 M Tris HCl (pH 9.0), and the final combined aqueous phases were re-extracted with 0.5 volumes of choloroform. The RNA was precipitated from the aqueous phase with ethanol and redissolved in acetate–NaCl–EDTA buffer (28).

Extraction of Post-Polysomal RNA

The post-polysomal supernatant was mixed with sodium dodecyl sulfate to a final concentration of 0.5 percent, and the RNA was extracted by the cholorform–phenol procedure described above for polysomal RNA.

Isolation of Poly(A)-Rich RNA

Binding of RNA containing poly(A)-rich sequences to nitrocellulose membrane filters (Millipore) was performed according to Lee et al. (19): 50-μl aliquots of chloroform–phenol extracted polysomal RNA containing equivalent amounts by optical density of RNA (16 μg) were diluted 30 times in 0.01 M Tris HCl (pH 7.6), containing 0.5 M KCl and 0.1 mM $MgCl_2$ incubated in ice for 10 min, and absorbed to Millipore filters. The filters were dissolved in 15-ml Aquasol cocktail (N.E.N.), and counted in a scintillation counter at 35 percent efficiency for tritium.

The total acid-insoluble radioactivity was measured by precipitating equal aliquots of RNA solution with 10 percent ice-cold trichloroacetic acid (TCA) collecting the precipitate on a Millipore filter, and counting as above.

Alkaline Hydrolysis of (A)-Rich RNA

Equivalent aliquots of chloroform–phenol-extracted polysomal RNA were tested for resistance to treatment with 0.3 N KOH at 100°C for 30 min. After exposure to alkali, the samples were neutralized, carrier calf thymus DNA was added (50 μg/ml), and TCA precipitable radioactivity was collected on Millipore filters and determined as above.

Ribonuclease Assay for Poly(A)

The RNase-resistant fraction of the RNA preparation was obtained by treatment with pancreatic (1.8 μg/ml) and T_1 (45 units/ml) ribonucleases in 50 mM Tris HCl (pH 7.6), containing 50 mM KCl and 1 mM $MgCl_2$ incubated at 30°C for 20 min according to Lee et al. (19). After incubation, 20 volumes of ice-cold 10 mM Tris HCl buffer (pH 7.6), containing 0.5 M KCl and 1 mM $MgCl_2$ were added. The diluted solution was kept on ice for 20 min, then filtered through a Millipore filter. The filters were dissolved in Aquasol and counted as above.

Ribonuclease Assay of [³H]Adenosine-Labeled RNA Not Adhering to Millipore Filters

The RNA retained on the filters was precipitated by ethanol in the presence of carrier poly(A) (20 μg/ml). The RNA precipitate was dissolved in 50 mM Tris HCl (pH 7.6), containing 50 mM KCl and 1 mM $MgCl_2$ and incubated with pancreatic (1.8 μg/ml) and T_1 ribonucleases (45 units/ml) at 30°C for 30 min. The RNase-resistant radioactive material was precipitated with cold 10 percent TCA, collected on Millipore filters, and counted in a scintillation counter as described above.

Assessment of Poly(A) Content by Hybridization with Radioactive Poly(U)

Poly(A) content of cytoplasm of WI-38 cells was assayed by the [³H] poly(U)–formamide system according to Gillespie et al. (15). Polysomal RNA extracted as described above was adjusted to a final concentration of 20 μg/ml in a solution consisting of 0.5 M KCl, 1 mM $MgCl_2$, and 10 mM Tris HCl (pH 7.6), and passed through Millipore filters (0.45 μm; 25 mm) at approximately 40 drops/min. After loading, the filters were cut in small pieces, dipped in 0.1 M Tris HCl (pH 9.0), made up to 0.5 percent with sodium dodecyl sulfate, and shaken at 15° for 30 min. The wash fluid was removed, and the filter pieces were washed again with 0.1 M Tris HCl (pH 9.0). The combined washes were chilled at 4°C for 3 min, centrifuged twice at 17,000 ×g for 10 min in a Sorvall Model RC-2 refrigerated centrifuge, made up to 0.1 M with NaCl, and precipitated by ethanol at −20°. The resulting precipitate was washed twice with 66 percent aqueous ethanol made up to 0.1 M (NaCl) and dissolved in water. Hybridization and assay for ribonuclease resistance of hybrid structures was carried out as described by Gillespie et al.

(15) in 250 μl of hybridization mixture containing 50 percent formamide, 3x SSC (0.15 M NaCl; 0.015 M Na citrate), 0.01 M Tris (pH 7.2), 2.5 μg [³H]poly(U), and 23 μg of RNA. The unhybridized poly(U) was digested with pancreatic ribonuclease in the presence of 0.5 M NaCl (15), and the ribonuclease-resistant poly(U) was precipitated and collected on filters as described by Gillespie et al. (15).

Chemicals

The chemicals used and their sources were: [³H]adenosine (18.3 Ci/mmole), (Schwarz/Mann); [³H]adenosine (31.2 Ci/mmole) (New England Nuclear); [³H]uridine (14 Ci/mmole) (New England Nuclear); [³H]poly-(U) (81.6 μCi/moles phosphorus) (Miles Laboratories); poly(A) (Miles Laboratories); RNase T$_1$ and pancreatic RNase, electrophoretically pure (Worthington); DNase A electrophoretically pure (Sigma); Triton X-100 (Sigma). All other chemicals were of reagent grade.

Results

Characteristics of Rapidly Labeled Polysomal RNA from WI-38 Cells: Evidence for the Presence of Poly(A)-Rich Sequences

Rapidly labeled polysomal RNA is defined here as polysomal RNA from WI-38 cells pulse-labeled for 1 hr with either [³H]adenosine or [³H]uridine. The characteristics of poly(A)-rich RNA from this rapidly labeled polysomal RNA are shown in Table 29-1. When [³H]adenosine rapidly labeled polysomal RNA was adsorbed to Millipore filters in the presence of 0.5 M KCl (19), 65 to 75 percent of the total radioactivity precipitable with TCA was retained on the filter.

Ribosomal RNA assayed under the same experimental conditions did not bind to Millipore filters to any appreciable extent (results not shown). Treatment of [³H]adenosine-labeled polysomal RNA with pancreatic and T$_1$ ribonucleases left a substantial fraction of radioactivity still able to bind to Millipore filters (16 to 22 percent), whereas the same treatment almost completely abolished the ability of [³H]uridine-labeled polysomal RNA to bind to the filter. Digestion with 0.1 N KOH solubilized 100 percent of the radioactivity, thus indicating the absence of labeled DNA. Finally, when [³H]adenosine-labeled RNA not adhering to nitrocellulose filters was treated with pancreatic and T$_1$ ribonucleases, 95 to 100 percent of the counts were rendered acid soluble (results not shown).

Table 29-1   Characteristics of WI-38 Rapidly Labeled Polysomal RNA

The WI-38 cells were incubated for 2 hr at 37° with 40 μCi/ml of either [³H]adenosine or [³H]uridine, harvested, lysed, and processed as described in the text. Then 50-μl aliquots of chloroform–phenol-extracted polysomal RNA containing equivalent amounts of RNA by O.D. (16 μg) were (a) directly precipitated with 10 percent TCA or bound to Millipore filter (first row); (b) digested with ribonucleases before being precipitated with 10 percent TCA or bound to Millipore filter (second row), or (c) hydrolyzed in alkali as described in the text.

	Adenosine labeled		Uridine labeled	
Treatment	Acid-precipitable radioactivity (cpm)	Millipore-bound radioactivity (cpm)	Acid-precipitable radioactivity (cpm)	Millipore-bound radioactivity (cpm)
None	1,300 ± 200[a]	920 ± 30	880 ± 30	350 ± 40
RNase (pancreatic + T₁)	360 ± 40	310 ± 30	12 ± 0.3	10 ± 0.4
0.1 N KOH (100°C, 30 min)	0		0	

[a] ± represents standard deviations.

Incorporation of [³H]Adenosine into the Acid-Soluble and Acid-Insoluble Fractions of WI-38 Cells at Various Intervals after Stimulation by a Change of Medium

The incorporation of [³H]adenosine into the acid-soluble and acid-insoluble fractions of total cellular lysates at various intervals after stimulation is shown in Figure 29-1. At 1 hr after stimulation, the acid-soluble radioactivity was 75 percent above control values, then it increased sharply (250 percent) by 3 hr after stimulation, well above the 165 percent increase in the corporation of [³H]adenosine into the acid-insoluble fraction. From 9 to 30 hr after stimulation, the incorporation of radioactivity into both fractions increased only slightly. But, the incorporation of [³H]adenosine into the acid-insoluble fraction was constantly higher than the uptake into the acid-soluble fraction.

Incorporation of [³H]Adenosine into Rapidly Labeled Poly(A)-Rich Polysomal RNA at Various Intervals after Stimulation by a Change of Medium

The percentage increase above control values in the incorporation of [³H]adenosine into rapidly labeled polysomal RNA at various intervals after stimulation is shown in Figure 29-2 (after corrections due to changes in the

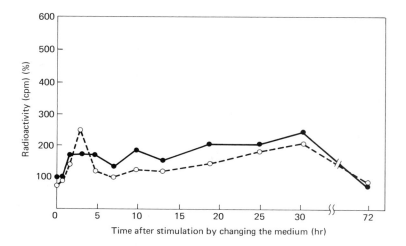

Figure 29-1. Percentage increase above control values of [³H]adeno-
sine incorporated into (O———O) the acid-soluble fractions and
(●———●) the acid-insoluble fractions of total cellular lysates of
WI-38 cells at intervals after stimulation by a change of medium.
At the times after stimulation indicated on the abscissa, cells
were labeled for 1 hr with 40 μCl/ml [³H]adenosine. Cells were then
harvested and lysed. Aliquots of total cellular lysates were washed
twice with ice-cold 0.3 N perchloric acid and centrifuged, and the
residual pellet was digested with 1.0 N NaOH at 100° for 30 min.
Radioactivity of each point (average of two determinations or more)
is expressed as percentage of control values.

uptake of the labeled precursor, see above). There are two sharp peaks of
increase in [³H]adenosine incorporation, respectively, at 3 and 24 hr after
stimulation. By 72 hr, incorporation of [³H]adenosine into poly(A)-rich cytoplasmic RNA had returned to control levels. Similarly, [³H]adenosine incorporation into poly(A) sequences (closed circles in Fig. 29-2) increased within
1 hr after stimulation with a smaller peak at 3 hr followed by a higher one at
24 hr. By 72 hr, the amount of RNase-resistant radioatcivity retained on the
filter had returned to control values.

Correlation between Stimulation of DNA Synthesis and Incorporation of [³H]Adenosine into Poly(A)-Rich Rapidly Labeled Polysomal RNA in WI-38 Cells Stimulated To Proliferate by a Change of Medium

Rovera and Baserga (30) have shown that the extent of stimulation of
DNA synthesis in WI-38 cells was highest with fresh medium containing 10

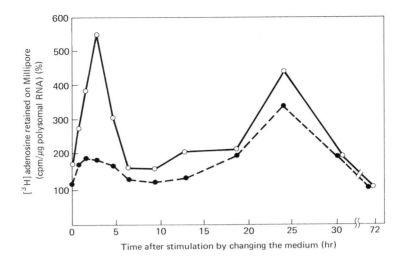

Figure 29-2. Percentage increase above control values of [³H]adenosine incorporated into rapidly labeled polysomal RNA (○——○) retained by Millipore filters or (●---●) resistant to RNase, at intervals after stimulation by a change of medium. The WI-38 cells were stimulated to proliferate and labeled as indicated in Figure 29-1. Cells were then harvested, lysed, and processed. Equal aliquots of chloroform–phenol-extracted polysomal RNA containing equivalent amounts of RNA by O.D. were adsorbed on Millipore filters (19) or digested by ribonucleases and bound to Millipore filters. Radioactivity of each point was corrected for uptake into the acid-soluble fraction, divided by the amount (μg) of pelleted polysomal RNA, and expressed as percentage of control values.

percent serum and considerably lower when 10 percent serum was added to the conditioned medium. Replacement of the old medium with fresh medium containing 0.3 percent serum caused only minimal stimulation. The incorporation of [³H]adenosine into rapidly labeled poly(A)-rich polysomal RNA was assayed under the same experimental conditions. As shown in Table 29-2, fresh medium containing 10 percent serum increased the incorporation of [³H]adenosine into poly(A)-rich polysomal RNA up to 250 percent of control values, whereas 10 percent serum added to the conditioned medium, or 0.3 percent serum in fresh medium, were less effective, inducing an increased incorporation of [³H]adenosine of 138 percent and 120 percent, respectively. These results parallel the changes in chromatin template activity reported under the same experimental conditions by Rovera and Baserga (30).

Table 29-2   Effect of Nutritional Changes on [³H]Adenosine Incorporation
into Rapidly Labeled Poly(A)-Rich Polysomal RNA
of the WI-38 Cells

The WI-38 cells were stimulated to proliferate as described by Rovera and Baserga (30),
and, 40 min later, cells were labeled for 60 min with 40 μCi/ml of [³H]adenosine,
harvested, lysed, and processed as described in the text. Aliquots of chloroform–phenol-
extracted RNA containing equivalent amount of RNA were precipitated with TCA or
bound to Millipore or digested with ribonucleases and bound to Millipore as described
in the text.

| | Acid insoluble[a] | | Bound to Millipore[a] | | RNase resistant bound to | |
| | Total cpm ($\times 10^{-3}$) | Polysomal RNA (cpm/μg) | Total cpm ($\times 10^{-3}$) | Polysomal RNA (cpm/μg) | Millipore[a] Total cpm ($\times 10^{-3}$) | Polysomal RNA (cpm/μg) |
Treatment						
Unstimulated cells	248±2	479.0±52	131±2	179.2±44	49±2	66.4±2.0
Fresh medium +0.3% serum	287±2	564.9±64	160±1	265.0±22	42±2	69.7±2.3
Conditioned medium +10% serum	402±3	715.0±81	181±2	254.0±61	60±2	84.2±4.1
Fresh medium +10% serum	480±4	337.0±47	301±3	462.0±56	63±1	93.6±3.1

[a] ± are standard deviations.

Presence of Rapidly Labeled Poly(A) Containing RNA in the Post-Polysomal Supernatant

RNA in the post-polysomal supernatant was assayed for poly(A)-rich
sequences according to Lee et al. (19). When [³H]adenosine rapidly labeled
RNA was adsorbed to Millipore filters in the presence of 0.5 M KCl, 10 to
15 percent of the total radioactivity precipitable by TCA was retained on the
filter. Treatment with pancreatic and T_1 ribonucleases left 4 to 9 percent of the
total radioactivity still able to bind to Millipore filters. Stimulation of cell proliferation by a change of medium induced a biphasic increase in the incorporation of [³H]adenosine into poly(A) containing post-polysomal RNA and its
poly(A) sequences (not shown). One hour after stimulation, the amount of
[³H]adenosine from post-polysomal RNA retained on Millipore filters was
210 percent of the controls. It decreased to 170 percent 6 hr after stimulation
and began to increase again 3 hr later, paralleling the pattern of retention on
Millipore filter of [³H]adenosine incorporated into rapidly labeled polysomal
RNA.

Effect of Actinomycin D

Actinomycin D at a concentration of 0.09 g/ml decreased the incorporation of [³H]adenosine into poly(A)-rich polysomal RNA by about 50 percent, both in control and in stimulated cells (Table 29-3). The incorporation of [³H]adenosine into poly(A) tracts was also reduced but to a lesser extent (25 percent inhibition). Administration of actinomycin D markedly influenced poly(A)-containing RNA in the post-polysomal fraction. The amount of [³H]adenosine retained on Millipore filters was sharply reduced both in

Table 29-3   Effect of Actinomycin D on [³H]Adenosine Incorporation into Rapidly Labeled Poly(A)-Rich Polysomal and Post-Polysomal RNA of Quiescent WI-38 Cells and WI-38 Cells Stimulated to Proliferate by a Change of Medium

Here the WI-38 cells were incubated for 40 min at 37° with 0.09 μg/ml of actinomycin D (32), stimulated to proliferate as described in the text, and labeled for 60 min at 37° with 40 μCi/ml of [³H]adenosine. Cells were then harvested, lysed, and processed as described. Equal aliquots of chloroform phenol-extracted RNA containing equivalent amounts of RNA (12 μg/ml polysomal RNA; 5 μg/ml post-polysomal RNA) were directly bound to Millipore (19), or digested by ribonuclease and bound to Millipore as described.

	Poly(A)-rich polysomal RNA		Poly(A) containing post-polysomal RNA	
	Bound to Millipore[a,b]	RNase-treated bound to Millipore[a,b]	Bound to Millipore[a,b]	RNase-treated bound to Millipore[a,b]
	Total cpm	Total cpm	Total cpm	Total cpm
None	11,200±223 (100)	3,060±45 (100)	3,360±143 (100)	2,470±87 (100)
Unstimulated cells treated with actinomycin D	5,190±134 (46)	2,280±86 (74)	1,940±106 (58)	1,480±42 (60)
Cells stimulated by 10% serum in fresh medium	19,090±264 (100)	3,480±102 (100)	6,820±118 (100)	4,330±104 (100)
Cells stimulated by 10% serum in fresh medium in the presence of actinomycin D	8,620±84 (45)	2,630±27 (75)	2,420±92 (35)	2,240±67 (52)

[a] ± Are standard deviations.

[b] The numbers in parentheses are values obtained in the presence of actionomycin D, expressed as percent of the values obtained without actinomycin D.

control and in stimulated cells, and consisted almost entirely of RNase-resistant segments (Table 29-3).

Assessment of Poly(A) Content of Stimulated Cells by Hybridization with [³H]Poly(U)

Polysomal RNA was isolated from quiescent WI-38 cells and WI-38 cells stimulated for 3 hr by 10 percent serum in fresh medium, and its poly(A)-rich sequences were obtained by filtration through Millipore filters. The amount of RNA recovered from the filter was 27 percent of input in control cells, and 34 percent in stimulated cells. Equivalent amounts of Millipore-bound RNA (23 μg) either from quiescent or stimulated WI-38 cells were incubated with 2.5 μg of [³H]poly(U) in 250-μl hybridization mixture (15), digested with ribonuclease, and the ribonuclease-resistant [³H]poly(U) was precipitated and collected on filters (15). Under these experimental conditions, polysomal RNA from stimulated WI-38 cells had an increased ability to bind [³H]poly(U), this being about 48 percent above control levels. The amount of [³H]poly(U) hybridized with polysomal RNA was 1.2/μg of RNA in quiescent cells and 1.8 ng/μg of RNA in WI-38 cells stimulated to proliferate.

Discussion

Several observations made in this laboratory have shown that shortly after WI-38 cells are stimulated to proliferate by a change of medium, there is activation of the genome (5). The template activity of chromatin increases as early as 1 hr after stimulation and is paralleled by an increase in synthesis of total RNA (11). That gene activation may play an important role in stimulating G_0 cells to enter DNA synthesis and cell division has already been reported for several models of stimulated DNA synthesis (1,4,7,20). An increased chromatin template activity in the very early prereplicative phase has been reported in lymphocytes stimulated to divide by phytohemagglutinin (16), in rat liver cells stimulated to divide by partial hepatectomy (2,24,37), in the isoproterenol-stimulated salivary glands (26), and in estrogen-stimulated rat uterus cells (3,36). Our experiments were carried out to determine whether stimulation of cell proliferation would cause changes in poly(A)-rich cyto-plasmic RNA, which is presumably *m*RNA (see introduction). Our findings show that stimulation of cell proliferation by a change of medium induces a biphasic increase in the incorporation of [³H]adenosine into poly(A)-rich polysomal RNA. Similar results have been obtained by Rosenfeld *et al.* (29) in phytohemagglutinin-stimulated lymphocytes. Since the increase in the incor-poration of [³H]adenosine into poly(A)-rich polysomal RNA constantly exceeds the increase in the amount of radioactivity incorporated into total

Growth Regulation of
Human Acute Leukemia Cell Populations

A. M. Mauer and S. B. Murphy

Introduction

It was long held that the primary feature of cancer was rapid and uncontrolled growth. In recent years, however, it has become apparent from studies of both animal and human tumors that malignant cell growth is not necessarily more rapid than its normal tissue counterpart. In fact, a general characteristic of the malignant cell mitotic cycle is that it is longer than the mitotic cycle of the normal cell counterpart. Furthermore, it has become evident from animal tumor models in both transplanted and autochthonous form that tumor growth regulatory mechanisms exist (2,7). The characteristic feature of growth regulation is that as the tumor grows in mass, a progressively greater number of cells go out of the cell cycle and become resting cells. These resting cells, however, retain the capacity to return to the mitotic cell cycle upon reimplantation. In many respects, growth in animal tumor models resembles that of cells in a tissue culture having regulatory mechanisms that appear to be density dependent.

Evidence that Growth Regulatory Mechanisms Are Operative
in Human Acute Leukemia

An understanding of growth regulatory mechanisms for leukemic cells would be of general interest in understanding the pathophysiology of that disease. Furthermore, there is some indication that the proliferative characteristics of the leukemic cell population can be perturbed by chemotherapy. Many of the chemotherapeutic agents in current use are maximally effective during some stage of the mitotic cycle. Techniques for increasing the proportion of the leukemic cell population in active cell division would, therefore, be of potential value. An understanding of growth regulation might be helpful in achieving this end. Finally, it will be important to determine the degree of overlap between growth regulation for the normal cell and the malignant cell population. If growth regulatory mechanisms were sufficiently different, inhibition

Fundamental Aspects of Neoplasia,
edited by A. Arthur Gottlieb, Otto J. Plescia, and David H. L. Bishop.
© 1975 by Springer-Verlag New York Inc.

of the leukemic cells, or stimulation with consequent chemotherapeutic advantage, might be selectively effected without alteration of normal cell growth responses.

The currently available evidence for growth regulation in leukemic cell populations will be presented in the following section. The types of observation vary according to the kind of leukemia and, therefore, the evidence will be separately presented for acute lymphoblastic leukemia (ALL), acute myeloblastic leukemia (AML), and erythroleukemia.

The length of the mitotic cycle in ALL has generally been reported as between 50 to 70 hr. The leukemic cell population in bone marrow has been the major proliferative compartment, with activity generally being much less in peripheral blood. Little is known about the proliferative activity of the leukemic lymphoblast at other tissue sites. Only a portion of the leukemic cell population of the bone marrow is in an active proliferative state with usually a majority of the cells being in a resting interphase state, as determined by inspection of autoradiographs obtained after *in vitro* incubation of bone marrow samples with tritiated thymidine ($[^3H]$Tdr). The percent of cells labeled with $[^3H]$Tdr, the labeling index, is a flash index of the percent of cells in DNA synthesis at any one time, i.e., in the S phase of the cell cycle. Other components of the cell cycle are: G_1, the interval following mitosis prior to the onset of DNA synthesis; G_2, the interval following DNA synthesis prior to the onset of mitosis; and, M, the interval of mitosis. Since there is relatively little variation reported for the lentgh of $S + G_2 + M$ in populations of leukemic lymphoblasts undergoing division, most of the variation in proliferative activity observed in ALL must take place by changes in the proportion of dividing and resting cells.

Simultaneous sampling of different marrow sites in the same patient with ALL reveals the same degree of proliferative activity in all sites sampled (13), suggesting that the proportion of dividing and resting cells is under a systemic rather than a local control. Such systemic control may be analogous to the humoral regulation observed for normal marrow cell populations.

A steady state of marrow proliferative activity lasting as long as 9 days has been observed in a child with untreated ALL (16). The mitotic index and percent of proliferative blasts as judged by cell size and nuclear chromatin characteristics were unchanged during the period of observation, suggesting that the cell population was sensitive to some growth regulatory mechanism determining the proportions of dividing and resting cells.

The leukemic cell population may also respond to some normal growth regulatory factors as well. In normal human bone marrow cell populations, there is a circadian rhythm for mitotic activity. The least number of mitotic figures are seen in the early morning hours with the greatest number being found during the evening hours. In four out of six patients with acute leukemia, a similar variation was found with significantly greater numbers of mitotic figures being found in the evening hours in bone marrow samples (13).

In animal tumor models, the proportion of resting cells increases with growth of the tumor. Measuring proliferative activity as a function of cell mass or duration of growth is not strictly possible in acute leukemia. An attempt to relate proliferative activity to duration of leukemic cell growth, however, has been made by comparing the proliferative activity at the time of diagnosis and the activity during a subsequent relapse. At the time of diagnosis, the patient has usually had symptoms for several weeks. Blood count changes are generally marked, with anemia, thrombocytopenia, and neutropenia indicating advanced marrow failure secondary to replacement by the leukemic cell population. After diagnosis, the patient is started on therapy and subsequently seen at close intervals. At the first indication of return of disease activity, a bone marrow sample is obtained. It is likely that cells obtained from patients in relapse have been growing for a shorter period of time than the cell population observed at diagnosis. Therefore, if the leukemic cell population is similar in this respect to animal tumor models, one would expect proliferative activity to be greater at the time of a relapse than at the time of diagnosis. This, in fact, was observed. Changes in the [^{3}H]Tdr-labeling index of leukemic cells obtained from eight of ten patients showed an increase in relapse as compared to diagnosis (13). Therefore, it is reasonable to conclude that one mechanism for regulation of growth is responsive to population density or to duration of malignant cell growth.

Extensive data obtained from culture of human marrow in agar semi-solid systems suggest that the growth of leukemic cells *in vitro* in AML depends on and is responsive to appropriate stimulation by colony-stimulating activity, reinforcing the concept that these leukemic cells are not autonomous (14,17). When assayed by standard techniques, colony formation by bone marrow cells from patients with AML in relapse is absent, or reduced, or limited to an abortive cluster formation. Colony formation shows a return to normal values when remission is achieved, and serial *in vitro* bone marrow culture has been proposed to monitor remission–relapse status in AML and ALL. Similar disorders of colony formation, as well as delayed maturation of cells in liquid suspension cultures, has been observed in preleukemia, again suggesting the possibility that AML represents a primary disturbance of cell maturation. It has also been shown that peripheral blood and bone marrow cells from some patients with AML can be stimulated to divide *in vitro* and give rise to small colonies of morphologically normal mature granulocytes by appropriate stimulation. Interpretation of these results is made difficult by uncertainty over whether growth represents that of normal colony-forming cells coexistent in the marrow with the leukemic cells but suggests that *in vitro* maturation and differentiation of leukemic cells is occurring.

Sera from patients with acute leukemia shows variable colony stimulating activity due to the presence or absence of infection, serum inhibitors and other unknown factors. Generally colony-stimulating activity factor is normal or low in leukemic sera. This factor is excreted through the kidneys, and abnormally large amounts of the factor are detected in about one-half of the urines from patients with ALL.

In erythroleukemia, the abnormal erythroid precursors are nevertheless still responsive to the physiologic control mechanisms of serum erythropoietin levels and the severity of the anemia. Suppression of erythropoiesis can be achieved with blood transfusion (1).

Further investigations will be required to establish the *in vivo* significance of the abnormal colony formation and abnormal colony-stimulating activity so frequently observed in AML. Their presence, however, is evidence of a disturbed responsiveness to normal hemopoietic regulatory mechanisms. The remarkable feature of the response observed in AML and erythroleukemia is that it occurs at all.

Possible Nature of Growth Regulatory Mechanisms

The possible nature of the growth regulation observed in leukemic cell populations is unclear at present and likely to be complex and multifactorial. Such factors as cell density, body burden of leukemic cells, supply of oxygen and other nutrients, serum inhibitory or stimulatory substances, cell–cell contact and inductive interaction between stem cells, and the microenvironment all may influence the maintenance of leukemic relapse or remission. The specific growth rate of leukemic cell populations is observed to undergo decay during growth, which may be due to cell loss or death, decrease in the growth fraction, and/or an increase in the generation time as growth continues. *In vitro* study of the proliferation kinetics of SK-L7 cells, a long-term suspension culture of cells derived from the peripheral blood of a child with AML, exhibited alterations in the cell cycle during different phases of cell growth (18). As the population changed from logarithmic to stationary growth, the S, G_2, and G_1 phases of the cell cycle became longer and more variable. The G_1 phase was the most strongly affected, with an increased proportion of cells remaining in that phase. The changes were reversible upon reduction of population density and increase in nutrient supply.

No clear picture has yet emerged of the *in vivo* interplay of factors regulating growth in leukemia. Burke et al. (3) demonstrated factors in human sera obtained during a period of drug-induced marrow aplasia; these factors stimulated [^{3}H]Tdr incorporation by a variety of target cells, including human leukemic cells, during an 18-hr *in vitro* culture period. It was suggested that these changes might be due to removal of a negative feedback inhibition. Such results are somewhat añalogous to the findings of Houck and Rytömaa and other workers in their studies of the lymphocytic and granulocytic chalones, which have been proposed as tissue-specific endogenous mitotic inhibitors (10,15). Extracts of major lymphoid tissue, such as spleen, thymus, or lymph node, inhibit the uptake of thymidine by phytohemagglutinin (PHA) stimulated normal lymphocytes and human leukemic lymphocytes *in vitro*. *In vivo*, such extracts are immunosuppressive. An extract of granulocytes has been shown to specifically reduce thymidine incorporation by granulocyte precursors in the marrow, as assessed by autoradiography, and to inhibit granulocyte proliferation in diffusion chambers. Furthermore, treatment of rats with chloroleukemia with injections of granulocytic chalone causes regression of these leukemic tumors. The effect of chalones extracted from leukocytes is somewhat paradoxical in view of the stimulation of cell growth observed with various "conditioned media" or feeder layers of leukocytes; growth regulation, however, may depend on a balance between stimulatory and inhibitory influences. The effects observed appear to depend greatly on the assay system employed and the concentrations of cells and sera. Like the situation with colony-stimulatory activity, the lack of pure, fully characterized chalones clouds interpretation of their nature, specificity, and mechanism of action. Further studies will be necessary to elucidate their *in vivo* significance.

The importance of cell to cell interaction in growth regulation may be suspected by drawing an analogy to known T and B cell interactions observed in lymphocytes. T cells have been shown to secrete a lymphocyte mitogenic factor, which effects B cell proliferation under certain conditions (8). A proliferation inhibitory factor also exists for lymphocytes.

The density of a cell population also clearly depends upon the supply of oxygen and other nutrients and the build-up of toxic end products. As these factors become limiting, the cells may switch over to resting periods in their cell cycle as an adaptive survival mechanism under unfavorable environmental conditions. Support for the operation of this general mechanism is the aforementioned observation that the labeling index of cells present at diagnosis of leukemia is generally lower than at subsequent relapse, suggesting that the duration of population growth exerts an inverse effect on numbers of proliferating cells. Furthermore, the large amount of data available on perturbations of the cell cycle induced by chemotherapy provides further evidence that the equilibrium between resting and proliferating cells can be altered by the effect of treatment, which reduces population density by killing cells.

Drugs used in the treatment of acute leukemia exert their effects at different phases of the cell cycle. In addition to the specific therapeutic effect achieved, it has been possible, by appropriate manipulation, to allow cells in a certain phase of the cell cycle to accumulate, with their subsequent release as a cohort. Thus, patrial synchronization of the leukemic cell population may be achieved. Drugs may also stimulate an accelerated reentry of resting or nonproliferating cells into the proliferative compartment, i.e., recruitment (11).

For example, when cytosine arabinoside is given as a single intravenous injection of 5 mg/kg to patients with acute leukemia in relapse, one observes a marked decrease in incorporation [^{3}H]Tdr into leukemic blast cells and a decrease in numbers of observable mitotic figures within 1 to 4 hr following drug administration. Pretreatment levels are regained at approximately 24 hr, and a roughly twofold overshoot in these proliferative indices is observed at 48 hr. Recovery of the mitotic index lags behind recovery of the labeling index. The combination of cytosine arabinoside with a second cycle specific agent at a time when the cells are maximally synchronized results in further alteration of the cell cycle. When vincristine is administered following cytosine arabinoside, there results a prolonged increase in the labeling index and mitotic index lasting 72 to 96 hr. When subsequent sequential 12-hr infusions of cytosine arabinoside are repeated every 18 to 24 hr after the initial synchronizing injection, further increases in both the labeling index and the mitotic index may be observed.

Although it is true that an element of synchronization and recruitment may be introduced into leukemic cell populations with optimal use of chemotherapeutic agents, and that improvement of results of treatment may be anticipated with appropriate scheduling, it is unlikely that cytokinetically directed chemotherapy alone will ever produce a uniform cure of leukemia. Reasons for this pessimism are, (a) it has so far been impossible to achieve perfect synchrony of mammalian cell systems *in vitro* or *in vivo*. The coefficient of variation in cell cycle length observed allows for only partial synchronization at best, with loss of synchrony after one mitotic division, and (b) success of therapy directed at synchronizing cells in cycle depends on simultaneously not synchronizing normal hemopoietic cells and other rapidly dividing tissues, such as epithelia. Otherwise, no improvement in the therapeutic index is achieved.

Also of enormous importance in the treatment of leukemia is the resting or nonproliferating cell population that is insensitive to cell cycle specific therapy. By means of continuous infusion of [^{3}H]thymidine in patients with ALL, it has been shown that a small but significant fraction of the leukemic cell population may remain dormant for at least 10 to 20 days (5). These cells retain the capacity for reentry into the cell cycle. Such reentry may be stimulated to an extent by chemotherapy, but it also takes place spontaneously. Details of this reversibility and regulation of the reversion are unknown.

As alluded to earlier, the leukemic cell population may be divided into proliferating and nonproliferating compartments on the basis of size and characteristics of nuclear chromatin. The dividing cells are large, have fine nuclear material, and are the only cells initially found to be labeled after an intravenous injection of [³H]Tdr. The nondividing cells are small, have dense coarse nuclear chromatin, and, initially, are unlabeled. Large cells divide to become small cells, and, conversely, the large cell proliferating compartment is apparently replenished from the small cells.

Evidence supporting the reentry of small leukemic cells into a proliferative phase has been obtained in a study of a 3-year-old child with untreated ALL by observing the rate of change of proportions of large and small labeled cells after [³H]Tdr injections (16).

During the steady state study period, initially 75 percent of the large and 10 percent of the small cells were labeled. The percentage of large cells labeled decreased in the next 24 to 48 hr, as some labeled large cells divided to form small cells. After subsequent serial injections of [³H]Tdr when 93 percent of the large and 72 percent of the small blasts had become labeled, there was only a slight change in the labeling of the large proliferating cells, indicating that the proliferating compartment was being maintained by a source of labeled cells, i.e., by reentry of small blast cells. Parenthetically, this provides evidence that the total leukemic cell population is capable of self-maintenance and does not depend upon continued leukemic transformation of normal cells for its perpetuation. The conditions that allowed the return of the small cells to a proliferative phase were not apparent from the study. Cell volume may play a determining role in triggering cell division, with a continuous interconversion of large and small cells on the basis of cell growth followed by reduction of volume upon division.

No hard information is presently available on the rate of cell loss or cell death in the marrow or at extramedullary sites. Calculations based on the observed discrepancy between estimated generation times and apparent population doubling times suggest that cell loss may be considerable. Death of cells may occur in the marrow due to ineffective leukopoiesis and probably also takes place through cell aging. Cell loss occurs through release of cells to the peripheral blood. From studies in which the rate of disappearance of the most highly labeled blasts in the blood was followed after a single injection of [³H]Tdr in patients, the half-time of disappearance of leukemic cells from the circulation was approximately 25 hr and the upper limit of the mean transit time was 36 hr (4). Reinfused circulating leukemic cells, which had been labeled *in vitro* with [³H]-uridine, in patients with AML or ALL were followed by periodic sampling of blood and showed half-times of disappearance in the same range, i.e., 28 and 32 hr (4). Recovery of labeled cells immediately after reinfusion is only one-quarter to one-fifth that anticipated relative to the absolute number reinfused. The discrepancy is likely to be due to margination on vessel walls and/or rapid loss into tissues. Of leukemic cells that enter the bloodstream, most probably die, a small fraction may return to the marrow, and some may multiply at such extramedullary sites as liver, spleen, meninges, and testicle. Relapse of disease from these so-called sanctuary areas implies that these leukemic cells retain proliferative potential. More precise details of the proliferative activity of leukemic cells in these extramedullary sites are currently unavailable.

Phases of the Cell Cycle where Growth Regulatory Factors May Exert Population Control

Once a cell initiates DNA synthesis it appears to be committed to progress through S, G_2, and M. Therefore, the immediate postmitotic events appear to be crucial in determining which cells will reenter another cycle of cell division, remain dormant, or differentiate. Cells that remain in a state of no cycle (G_0) have an intact and unlimited proliferative potential and at any time may be triggered to enter the cycle again. The triggering is random, and the statistical probability for it depends on the degree of population turnover (6). The existence of a true G_0 state for human acute leukemia cells, as distinct from a state of extremely prolonged G_1, has not strictly been demonstrated.

Clarkson and Fried (5) have represented human acute leukemia cell proliferation as intermediate between maximum logarithmic growth, on the one extreme, and the steady state characteristic of normal hemopoiesis, on the other (13). Only a fraction of the population has the essential characteristics of stem cells; and, in fact, it is considered likely that leukemic stem cells probably have varying degrees of "stemness." In their model, a fraction of the cells are committed to maturation and death. Observations of the partially mature cells, which have lost the potential to divide, seen in acute monocytic and acute myelomonocytic leukemia support their scheme.

In order to further explore the characteristics of the leukemic cell population with respect to proliferation, a computer-simulated model was constructed (12). Discrete modeling techniques were used so that representation of individual cells going through the mitotic cycle could be reproduced. By means of this model, the passage of cells through the mitotic cycle with the appropriate delayed times could be studied. After mitosis it was possible to direct the simulated cells either back into another phase of cell division or into a resting phase both of which occur in the actual leukemic cell population. With this model, therefore, it was possible to look at the sensitivity of the simulated cells to alterations of various aspects of the cell cycle.

In studying the effect of alteration of duration of the various parts of the cell cycle, it was found that only relatively minor alterations of growth rates could be achieved by increasing the time required to complete the phases of the mitotic cycle. A most important determining factor was the "decision" of the cell after completion of mitosis to enter the resting phase or to return to active cell division. For example, increasing the percent of cells returning to the mitotic cycle from 50 to 80 percent reduced the doubling time by about one-half. Therefore, it would seem that the cell after mitosis would be most susceptible to growth regulatory mechanism affecting the proportion of resting and dividing cells.

Another feature that could be studied on the computer-simulated model was the role of cell death in growth regulation. Unfortunately, this feature of the leukemic cell population cannot be quantitiated at the present time in patients. But, by computer simulation, cell death can play a major role in determining the population doubling time. In fact, models that did not include cell death displayed a rapid growth rate, which from a clinical point of view, appeared unrealistic.

As has already been mentioned, under conditions of chemotherapy perturbation, it appears to be possible to achieve an accelerated delivery of resting cells into the proliferating compartment. This feature could also be simulated on the computer model, matching the experimental data. Regulatory mechanisms underlying the conversion of resting cells into ,a state of proliferation are unknown. Such alterations might have real significance in the potentiation of cycle-dependent chemotherapeutic agents.

Concluding Remarks and Areas of Future Investigation

There is a precedent for the crucial role of viruses in inducing alterations in regulation of growth. For example, it is generally recognized that Epstein–Barr virus (EBV) has a lymphoproliferative effect. Leukocytes obtained from persons with previous infection with EBV, as evidenced by presence of EBV antibodies, display metabolic and morphologic characteristics of a long-term lymphoblastoid culture *in vitro*, becoming autonomous after 30 to 60 days and exhibiting an apparently unlimited growth potential. Maintenance of the transformed state seems to depend on continued presence of the EB viral genome (9). Conclusive evidence that viruses are the causative agents of human acute leukemia will not, however, per se advance our understanding of the disturbances of growth regulation observed in leukemic cell populations nor provide us with the molecular answers as to why leukemic cells have lost the ability to mature normally. Presumably, however, these effects will turn out to be mediated by viral-induced regulation and/or depression of the host's genome.

Future studies will be necessary to elucidate differences between the actively proliferating and the dormant cell populations in acute leukemia. Differences in nuclear chromatin, surface membrane characteristics, and synthesis of DNA, RNA, and proteins in relation to the cell cycle and factors that regulate these differences must be sought. Established methods of density-dependent cell separation may be used to separate light, actively proliferating cells from the smaller, more dense nonproliferating cells. The effects of possible serum regulatory factors that stimulate or inhibit cell division may be assayed in cell culture. New techniques will be necessary for the investigation of currently unknown variables, such as the event of cell death, the total body burden of leukemic cells, and the proliferative potential of leukemic stem cells present in small numbers, e.g., in drug-induced remissions.

Study of leukemic cell kinetics has thus far shown that leukemic cells divide more slowly, on the whole, than their normal counterparts and that, at any one time, a large proportion of the cells are not dividing. Spontaneous shifts in leukemic cell populations, as well as perturbations induced by chemotherapy, have been demonstrated, and some insight has been gained into how chemotherapeutic agents may be used more advantageously. Significant advances in understanding the pathogenesis and improving the management of leukemia, however, are only likely to be achieved by further insight into the disturbances of growth regulation and differentiation observed.

REFERENCES

1. Adamson, J. W. and Finch, C. A. Erythropoietin and the regulation of erythropoiesis in Di Guglielmo's syndrome. Blood, 36:590, 1970.

2. Baserga, R. Mitotic cycle of ascites tumor cells. Arch. Pathol., 75:156, 1963.

3. Burke, P. J., Diggs, C. H., and Owens, A. H. Factors in human serum affecting the proliferation of normal and leukemic cells. Cancer Res., 33:800, 1973.

4. Clarkson, B. D. Review of recent studies of cellular proliferation in acute leukemia. Natl. Cancer Inst. Monogr., 30:81, 1969.

5. Clarkson, B. D. and Fried, J. Changing concepts of treatment in acute leukemia. Med. Clin. North Am., 55:561, 1971.

6. Epifanova, O. I. and Terskikh, V. V. On the resting periods in the cell life cycle. Cell Tissue Kinet., 2:75, 1969.

7. Frindel, E., Malaise, E. P., Alpen, E., and Tubiana, M. Kinetics of cell proliferation of an experimental tumor. Cancer Res., 27:1122, 1967.

8. Geha, R., Schneeberger, E., Rosen, F., and Merler, E. Interaction of human thymus derived and non-thymus derived lymphocytes *in vitro*. Induction of proliferation and antibody synthesis in B lymphocytes by a soluble factor released from antigen-stimulated T lymphocytes. J. Exp. Med., 138:1230, 1972.

9. Gerber, P. and Deal, D. R. Studies on oncogenic properties of Epstein–Barr virus.

In Dutcher, R. M. and Chieco-Bianchi, L., eds. Unifying Concepts of Leukemia. Bibl. Haemat., No. 30. Basel, Karger, 1973.

10. Houck, J. C. and Irasquin, H. Some properties of the lymphocyte chalone. Natl. Cancer Inst. Monogr., 38:117, 1973.

11. Lampkin, B. C., McWilliams, N. B., and Mauer, A. M. Cell kinetics and chemotherapy in acute leukemia, Sem. in Hematology, IX:211, 1972.

12. Mauer, A. M., Evert, C. F., Lampkin, B. C., and McWilliams, N. B. Cell kinetics in human acute lymphoblastic leukemia: Computer Simulation with Discrete Modeling Techniques. Blood, 41:141, 1973.

13. Mauer, A. M., Saunders, E. F., and Lampkin, B. C. Possible significance of non-proliferating leukemic cells. Natl. Cancer Inst. Monog., 30:63, 1969.

14. Metcalf, D. Human leukaemia: Recent tissue culture studies on the nature of myeloid leukaemia. Br. J. Cancer, 27:191, 1973.

15. Rytomaa, T. Chalone of the granulocyte system. Natl. Cancer Inst. Monogr., 38:143, 1973.

16. Saunders, E. F. and Mauer, A. M. Re-entry of non-dividing leukemic cells into a proliferative phase in acute childhood leukemia. J. Clin. Invest., 48:1299, 1969.

17. Stohlman, F., Quesenberry, P. J., and Tyler, W. S. The regulation of myelopoiesis as approached with *in vivo* and *in vitro* techniques. Prog. Hematol., VIII:259, 1973.

18. Todo, A., Strife, A., Fried, J., and Clarkson, B. D. Proliferative kinetics of human hematopoietic cells during different growth phases *in vitro*. Cancer Res., 31:1330, 1971.

Tumor Angiogenesis:
Effect on Tumor Growth and Immunity

J. Folkman and M. Klagsbrun

Introduction

A profitable approach to an understanding of tumor biology would be a study of how tumors reorganize their local environment to facilitate tumor growth. For example, Reich has suggested that proteases secreted by malignant cells may increase the permeability of neighboring vessels to allow increased uptake of proteins and amino acids by the tumor (20). Gullino has shown that, while the collagen within a tumor is produced by the host, the content of collagen is controlled by the tumor cells (15).

Recently, another phenomenon has been elucidated, i.e., tumor angiogenesis, the capacity of malignant tumors to continuously stimulate proliferation of new capillaries. Several experiments suggest that tumors stimulate neovascularization by releasing a diffusible material (14), which can be isolated from tumor cells in both the solid and the ascites form (5). This material, tumor angiogenesis factor (TAF), has been found in tumor cytoplasm and nucleus (24), but has not been found in normal tissue, such as liver. It has also been isolated from tumor cells in culture (6). Recently, Klagsbrun et al. have extended these observations and have demonstrated TAF activity in a variety of neoplastic cells in culture and in two established non-neoplastic cell lines but not in primary cell cultures, such as mouse embryo fibroblasts and human skin fibroblasts (17) (Table 31-1).

Bioassay and Biology of TAF

The chorioallantoic membrane (CAM) of the 10 to 11-day-old chick embryo and the rabbit cornea are both used as bioassays for TAF. Tissues to be tested for TAF activity are implanted in the CAM, and the intensity of new vascular proliferation converging on the implant is recorded at 48 to 72 hr on a scale of 1+ to 5+. Soluble fractions of TAF to be tested are absorbed by pieces of Millipore filter placed on the CAM. At this writing, however, we have also

Fundamental Aspects of Neoplasia,
edited by A. Arthur Gottlieb, Otto J. Plescia, and David H. L. Bishop.
© 1975 by Springer-Verlag New York Inc.

Table 31-1   Tumor Angiogenesis in Neoplastic and Non-Neoplastic Cell Lines

(A)

Species	Cells giving positive TAF response[a]	Minimum number of cells to obtain positive assay
Mouse	BALB/c-3T3 embryo[b]	3×10^6
	BALB/c-SVT2 (SV40 virus transformed 3T3)	3×10^6
	B-16 melanoma	5×10^6
Rat	Walker 256	6×10^6
Human	WI-38 embryonic lung (passage 24)	4×10^6
	SVWI26 (SV40 virus transformed WI26)	4×10^6
	Glioblastoma	1×10^6
	Meningioma	1×10^5
	HeLa[c]	—

(B)

Species	Cells giving negative TAF response	Maximum number of cells tested which still gave a negative response[e]
Mouse	BALB/c primary embryo	$>6 \times 10^6$
Human	Skin fibroblast (passage 11)	$>10^7$

[a] As measured by bioassay on chick embryo chorioallantoic membrane. Cells are exponentially growing in T-75 tissue culture flasks.

[b] Contact inhibited cell line but grows as tumor on CAM.

[c] Positive for cells grown in suspension but negative for cells grown as monolayer.

[d] No data.

[e] Might be higher but not tested.

found that fractions of TAF can be dissolved into tiny discs of Hydron* polymer. When these discs are placed upon the CAM, TAF is released slowly. When the cornea is used for bioassay, 1-mm pieces of tissue are implanted into a corneal pocket 1.5 by 2 mm (11). The TAF fractions are dispersed either in Hydron polymer or in acrylamide, which is then implanted into the corneal pocket. The TAF diffuses into the cornea, and new vessels grow from the limbal edge toward the implant. The number of new vessels and their rate of growth are used to grade the intensity of angiogenesis activity.

A variety of normal tissues, including mouse placenta, mouse liver, myo-

* Hydron, hydroxy-ethyl methacrylate, courtesy of Alza Corporation, Palo Alto, California.

cardium, and skeletal muscle, do not stimulate angiogenesis. Lymph node allografts may produce delayed hypersensitivity with neovascularization (2), but nodes from the same rabbit give no angiogenesis activity.

Tumor cells appear capable of synthesizing TAF in the absence of cell division. Auerbach (1) has shown that explants of V-2 carcinoma cells previously irradiated *in vitro* with 4,000 R elicit new vascularization in the rabbit cornea for 3 to 4 weeks, although the tumor fails to grow. Furthermore, Klagsbrun et al. (17) were able to demonstrate TAF activity in extracts of cultured SVT2 cells after inhibition of protein synthesis by exposure to cyclohexamide for 24 hr. When SVT2 cells in culture were fed ^{14}C-labeled uridine, lysine, and arginine and ^{3}H-labeled thymidine, extracts with TAF activity contained labeled RNA and protein, but no DNA. Tuan (24) found that nuclear DNA of tumor cells had no TAF activity.

Angiogenesis capacity may appear early during the conversion of normal to malignant tissue. Gimbrone and Gullino (12) studied a variety of mammary tissues from a strain of mice with a high spontaneous incidence of mammary carcinoma. These tissues were implanted into the rabbit iris, and the neovascular response was measured. Only 4 percent of the "normal" mammary tissues induced neovascularization of the iris, whereas 37 percent of nontransplantable hyperplastic nodules and 60 percent of transplantable hyperplastic nodules had angiogenesis capacity. When mammary carcinomas finally developed, 97 percent induced neovascularization. Thus, the capacity to stimulate neovascularization arose months before malignancy was recognizable, either by histologic abnormalities or other manifestations of a neoplasm.

Purification of TAF

At the current writing, TAF is being purified from crude preparations extracted from cultures of Walker tumor cells and SVT2 cells. After cells have grown to near confluence, the media is drained, and the cells are washed in Ringer's solution for 3 hr at 4°C. The Ringer's solution is removed, and the cells are re-fed with fresh medium and incubated at 37°C. The Ringer's solution is dialyzed against distilled water and lyophilized. Approximately 1 to 3 μg of protein, with TAF activity, are released from 1×10^7 cells when roller bottles are used, and slightly higher protein yields are obtained from flat monolayer cultures. Approximately 30 to 100 μg of this crude material is required to demonstrate angiogenesis activity on the CAM and much less in the corneal pocket. This crude material is then subjected to further purification by Sephadex chromatography. Purification and characterization are tedious because of the lack of an *in vitro* assay.

Avascular and Vascular Phases of Tumor Growth

The capacity of solid tumors to produce TAF, in effect, dissociates their growth into two phases, the *avascular phase* and the *vascular phase* (6). Each phase has unique properties. The avascular phase is characterized by initial slow growth followed by a dormant state if the tumor mass has not been penetrated by new capillaries by the time it has grown to approximately 1 to 2 mm diameter. Under usual conditions, the avascular phase is imperceptible, because most animal tumors become vascularized within a few days of implantation. To prolong the avascular phase so that it can be studied in more detail, vascularization must be delayed experimentally. For example, if tumor implants are kept suspended in the aqueous humor of the anterior chamber of the rabbit eye, new blood vessels in the iris cannot traverse the aqueous humor, and the floating tumor spheroid remains avascular. In the avascular state, it will not grow beyond 1 mm in diameter. When tumors are implanted in the CAM, there is a 72-hr period before new host vessels have penetrated the tumor (18). During this avascular phase, tumors originally smaller than 1 mm grow up to this diameter, before they stop enlarging, whereas tumor implants initially larger, shrink toward the 1 mm diameter. There are some clinical situations in which the avascular state is visible and occasionally prolonged. Carcinoma-in-situ of the cervix, certain early carcinomas of the bladder, superficial cutaneous melanomas, and vitreous metastases of retinoblastoma are some examples. In one of our cases, a rhabdomyosarcoma was found to be metastatic to the skin of an infant terminally ill from widespread malignancy. At postmortem, these multiple skin metastases were measured and histologic sections were made. There were no capillaries within tumor nodules of a diameter 1.5 mm or less, but larger tumors were completely vascularized (7).

Therefore, a major characteristic of the *avascular* phase is that tumor growth is limited to a diameter of approximately 1 to 2 mm and that, if the avascular period is prolonged, tumors become dormant at approximately this diameter.

By contrast, the identifying characteristic of the *vascular* phase is rapid tumor growth. Once the tumor implant has been penetrated by new capillaries, rapid tumor growth (in some instances, exponential growth) begins. In the anterior chamber, a Brown–Pearce tumor spheroid implanted among iris vessels is penetrated by new capillaries within 5 to 6 days (13). Exponential growth follows; the tumor reaches maximum size of up to 16,000 times its original volume in less than 2 weeks. Knighton (18) has shown a similar rapid growth phase following vascularization of Walker carcinoma implanted on the CAM of 5-day-old chick embryos. Implants that maintained a mean diameter of 0.93 mm $\pm$ 0.29 mm during the avascular phase began rapid growth 24 hr after vascularization and reached a mean diameter of 8.0 $\pm$ 2.5 mm over a

7-day period. It is also possible that the vascular phase is primarily responsible for local invasiveness, shedding of metastases, and malignant drift (6),
although the experiments to establish this have not been carried out.

Mechanism of Dormancy in the Avascular Phase

It was not immediately obvious to us why tumor growth should become
dormant when the avascular stage was prolonged. Therefore, tumors were
grown in soft agar to simulate the environment of an avascular tumor (10).
Tumor cells suspended in soft agar grow into spheroids, which eventually stop
enlarging at a diameter of a few millimeters, despite frequent changes of
medium. Cells at the periphery of each spheroid incorporate [³H]thymidine,
and continue to proliferate, but cells deep in the center die and are lysed, so
that their disappearance balances the rate of proliferation of peripheral cells.
The most probable explanation is that, as the volume of cells expands, a
critical diameter is reached at which the surface area of the spheroid becomes
insufficient for nutrient absorption and waste release. Possibly, the same
mechanism operates for the avascular tumor nodule *in vivo*. Even though such
a nodule would be surrounded by vessels, its surface area would still limit the
the absorption of nutrients and release of wastes until the nodule was actually
penetrated by new capillaries. In both the avascular tumor spheroids suspended in the anterior chamber and in the avascular phase of tumor growth on
the CAM, there was a similar histologic pattern. Only cells at the outer
periphery incorporated [³H]thymidine, whereas those in the center were
necrotic.

Are Tumor Immunity and Tumor Angiogenesis Related?
A Hypothesis

The idea that solid tumors pass through an avascular phase and a vascular
phase prompted us to look at the possible relationship of tumor immunity and
tumor angiogenesis. Tumor angiogenesis seems to proceed independently of
the immune system. Evidence for this statement is found in the 3-day-old
chick embryo, where tumor implants will stimulate neovascularization (18),
yet no significant humoral or cellular immunocompetence develops until approximately the 14th day (22). Also, large vascularized tumors develop in con-
genitally athymic mice. Furthermore, the onset and progression of tumor-
induced angiogenesis in the rabbit cornea is the same whether the animal has
been sensitized or not.

On the other hand, the type of immune reaction against tumor may be
influenced by the state of tumor vascularization. The evidence for this state-

405

ment is preliminary, but we believe it is now sufficient to set forth a hypothesis. The hypothesis is based on the following observations:

1. A Brown–Pearce tumor implanted in a corneal pocket of the rabbit eye (3) will grow slowly as a plate two or three cell layers thick (Fig. 31-1,A). When one edge of the tumor grows to within 2 mm of the limbus,** new capillaries are stimulated. After about 2 weeks, these capillaries approach the edge of the tumor. If the animal has not been previously immunized against the tumor, the capillaries penetrate the tumor plate; immediately there is rapid tumor growth and, the vascularized portion of tumor becomes exophytic (Fig. 31-1,B). There follows a first-set rejection of only the vascularized portion of the tumor (Fig. 31-1,C). That sector of the tumor and its corresponding vessels regress. Histologic sections show an infiltrate of mononuclear cells with necrotic tumor cells. But the rejection is localized, as if the immune cells were unable to traverse the whole tumor plate. The rejection process terminates when the capillaries in that sector regress and are no longer able

** The tumor-to-limbus distance of about 2 mm is similar for a variety of tumors and for fractions of TAF inserted into a corneal pocket. This implies that effective diffusion of TAF in the cornea is limited to this range.

Figure 31-1 (opposite). Sequence of vascularization and rejection of Brown-Pearce tumor implanted into rabbit cornea. (A) Capillary proliferation at the limbus does not begin until one edge of tumor has advanced within 2 mm of the limbus (4 days after implant). (B) By approximately 3 weeks, one portion of the tumor is vascularized and beginning rapid growth. (C) At 5 weeks, first-set rejection begins, and the vascularized region of the tumor regresses and the tumor vessels also fade away. The opposite edge of the tumor continues to grow. Had the initial tumor been implanted 2 mm from the limbus instead of 5 mm, it would be completely destroyed by the first-set rejection because the opposite pole of the avascular implant would not have had time to grow beyond the range of immune cells delivered during the first-set rejection. (D) Six weeks after implant, as the opposite edge of tumor advances within 2 mm of the limbus, new vessels appear. (E) A second-set rejection occurs when vessel tips are approximately 0.5 mm from the tumor edge (8 weeks). Tumor regression begins; the vessels never penetrate the tumor as in (B). In several animals, other regions of an avascular tumor continued to grow toward the limbus and were rejected in a series of second-set responses until the cornea was completely cleared of tumor. Solid tumor cell immunity can be further demonstrated in these animals by implanting tumor subcutaneously, where it will fail to grow. Also, fresh tumor implanted in the other eye will be rejected by a second-set response. The time periods are approximate and represent an average of observations on 15 animals.

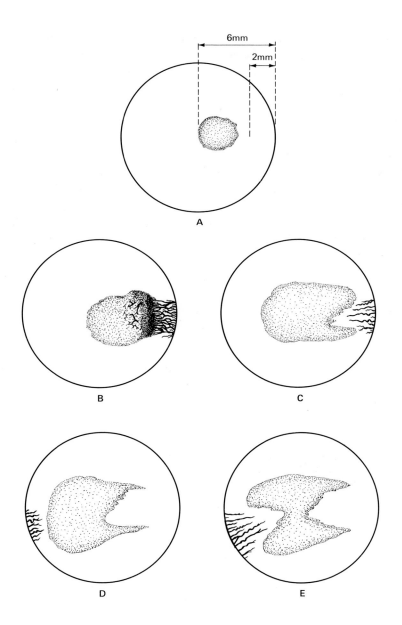

A

B

C

D

E

to carry fresh immune cells to the tumor. Meanwhile, residual tumor continues to grow and will eventually elicit new vessels in a different sector (Fig. 31-1,D). This time there is no exophytic tumor growth because rejection begins *before* the capillaries have penetrated the tumor. The animal has been immunized during the previous rejection. A white infiltrate is observed just in front of the capillary tips when they have arrived within 0.5 mm of the edge of the tumor. Tumor regression begins again. That this rejection occurs *before* penetration by capillaries, implies that immune leukocytes can be delivered from capillary tips to a target over short distances of approximately 0.5 mm or less, but not over long distances. By this definition, a tumor graft in the cornea is "privileged" from the efferent rejection process only when it lies beyond the range that immune cells can travel to it from remote capillary tips (4).

2. Another example is the rejection of a corneal allograft. Ophthalmologists have observed, in both experimental and clinical keratoplasty, rejection of a corneal graft starting at a single point in its circumference adjacent to a capillary loop that had not yet made intimate contact with the graft (16).

3. A third piece of evidence is found in recent clinical experiments with BCG treatment of intradermal melanomas (19). Injection of BCG into a single intradermal melanoma will cause regression (apparently on an immune basis) of distant intradermal tumors. But, subcutaneous and visceral melanomas in the same patient continue to grow. Generally, these intradermal tumors are avascular. Dermal capillaries may be found contiguous to the tumor, but have not *penetrated* it. By contrast, the subcutaneous and visceral nodules are usually well vascularized.

4. Tannock has shown that most cells within a vascularized tumor lie within 100 μ or less from the nearest open capillary (23). Compare this to an avascular tumor of approximately 2 mm diameter with contiguous capillary tips that might be 0.5 mm away from the tumor edge. The shortest distance from a tumor cell to an open capillary in such a tumor would be in the range of 500 μ, while the greatest distance would be roughly 1,500 μ.

5. In our laboratory, India ink was injected into a corneal pocket containing an implant of V-2 carcinoma (9). Particles of India ink average 25 μ in size and will not diffuse through the normal rabbit cornea (21). In our rabbits, India ink remained trapped in the tumor pocket and never diffused into the cornea beyond the edge of the avascular tumor. Once the tumor was vascularized, large areas of India ink quickly disappeared, presumably into the circulation and into regional lymphatics, until, after a short period, no ink remained in the cornea. These experiments seem to demonstrate that large molecules or aggregates of antigenic material may be released into the circulation only *after* tumor vascularization.

From these observations, we propose the following hypothesis:

In terms of the proximity of a tumor population to capillaries, there may be three general patterns, each of which would influence the host's immune response in a different way.

1. Avascular Tumor with *Remote* Capillaries (Fig. 31-2,A)

This tumor population would be so far from the nearest capillary (for example 2,000 to 5,000 μ), that immunocompetent cells could not be delivered in sufficient numbers to cause rejection. Examples would be vitreous metastases from a retinoblastoma (8), tumor spheroids in the aqueous humor of the anterior chamber (13), and Brown–Pearce or V-2 carcinomas implanted in the central portion of the rabbit cornea. It might also be impossible for such a tumor to be "blocked" or enhanced. Whether the phenomenon of "blocking" operates through the release of large quantities of antigenic material from the tumor into the circulation or by the coating of tumor cells with circulating antibody, both processes would be unlikely in an avascular tumor. It seems not unreasonable to assume that the diffusion of antibody into an avascular tumor spheroid would be limited in the same way that the diffusion of wastes and nutrients are limited.

Figure 31-2. Illustration of a hypothesis that the proximity of a tumor population to its vessels may exist in three general patterns. (A) The avascular tumor with remote capillaries, for example, the tumors suspended in the aqueous humor in the anterior chamber. (B) The avascular tumor with contiguous capillaries, for example, most tumor implants in experimental animals prior to vascularization. (C) The vascular tumor penetrated by capillaries, for example, the majority of palpable experimental and clinical tumors.

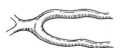

A Avascular (<u>remote</u> capillaries)

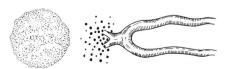
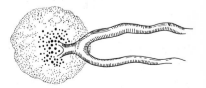

B Avascular (<u>contiguous</u> capillaries)   C Vascular (<u>penetrating</u> capillaries)

2. Avascular Tumor with *Contiguous* Capillaries (Fig. 31-2,B)

Capillaries might be less than 500 μ from the periphery of such an avascular spheroid. Examples would be the tumor implant in the chorioallantoic membrane during the first 72 hr before penetration by capillaries, the intracorneal tumor with contiguous vessels (Fig. 31-1,D), or most tumor implants in experimental animals, prior to vascularization. Clinical examples would be intradermal melanomas and possibly other tumors, such as early carcinoma of the bladder, before vascularization. These tumors might be accessible to immune cells but might not be susceptible to "blocking," for the reasons given above. Thus, such a tumor might be exposed to the full force of cell-mediated rejection without interference by "blocking" or enhancement. In a sensitized host, such a tumor would be especially vulnerable to immune rejection, since this particular vascular pattern would, in effect, dissociate cell-mediated immunity from humoral immunity. This might help explain why the intradermal melanomas regress after BCG therapy. The white skin graft that fails to vascularize during a second-set rejection might also be explained by this vascular pattern.

3. Vascularized Tumor *Penetrated* by Capillaries (Fig. 31-2,C)

In a well-vascularized tumor, most tumor cells would lie less than 100 μ from the nearest open capillary. Immune cells could easily be delivered into the tumor in large numbers, but "blocking" might also be facilitated because (a) a vascularized tumor can not only shed large quantities of material into the circulation, but it also grows faster than an avascular tumor and (b) the diffusion of circulating antibodies into a vascularized tumor should be more efficient than that into an avascular tumor. Examples might be the V-2 carcinoma in the rabbit cornea, which becomes large and exophytic and is almost never rejected before it kills the rabbit, possibly the majority of clinical solid cancers, and, especially, the subtaneous and visceral melanomas that continue to grow in the same patient who rejects intradermal melanomas.

In a previous report (7), we suggested that if tumors could be kept in the avascular stage, they might be more vulnerable to immunotherapy than vascularized tumors. Once it becomes possible to inhibit TAF or otherwise prevent tumor vascularization, "anti-angiogenesis" might be used as a therapeutic adjunct to synergize immunotherapy. The present hypothesis is a further refinement of this idea and is based upon additional evidence not previously available.

Summary

In summary, there is evidence that solid tumors stimulate new capillary proliferation by releasing a diffusible mediator, TAF and, thus, modify the local environment to their own advantage.

Although TAF has been only patrially purified, it is apparent that TAF synthesis can occur in tumor cells from solid tumors or in culture, that its production is not dependent upon cell division (mitosis), and that it makes its appearance early in the sequence of events following transformation of normal tissue to the neoplastic state.

We have shown that, prior to vascularization, solid tumors may exist for a time in an avascular state, which, if prolonged, limits growth to 1 to 2 mm diameter, so that the avascular state is predominantly one of population dormancy due to limits of diffusion of nutrients and wastes in a three-dimensional or spheroidal tumor population.

Subdivision of the tumor growth curve into an avascular and a vascular phase may increase our understanding of tumor biology in both animals and man. A new hypothesis relating tumor immunity and tumor angiogenesis is introduced to illustrate this.

This hypothesis states that although tumor angiogenesis can operate independently of the immune system, the type of immune reaction against a tumor is influenced in a major way by the state of tumor vascularization. In terms of the proximity of a tumor population to capillaries, there may be three general patterns, each of which would influence the host's immune response in a different way.

ACKNOWLEDGMENTS

We wish to acknowledge the many helpful discussions with Dr. Robert Auerbach, the work of Dr. Dianna Ausprunk and Henry Brem, and Mrs. Breen for typing the manuscript.

Supported by USPHS Grant #5-RO1-CA14019-02, a grant from the American Cancer Society #IC-28, and a gift from Alza Corporation.

REFERENCES

1. Auerbach, R., Arensman, R. Kubai, L., and Folkman, J. Tumor angiogenesis: Lack of inhibition by irradiation. Unpublished data.

2. Auerbach, R. Unpublished data.

3. Ausprunk, D. and Folkman, J. Unpublished data.

4. Billingham, R. E. and Boswell, T. Studies on the problem of corneal homografts. Proc. Roy. Soc., Lon. [Biol.], 141:392, 1953.

5. Folkman, J., Merler, E., Abernathy, C., and Williams, G. Isolation of a tumor factor responsible for angiogenesis. J. Exp. Med., 133:275, 1971.

6. Folkman, J. Tumor angiogenesis. *In* Klein, G. and Weinhouse, S., eds. Advances in Cancer Research. New York, Academic Press, 1974, Vol. 19, pp. 331–357.

7. Folkman, J. Anti-angiogenesis: New concept for therapy of solid tumors. Ann. Surg., 175:409, 1972.

8. Folkman, J. Tumor angiogenesis factor. Cancer Res., 34:2109, 1974.

9. Folkman, J., Brem, H., Tyler, K., and Zahniser, D. Unpublished data.

10. Folkman, J. and Hochberg, M. Self-regulation of growth in three dimensions. J. Exp. Med., 138:745, 1973.

11. Gimbrone, M. A., Cotran, R. S., Leapman, S. B., and Folkman, J. Tumor growth and vascularization: An experimental model using the rabbit cornea. J. Natl. Cancer Inst., 52:413, 1974.

12. Gimbrone, M. A. and Gullino, P. M. Neovascularization induced by intraocular xeno-grafts of normal, pre-neoplastic and neoplastic mouse mammary tissues. Fed. Proc., 33:396 (Part I, Abs. #2174), 1974.

13. Gimbrone, M. A., Leapman, S. B., Cotran, R. S., and Folkman, J. Tumor dormancy *in vivo* by prevention of neovascularization. J. Exp. Med., 136:261, 1972.

14. Greenblatt, M. and Shubik, P. Tumor angiogenesis: Trans-filter diffusion studies in the hamster by the transparent chamber technique. J. Natl. Cancer Inst., 41:111, 1968.

15. Gullino, P. M., Grantham, F. H., and Clark, S. H. The collagen content of transplanted tumors. Cancer Res., 22:1031, 1962.

16. Khodadoust, A. A. and Silverstein, A. M. Transplantation and rejection of individual cell layers of the cornea. Invest. Ophthalmol., 8:180, 195, 1969.

17. Klagsbrun, M., Knighton, D., and Folkman, J. Unpublished data.

18. Knighton, D., Ausprunk, D., Tapper, D., and Folkman, J. Study of the avascular and vascular phases of tumor growth in the chick embryo. Submitted for publication.

19. Nathanson, L. Regression of intradermal malignant melanoma after intralesional injec-tion of mycobacterium bovis strain BCG. Cancer Chemother. Rep., 56:659, 1972.

20. Reich, E. Tumor-associated fibrinolysis. *In* Clarkson, B., and Baserga, B., eds. Control of Proliferation in Animal Cells. Cold Spring Harbor Conferences on Cell Prolifera-tion, Cold Spring Harbor Laboratory, New York, 1974, Vol. 1, pp. 351–355.

21. Smolin, G. and Hyndiuk, R. A. Lymphatic drainage from vascularized rabbit cornea. Am. J. Ophthalmol., 72:147, 1971.

22. Solomon, J. B. Foetal and neonatal immunology. *In* Frontiers of Biology. Amsterdam, North-Holland/Elsevier, 1971, Vol. 20, 364 pp.

23. Tannock, I. F. and Steel, G. G. Quantitative techniques for the study of the anatomy and function of blood vessels in tumors. J. Natl. Cancer Inst., 42:771, 1969.

24. Tuan, D., Smith, S., Folkman, J., and Merler, E. Isolation of the non-histone proteins of rat Walker carcinoma 256. Their association with tumor angiogenesis. Biochemistry, 12:3159, 1973.

Epilogue:
On the Planning of Science

Lewis Thomas

If there are, as is sometimes claimed, certain matters that human beings are better off for not knowing about, or things that we ought not to be trying to understand, I cannot imagine what these might be. Therefore, I do not propose to get into this line of argument beyond acknowledging that the argument does exist. I take it as axiomatic that science is a useful, intelligent, and productive sort of human behavior, and, as our collective social activities go, it has a considerably better record than most. Moreover, I doubt that it will make a great deal of difference, in the very long run, whether any or even all of us were to decide that science was, for one reason or another, a bad thing and should be voted away. It is now a permanently established part of our social structure, and it will not go away. To be sure, it has only become a dominant part of human behavior during the last 300 years or so, but it represents an explosively successful expression of the most fundamental of all human urges, which is to find out about things. We are not, of course, unique among animals for curiosity in general, but our kind of incessant, compulsive, insatiable need to reach an understanding of nature, and, above all, our instinctive drive to make some kind of sense out of it, surely sets us apart from other forms of life. We seem to have agreed, informally, a few centuries ago, that we were not likely ever to find all the meaning we need by making it up out of our own heads, so we set about doing science, and I believe we will keep at it, for a long time to come.

I believe that science is a good thing for the human mind, and as important for the development of collective human thought as any of the other forms of art that seek meaning. I don't think its influence has yet penetrated the inner layers of our consciousness to the extent that literature has, or painting, or sculpture, but perhaps this is because science is still only beginning. I cannot imagine any terminal point in its future, nor any line of inquiry that will prove inaccessible.

I am aware of the dangers of hubris in this line of thinking. We do run certain risks, especially in biologic science, and all of us are aware of them.

Fundamental Aspects of Neoplasia,
edited by A. Arthur Gottlieb, Otto J. Plescia, and David H. L. Bishop.
© 1975 by Springer-Verlag New York Inc.

The new technology that permits the stitching together of DNA from different sources, bacterial, viral, even human, and the possible hazards to life posed by the resulting man-made micromonster, have sent a chill through the microbiologic community, but, by and large, the people who work in this field are sensible and trustworthy, as are the people who support the laboratories concerned, and I am sure that these hybrids will not be handled until there is certainty about their safety. Incidentally, hubris is a peculiarly appropriate and perhaps prophetic word here, since it is the etymologic source of the word hybrid. Hubris was constructed from two Indo-European roots signifying outrage, and hybrid was originally used to describe the inappropriate offspring of the wild boar and domestic sow. Like many of our oldest words, it carries its own warning.

There are, of course, other kinds of hazards ahead. The press has caught sight of some of them, and we are entering what I hope will be a temporary phase in which science is considered too risky for words. Along with oil spills, strip-mining, and herbicidal warfare, for which science gets blamed, we are also suspected of making plans to clone prominent politicians from bits of their own notable cells, or transplanting heads, or devising drugs to control human behavior to our personal liking. People are becoming fearful of science, and I would too if I thought such things were likely to happen. But I do not.

Set against the possible hazards of new and better science are the self-evident benefits. There are three general categories of benefit, which I would list in the order of their importance to humanity as follows: First, a more comprehensive understanding of nature, and a consequent enrichment of the human spirit. Second, more information that can be used to solve major human problems in the future, and especially problems relating to human disease. Third, a kind of information that can be put to use directly, the minute it is obtained, for practical and beneficial purposes.

The first category, that of understanding and meaning, I do not propose to deal with further here. Although it ranks at the top of my list (or perhaps *because* it is there), I could not possibly deal with it and still have time to discuss the other two categories. And it is these categories about which most of us are deeply worried today, and with which society's decisions about the planning of science are most directly concerned.

I intend to talk about the difference between basic and applied science, for this is actually the center of today's argument. It is a particularly agitated, and agitating, argument in the biomedical sciences, and this year—and I expect for some years to come—it is also, separately, an argument about how science should be carried out in dealing with the problem of cancer.

The great trouble with talking about basic and applied science is that people think you are arranging scientists into social castes, with differing and antagonistic customs and manners. The terms have become loaded with bogus meanings. Basic scientists are always delving into profundities, thinking every inch of the way, fishing up obscure bits of information for which there can be no conceivable use; they are ill-paid for their infinite pains. Applied scientists are well-off, athletic chaps, using other people's research to manufacture things that can be sold at a profit; they are superficial, unmeditative.

Because of labels like these, the terms basic and applied have lost much of their usefulness, and when they come into general conversation they tend to cause more trouble than they are worth. Nevertheless, I would like to use them for this discussion, on condition that I can make them mean exactly what I want them to mean. They are necessary if you are going to consider the planning of science, and, most especially, the funding of science, whether by government, or foundations, or universities, or research institutes. They are, in fact, two entirely different kinds of scientific effort, and it is perfectly fair to call one basic and the other applied, if you're scrupulously fair-minded about values. Unless you manage to keep them separate in your mind, and plan for them as quite different kinds of activity, you run the danger of ending up with no good science at all.

Applied science, then, according to my definition, is the kind of scientific activity that you must engage in when you are almost entirely certain how an experiment, or a chain of experiments, is going to turn out. The potential usefulness or profitability of the outcome has nothing to do with the matter; the outcome could simply be entertaining or philosophically illuminating, and it would still be applied science if you start out with a very high degree of certainty. To become engaged in this kind of work you have to start out with an orderly and abundant array of indisputable facts, better still, a redundant array, and these facts inform you that the outcome is not just a possibility, or even a probability, but a dead certainty.

There are several outstanding examples of this sort of applied science in biology. The Salk vaccine is a particularly instructive one. The indisputable facts at hand were that there were three types of polio virus, and no more, that all three were good antigens, and that they could be provided in infinite quantities in tissue cultures. Once these things were known, it was an absolute certainty that a vaccine against poliomyelitis could be made for use in humans. This is not to suggest that the work would be easy, or undemanding of high immunologic skill, or any less rigorous and sophisticated than any other set of experiments in biomedical science. Just that it was a certainty, and the work that was then performed by Salk and his associates was a masterpiece of elegant applied science.

The development in the past several years of better and constantly more effective chemotherapy against acute childhood leukemia is another example.

415

It became a certainty, or a near-certainty, that if the right combinations of certain drugs could be worked out, and their administration timed and monitored correctly, the disease could be cured in more children, and the rate of sustained remissions rose from around 20 percent to around 80 percent or higher. The work required meticulous attention and great caution, involving a large number of skilled clinical investigators, and the outcome was as had been predicted by the most knowledgeable people in the field. Something like this has also happened in the therapy of Hodgkin's disease and certain other lymphomas and, most spectacularly, in a number of the solid cancers of childhood.

In some respects, this kind of applied research resembles the moon shot, or the proximity fuse, or the hydrogen bomb, and it is fair enough to draw analogies between the planning of biomedical and physical science when you are working at this level. You obviously need a high degree of organization. Management skills are indispensable in both the planning and the doing of the science. The logic of systems analysis may be invaluable. All of the scientists involved are under an obligation to work together in team-fashion, and everyone must stick closely to an agreed schedule.

It is a distinguishing characteristic of any really great piece of applied science that, if it doesn't turn out the way it is supposed to, this comes as a shock and a surprise. Something really quite awful must have gone wrong.

In basic science, everything is precisely the opposite. The shock, and the surprise, come when the experiment *does* turn out as you hoped. Instead of certainty about the outcome, you start out with a very high degree of uncertainty. It is all right to pretend confidence, and to go around your laboratory bragging that this or that experiment is fated to come out as you predict, but if you always have the nagging, uncomfortable hunch that you're on the wrong track, you're doing basic science, under my classification.

Generally speaking, the uncertainty of basic science is due to the fact that what is being looked for is really an idea that will fit with another idea, a connection and a meaning, perhaps a mechanism, and when you are dealing with work of this kind you have to rely on your imagination. It is a form of gambling, but the great difference from real gambling is that if you are lucky, and win, your first thought has to be that maybe you're wrong after all.

You can measure the quality of the work by the intensity of your own surprise. Any really significant piece of new information about nature is bound to be a surprise. Sometimes, if you have a winning streak, the surprise will simply be your own astonishment at being right. At other times, it will be surprise that something else turned up; instead of coming out the way you hoped, the experiment revealed something else, totally unexpected, unpredicted and unpredictable. There are, of course, two ways of looking at this kind of event: one is to persuade yourself that the unexpected information is, in fact, an irrelevant triviality; the other is to realize that your whole program has just been derailed and you are now entrapped in a completely new approach. Whichever, you can't leave it there, sitting in your notes; you are now obliged to run it down.

Well, how do you plan and organize this kind of science? I really have no answer for this, except that I am absolutely certain that you can't turn it, just by wishing, into what is primarily a management problem, with the solutions now dependent upon the proper kind of organization charts, team deployment, systems analysis, and neat labels inside sequentially arranged boxes with big arrows and little arrows running back and forth between them. The way you do it, I suspect, is to find a bunch of very bright and very imaginative investigators, pack them together in quarters as crowded as possible, consistent with free breathing, and hope for the best. It may be very important to pay more attention to the design of the corridors than has been customary for most institutions. Corridors should have reasonably comfortable structures to lean against or sit on, and plenty of blackboard with inexhaustible chalk supplies. I sometimes wonder if we are in need of so many clocks in our hallways, or, for that matter, any.

You need skilled, hardworking committees to arrange the doing of applied science, and the success of the outcome may very well depend on the quality of committee planning. On the other hand, committees, even small committees composed of the brainiest people in town, can be the death of basic science. Not always, of course; once in a while it happens that a committee member will cry out in anguish because a new idea has just fought its way up into his consciousness, but the chances are statistically better, in my opinion, that the idea would have come sooner and with greater clarity if he'd been away from the committee, stumbling down the corridor, or staring· out of his laboratory window, or maybe in the shower.

The really good ideas, the sudden intuitive perceptions of connections between seemingly unrelated bits of information, the sudden overwhelming revelations that make a scientist worry seriously about what would happen to the fate of the world if he were hit by a truck on his way to work, occur in individual minds, and they cannot be programmed or planned.

If I am right about these things, then the most important and difficult step in the planning of science is to decide where the problem stands on the issue of certainty. If you have lots of good hard facts, all pointing plainly to a predictable outcome, it makes no difference how difficult the technologic steps or how sophisticated the instruments required: if you line up the investigators in the right order and lay out the work in a properly systematic fashion, you get what you want, sooner or later. But if you make a mistake at the outset in your evaluation of the certainty of the position, and if what you are really in need of are good hunches and flashes of intuition, it will be a disaster. If you try to organize basic science in this manner you'll get nothing out of it except more uncertainty in an endless, impenetrable series of committee reports, all equally depressed and depressing.

I have a strong hunch that most of the important and interesting problems in biomedical science today, including the problem of cancer, are predominantly matters of high uncertainty. There is an abundance of new and fascinating information, and there are a good many enticing theories concerning the key issues of etiology, the fundamental mechanisms underlying neoplastic transformation, the possible role of immunologic reactants, the nature of viral transformation, and even new approaches to chemical control of neoplastic cells. But, despite the richness of the new information, and the increasing speed with which it is being accumulated, I do not sense any general feeling of certainty at this time about any fundamental aspect of the cancer problem. It seems to me a completely safe prediction that, if and when the time comes, when there is a general and comprehensive answer to the problem of cancer, this will be an event of overwhelming surprise; indeed, I would go so far as to predict that the first reaction of most of us in this room will be, "But that is impossible!" Needless to say, the almost immediate second reaction in some quarters may be, "Ah yes, that is really what my group has been saying for some time," but the very first response will be dumbfoundment. And how do we make plans for that?

Meanwhile, there are important parts of the problem that lend themselves nicely to the most exacting methods of applied science right now, and there will be more of these in the years just ahead, if we are lucky. We need to develop better techniques of assessment so that these can be recognized quickly, and capitalized on—like the childhood leukemia story, for example. But there are not many, not yet, and we must not make the mistake of trying to force them into existence before their time.

A similar situation exists for most of the other major human diseases. There is a limited number of problems where certainty has already led to major achievements in applied science; the outstanding example is, I suppose, the development of the whole field of antibiotic therapy for bacterial infections. For the most part, however, we are unknown territory, engaged in a running hunt, and we will have to rely on the same chaotic, disorderly, spontaneous, unmanageable, and uncontrollable manifestations of the human intellect that have brought the natural sciences to their present stature over the last couple of hundred years.

418

Even though it isn't yet clear just how it worked, it hasn't worked out all that badly. We stumbled our way into chemistry, and evolution, quantum mechanics, and relativity turned up, genetics evolved with a life of its own, microbiology blundered its way along from 1875 into the era of antibiotics, and, here today, all unplanned for and unpredicted, are molecular biology, immunology, neurophysiology, and, who knows, experimental psychology.

It is normal and healthy for scientists to be impatient, but impatience is a hazard for the planners and policy-makers who do their best work in an atmosphere of optimistic quiet. Perhaps the wisest thing of all for us to agree upon, for the time being, would be a public acknowledgment that our predecessors in science have started, long before our own time, a job that will never, ever be finished. Cancer will be solved, to be sure, as soon as the right ideas drift to the surface in the right minds, and we need to make sure that the right minds are there and ready, with an ample supply of even brighter young minds being trained to follow on, for there will always be more new things to find out about, and there will be no end to the enterprise.

We owe an enormous debt to the past, but we have an even greater obligation to the future. We must concede that the future exists, and that there is a tremendous amount of highly important work to be done, which we will never know anything about, and cannot even guess at today. This requires of us more humility than we are accustomed to display, and we must dig deep to find it.

In summary, I'd like to itemize a few matters that are at the top of my own list of things to be apprehensive about; where I think we might run into various sorts of trouble in the planning of science over the next few years. I should perhaps emphasize, for quite obvious reasons, that I am speaking now about biomedical science in general, and not necessarily about the cancer program or any of the other special research projects with which the federal government is currently concerned. Also, I wish to stipulate that these are my own views as a private citizen, and no other person or persons, or governmental body, living or dead, can be blamed for them.

Item: Committees should not be charged with a responsibility for generating research ideas. It is fitting and proper for committees to act as peer review bodies, to assess the quality of scientific ideas as well as scientific work, but it is a violation of nature for a committee to sit down and try to think up bright ideas for other scientists to work on.

Item: Before you organize scientists into interdisciplinary, inter-institutional, or international teams, with detailed instructions and protocols for each worker, you had better be absolutely certain that you have a solid, concrete objective in mind, and that all participants are in agreement about the value of the objective as well as its reachability. If you deploy teams of scientists, not as individuals but as teams, in a highly structured, systematic way, with the intention or even the hope that something now unforeseen will turn up, or that brand new ideas about brand new mechanisms will somehow come to light, you are committing everyone concerned to an entirely novel and still untested way of doing basic science, and you should know this. It worked marvelously well for landing on the moon, but I doubt that if you were starting from scratch it would have uncovered the syphilis spirochaete, or the function and structure of DNA, or even aspirin.

Item: Whatever you do, make sure that the scientists who are given responsibilities for solving significant problems are able to take pleasure from their work. This means accepting the fact that the exceptionally good ones, who will move things forward, are really wild men, involved in one of the wildest of all the instinctive activities that humans can become engaged in. It is a form of social behavior, subject to a certain kind of control, immensely responsive to encouragement and support, insatiable in its demands for ever-increasing sums of money, and incalculably productive when it goes well. But the transport of information from mind to mind is dependent on what we have always called trains of thought, and it is important to remember that these, like ordinary trains, can be stalled, derailed, or sent off to the wrong destinations or even lost altogether, depending upon the way the system is working. Therefore, before we permit major interventions and transformations of a system that has worked with reasonable success in the past, we should go cautiously and apprehensively, looking over our shoulders every step of the way.

Reasonable success, indeed. We are entitled to celebrate the body of science as one of the greatest of all human accomplishments, and we can do this without any risk of seeming to boast, provided we make it clear that we are describing the whole science, and all its history. Where we get ourselves into deep trouble is by seeming to claim that science is something we just invented, around, say, two decades ago, and, having invented it, we're about to figure out some really neat ways of doing it better and quicker. We didn't invent it, and we haven't really discovered any qualitatively different ways of doing it yet, and we certainly can't claim to understand how the system works. The best we can do, if we want to improve it, is to continue reminding ourselves of the principle features of the scientific structure that we have inherited from our forebears. It is a legacy passed straight down from the longer, more ancient tradition of *scholarship*, and it includes honesty, the endlessly rewarding and uniquely human gratification that comes with the opportunity to tell someone else everything you know about something new and important, the pleasure that comes from surprise, and certain congenial habits of work: these include meticulousness, self-criticism, skepticism, an obsession with making notes and references to the work of predecessors; in short, rigor. With these we obtained Faraday, Maxwell, Gibbs, Pasteur, Ehrlich, Metchnikoff, a tremendous list of today's luminaries too long to mention, and heaven knows who tomorrow. With so many other things in doubt, it is comforting to know that the tradition is so old and so powerful, and that, whatever today's weather, it is certainly here to stay.

Index

Index

1 3 6 1 7 2

8106042

3 1378 00810 6042